Contemporary Cardiology

Series Editor:

Peter P. Toth
Ciccarone Center for the Prevention of Cardiovascular Disease
Johns Hopkins University School of Medicine
Baltimore, MD
USA

For more than a decade, cardiologists have relied on the Contemporary Cardiology series to provide them with forefront medical references on all aspects of cardiology. Each title is carefully crafted by world-renown cardiologists who comprehensively cover the most important topics in this rapidly advancing field. With more than 75 titles in print covering everything from diabetes and cardiovascular disease to the management of acute coronary syndromes, the Contemporary Cardiology series has become the leading reference source for the practice of cardiac care.

More information about this series at http://www.springer.com/series/7677

Michael J. Wilkinson
Michael S. Garshick • Pam R. Taub
Editors

Prevention and Treatment of Cardiovascular Disease

Nutritional and Dietary Approaches

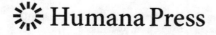 Humana Press

Editors
Michael J. Wilkinson
Division of Cardiovascular
Medicine, Department of Medicine
University of California San Diego
San Diego, CA
USA

Michael S. Garshick
Center for the Prevention of
Cardiovascular Disease and
Leon H. Charney Division of
Cardiology, Department of Medicine
New York University Langone Health
New York, NY
USA

Pam R. Taub
Division of Cardiovascular
Medicine, Department of Medicine
University of California San Diego
San Diego, CA
USA

ISSN 2196-8969   ISSN 2196-8977   (electronic)
Contemporary Cardiology
ISBN 978-3-030-78179-8   ISBN 978-3-030-78177-4   (eBook)
https://doi.org/10.1007/978-3-030-78177-4

This Humana imprint is published by the registered company Springer Nature Switzerland AG
The registered company address is: Gewerbestrasse 11, 6330 Cham, Switzerland

Contents

1 **Role of Dietary Nutrition, Vitamins, Nutrients, and Supplements in Cardiovascular Health**............... 1
Ryan Moran, Marsha-Gail Davis, and Anastasia Maletz

2 **Impact of Nutrition on Biomarkers of Cardiovascular Health**............................ 29
Cameron K. Ormiston, Rebecca Ocher, and Pam R. Taub

3 **The Mediterranean Dietary Pattern**...................... 47
Jessica K. Bjorklund, Carol F. Kirkpatrick, and Eugenia Gianos

4 **Dietary Approaches to Hypertension: Dietary Sodium and the DASH Diet for Cardiovascular Health**............. 61
Keith C. Ferdinand, Samar A. Nasser, Daphne P. Ferdinand, and Rachel M. Bond

5 **The Impact of Carbohydrate Restriction and Nutritional Ketosis on Cardiovascular Health**...................... 73
Dylan Lowe, Kevin C. Corbit, and Ethan J. Weiss

6 **Plant-Based Diets in the Prevention and Treatment of Cardiovascular Disease**............................ 95
Rajiv S. Vasudevan, Ashley Rosander, Aryana Pazargadi, and Michael J. Wilkinson

7 **Plant-Based Oils**...................................... 115
Katrina Han, Kelley Jo Willams, and Anne Carol Goldberg

8 **Prevention and Treatment of Obesity for Cardiovascular Risk Mitigation: Dietary and Pharmacologic Approaches**..... 129
Joanne Bruno, David Carruthers, and José O. Alemán

9 **Fasting for Cardiovascular Health**..................... 143
Elizabeth S. Epstein, Kathryn Maysent, and Michael J. Wilkinson

**10 Optimal Dietary Approaches for Those Living
with Metabolic Syndrome to Prevent Progression
to Diabetes and Reduce the Risk of Cardiovascular Disease** . . . 161
Melroy S. D'Souza, Tiffany A. Dong, Devinder S. Dhindsa,
Anurag Mehta, and Laurence S. Sperling

**11 Optimal Diet for Diabetes: Glucose Control,
Hemoglobin A1c Reduction, and CV Risk** 171
Wahida Karmally and Ira J. Goldberg

**12 Dietary and Lifestyle Cardiometabolic Risk Reduction
Strategies in Pro-inflammatory Diseases** 179
Ashira Blazer, Kinjan Parikh, David I. Fudman,
and Michael S. Garshick

13 Dietary Approaches to Lowering LDL-C 193
Parag Anilkumar Chevli and Michael D. Shapiro

14 Lifestyle Approaches to Lowering Triglycerides 211
Stephen J. Hankinson, Michael Miller,
and Andrew M. Freeman

15 Role of the Microbiome in Cardiovascular Disease 225
Thanat Chaikijurajai, Jennifer Wilcox,
and W. H. Wilson Tang

**16 Dietary and Nutritional Recommendations
for the Prevention and Treatment of Heart Failure** 251
Prerana Bhatia and Nicholas Wettersten

**17 Dietary Considerations for the Prevention
and Treatment of Arrhythmia** 265
Marin Nishimura and Jonathan C. Hsu

Index 273

Contributors

José O. Alemán Division of Endocrinology, Department of Medicine, New York University Langone Health, New York, NY, USA

Prerana Bhatia Division of Cardiology, University of California, San Diego, La Jolla, CA, USA

Jessica K. Bjorklund North Shore University Hospital, Manhasset, NY, USA

Zucker School of Medicine, Hempstead, NY, USA

Ashira Blazer Division of Rheumatology, Department of Medicine, New York University Langone Health, New York, NY, USA

Rachel M. Bond Dignity Health, Chandler Regional Medical Center, Chandler, AZ, USA

Creighton University School of Medicine, Omaha, NE, USA

Joanne Bruno Division of Endocrinology, Department of Medicine, New York University Langone Health, New York, NY, USA

David Carruthers Division of Endocrinology, Department of Medicine, New York University Langone Health, New York, NY, USA

Thanat Chaikijurajai Department of Cardiovascular Medicine, Heart, Vascular and Thoracic Institute, Cleveland Clinic, Cleveland, OH, USA

Department of Internal Medicine, Faculty of Medicine Ramathibodi Hospital, Mahidol University, Bangkok, Thailand

Parag Anilkumar Chevli Center for Prevention of Cardiovascular Disease, Section on Cardiovascular Medicine, Wake Forest University Baptist Medical Center, Medical Center Boulevard, Winston Salem, NC, USA

Kevin C. Corbit The Cardiovascular Research Institute, University of California, San Francisco, CA, USA

Marsha-Gail Davis Department of Family Medicine, UCSD/SDSU Preventive Medicine Residency, University of California, San Diego Health, San Diego, CA, USA

San Diego State University School of Public Health, San Diego, CA, USA

Devinder S. Dhindsa Emory Clinical Cardiovascular Research Institute, Division of Cardiology, Emory University School of Medicine, Atlanta, GA, USA

Tiffany A. Dong Department of Internal Medicine, Emory University School of Medicine, Atlanta, GA, USA

Melroy S. D'Souza Department of Internal Medicine, Emory University School of Medicine, Atlanta, GA, USA

Elizabeth S. Epstein Division of Cardiovascular Medicine, Department of Medicine, University of California San Diego, San Diego, CA, USA

Keith C. Ferdinand Gerald S. Berenson Endowed Chair in Preventive Cardiology, Tulane University School of Medicine, New Orleans, LA, USA

Daphne P. Ferdinand Healthy Heart Community Prevention Project, Inc, New Orleans, LA, USA

Andrew M. Freeman Division of Cardiology, Department of Medicine, National Jewish Health, Denver, CO, USA

David I. Fudman Division of Digestive and Liver Diseases, Department of Medicine, University of Texas Southwestern Medical Center, Dallas, TX, USA

Michael S. Garshick Leon H. Charney Division of Cardiology, Department of Medicine, New York University Langone Health, New York, NY, USA
Center for the Prevention of Cardiovascular Disease, New York University Langone Health, New York, NY, USA

Eugenia Gianos Zucker School of Medicine, Hempstead, NY, USA
Cardiovascular Prevention, Northwell Health, New Hyde Park, NY, USA
Western Region, Katz Institute Women's Heart Program, Manhasset, NY, USA
Women's Heart Program, Lenox Hill Hospital, New York, NY, USA

Ira J. Goldberg Division of Endocrinology, Diabetes and Metabolism, New York University Grossman School of Medicine, New York, NY, USA

Stephen J. Hankinson Division of Cardiology, Department of Medicine, University of Maryland School of Medicine, Baltimore, MD, USA

Jonathan C. Hsu Cardiac Electrophysiology Section, Division of Cardiology, Department of Medicine, University of California, San Diego, La Jolla, CA, USA

Wahida Karmally Columbia University, New York, NY, USA

Carol F. Kirkpatrick Idaho State University Wellness Center, Pocatello, ID, USA

Dylan Lowe The Cardiovascular Research Institute, University of California, San Francisco, CA, USA

Anastasia Maletz Department of Family Medicine, UCSD/SDSU Preventive Medicine Residency, University of California, San Diego Health, San Diego, CA, USA

San Diego State University School of Public Health, San Diego, CA, USA

Kathryn Maysent Division of Cardiovascular Medicine, Department of Medicine, University of California San Diego, San Diego, CA, USA

Anurag Mehta Emory Clinical Cardiovascular Research Institute, Division of Cardiology, Emory University School of Medicine, Atlanta, GA, USA

Michael Miller Division of Cardiology, Department of Medicine, University of Maryland School of Medicine, Baltimore, MD, USA

Ryan Moran Department of Medicine, University of California, San Diego Health, San Diego, CA, USA

Department of Family Medicine, UCSD/SDSU Preventive Medicine Residency, University of California, San Diego Health, San Diego, CA, USA

San Diego State University School of Public Health, San Diego, CA, USA

Samar A. Nasser Department of Clinical Research & Leadership, School of Medicine and Health Sciences, The George Washington University, Washington, DC, USA

Marin Nishimura Cardiac Electrophysiology Section, Division of Cardiology, Department of Medicine, University of California, San Diego, La Jolla, CA, USA

Rebecca Ocher Department of Medicine, University of California, Los Angeles, Los Angeles, CA, USA

Cameron K. Ormiston Division of Cardiovascular Diseases, Department of Medicine, University of California, San Diego, La Jolla, CA, USA

Kinjan Parikh Leon H. Charney Division of Cardiology, Department of Medicine, New York University Langone Health, New York, NY, USA

Aryana Pazargadi Division of Cardiovascular Medicine, Department of Medicine, University of California San Diego, San Diego, CA, USA

Ashley Rosander Division of Cardiovascular Medicine, Department of Medicine, University of California San Diego, San Diego, CA, USA

Michael D. Shapiro Center for Prevention of Cardiovascular Disease, Section on Cardiovascular Medicine, Wake Forest University Baptist Medical Center, Medical Center Boulevard, Winston Salem, NC, USA

Laurence S. Sperling Emory Clinical Cardiovascular Research Institute, Division of Cardiology, Emory University School of Medicine, Atlanta, GA, USA

W. H. Wilson Tang Department of Cardiovascular Medicine, Heart, Vascular and Thoracic Institute, Cleveland Clinic, Cleveland, OH, USA

Center for Microbiome and Human Health, Department of Cardiovascular and Metabolic Sciences, Lerner Research Institute, Cleveland Clinic, Cleveland, OH, USA

Pam R. Taub Division of Cardiovascular Medicine, Department of Medicine, University of California San Diego, San Diego, CA, USA

Rajiv S. Vasudevan University of California, San Diego School of Medicine, La Jolla, CA, USA

Ethan J. Weiss The Cardiovascular Research Institute, University of California, San Francisco, CA, USA

Nicholas Wettersten Division of Cardiology, University of California, San Diego, La Jolla, CA, USA

Section of Cardiology, San Diego Veterans Affairs Health System, San Diego, CA, USA

Jennifer Wilcox Center for Microbiome and Human Health, Department of Cardiovascular and Metabolic Sciences, Lerner Research Institute, Cleveland Clinic, Cleveland, OH, USA

Michael J. Wilkinson Division of Cardiovascular Medicine, Department of Medicine, University of California San Diego, San Diego, CA, USA

Role of Dietary Nutrition, Vitamins, Nutrients, and Supplements in Cardiovascular Health

Ryan Moran, Marsha-Gail Davis, and Anastasia Maletz

Regular supplement use has increased in the last several decades in USA, with now almost 50% of Americans reporting regular use. The primary reason or motivator for use of dietary supplements is to improve, supplement, or maintain health [1]. However, despite this, there remains uncertainty and misunderstanding regarding many of these supplements and their role in cardiovascular protection, namely because of the intense heterogeneity, availability, and dose variations of supplements. Because of the prevalence and interest in use, there has been a great interest in better understanding how micro- and macronutrients mitigate disease and potentiate health. Some of the most widely used supplements include multivitamins (MVI)—which include both varied and single vitamin formulations—mineral and elemental formulated supplements, and macronutrient compounds which have physiologic roles in pathways related to metabolism and homeostasis.

Multivitamin and B Vitamins

MVI and water-soluble vitamin supplementation has been a subject of interest for decades for cardiovascular disease (CVD) treatment or prevention, owing in part to the role of inflammation in the development of heart disease. Epidemiological studies have noted inverse relationships between diets high in vegetables, fruits, and whole grains and incident heart disease, and augmenting diets with substrates of these diets have been reasoned to have a role in atherogenesis [2]. However, single-pill MVI supplements have been a challenge to study, as well as to interpret across studies, owing to notable heterogeneity in inclusion constituents, doses, inclusion criteria, and endpoints. Despite this, pervasive evidence has not found that supplementation of combined MVI provides benefit for either primary or secondary cardiovascular prevention [3, 4]. In one large Euopean study, over 6000 healthy individuals were randomized to a combination of 120 mg ascorbic acid, 30 mg of Vitamin E, 6 mg of β-carotene, 100 µg of sele-

R. Moran (✉)
Department of Medicine, University of California, San Diego Health, San Diego, CA, USA

Department of Family Medicine, UCSD/SDSU Preventive Medicine Residency, University of California, San Diego Health, San Diego, CA, USA

San Diego State University School of Public Health, San Diego, CA, USA
e-mail: rjmoran@health.ucsd.edu

M.-G. Davis · A. Maletz
Department of Family Medicine, UCSD/SDSU Preventive Medicine Residency, University of California, San Diego Health, San Diego, CA, USA

San Diego State University School of Public Health, San Diego, CA, USA
e-mail: mdavis@health.ucsd.edu;
amaletz@health.ucsd.edu

M. J. Wilkinson et al. (eds.), *Prevention and Treatment of Cardiovascular Disease*, Contemporary Cardiology, https://doi.org/10.1007/978-3-030-78177-4_1

nium, and 20 mg of zinc for a median 7.89 years and found no cardiovascular benefit of supplementation [5]; more recently, a double-blinded study in USA evaluated that a combined MVI containing 32 different compounds in older men found a trend toward less myocardial infarction in those with established CVD at baseline, but no difference in the study's primary or secondary endpoints, and no difference in outcomes for primary prevention [6].

From a cardiovascular standpoint, three of nine B vitamins have a role in homocysteine metabolism (pyroxidine (B6), cyanocobalamin (B12), and folate (B9)), and given the proposed role of homocysteine in progression of atherogenesis, there has been considerable interest in evaluating supplementation in higher risk individuals to prevent disease progression [4]. Empirical support includes evidence that supplementing these three vitamins can decrease surrogate markers of risk, such as serum homocysteine concentrations [7], and that B supplementation may be associated with decreasing carotid intima media thickness progression [8]. However, interventional trials have generally failed to find support for routine supplementation in average or high-risk individuals for cardiovascular benefit. While one large study supplementing folate in middle aged Chinese hypertensive individuals did show decreased composite cardiovascular events [9], this has not been consistently found in other studies [10].

Vitamin B1 (*thiamine*) serves a variety of physiologic roles including as an essential cofactor in lipid metabolism as thiamin diphosphate, and deficiencies have been noted more commonly in patients with heart failure. Supporting this association, some evidence has found supplementation may have a role in left ventricular function [11, 12], although the clinical meaning is still unclear as data on functional improvement are lacking and the absolute difference—while significant—was relatively small.

Vitamin B5 (*pantothenic acid*) is metabolized into pantethine which has direct and indirect influences on lipid metabolism via inhibition of acetyl-coenzyme (CoA) carboxylase and 3-hydroxy-3-methyl-glutaryl-CoA reductase. Supplementation in high doses has been found to favorably alter both triglyceride and low-density lipoprotein (LDL) levels modestly in low and moderate risk individuals [13]. Long-term and outcome data, however, are lacking, though it is generally well tolerated and carries minimal risk.

Vitamin B3 (*niacin*, including *nicotinamide* and *nicotinic acid*) is metabolized to nicotinamide adenine dinucleotide (NAD) which is an important cofactor in enzymatic processes including in generation of adenosine triphosphate (ATP), a major cellular energy source. Supplementation of nicotinic acid in high-dose augments lipid profiles favorably, including increasing HDL and lowering LDL and triglycerides [14]. Outcome data, however, have been mixed: one randomized long-term (6.2 years) study using 3000 mg daily found fewer non-fatal MI compared with placebo, but increased rates of pulmonary thromboembolic events and arrhythmia events [15]. In addition, the study adherence was lower and dropout rate higher in the niacin arm (compared with placebo or fibrate) owing to the side effects of niacin including flushing, gastrointestinal side effects, and cardiovascular symptoms (including palpitations, headaches, increased heart rate, and low blood pressure). Interestingly, long-term (mean 15 years) follow-up to this noted decreased overall mortality rates in those in the niacin arm compared with placebo, though the mechanisms are not entirely clear but possibly related to the lipid profile benefits [16]. Several studies have found little evidence to support added benefit in addition to statin therapy, however, but have found increased side-effect profiles (especially at pharmacologic doses) and concerns for possibly increased all-cause mortality [17–19]. Thus, niacin is generally not recommended either for therapeutic benefit in secondary prevention, nor for primary prevention except in specific circumstances such as intolerance to safer options.

Vitamin C

Vitamin C (l-*ascorbic acid*) is an essential diet component with a wide range of physiologic activities including in the synthesis of collagen and some hormones, as well as an established antioxidant and pro-oxidant. In addition, it has a role in monocyte vascular adhesion and is thought to have a role in atherogenesis. Deficiencies are rare but are associated with blood vessel fragility and the clinical manifestation of scurvy. Higher intake of vitamin C has been noted to potentiate the antioxidant role of this compound, and epidemiological support exists for an inverse association with intake and incident heart disease [20–23]. Prospective studies however have found mixed results: in post-menopausal women, supplementation—but not dietary intake—was associated with decreased incident CVD [24], but high-dose supplementation in men without heart disease failed to find this and instead found a trend toward higher cardiovascular mortality [25]. A large pooled meta-analysis of prospective studies found high diet intake—but not supplement intake—inversely associated with CVD incidence [20]. Randomized trials have consistently found little evidence that supplementation of vitamin C is effective for either primary or secondary prevention of adverse cardiac events [26–28]. Therefore, a varied diet of fruits and vegetables, including those containing high amounts of vitamin C, are recommended rather than supplementation for heart health, as little evidence supports supplementation use to prevent heart disease [29].

Vitamin A

Vitamin A (*retinol, retinal, and retinyl esters*) is composed of a group of related hydrophobic compounds which have numerous physiologic roles and is consumed either as a provitamin A carotenoid compound or complete vitamin A compound which is then hydrolyzed in the intestinal lumen to be absorbed [30]. Once ingested, provitamin A or its active homolog is incorporated in the formation of bile acid micelles is solubilized and eventually is absorbed into enterocytes with dose- and concentration-independent mechanism, contributing to a potential for toxicity. Provitamin A (most commonly α-carotene, β-carotene, and β-cryptoxanthin) can be converted to retinol and enter the metabolic

pathway to becoming bioactive vitamin A. It is then esterified, incorporated into chylomicrons, secreted via lymphatic drainage, and eventually enter the bloodstream for storage (mainly in the liver) or for cellular distribution [31]. Retinoic acid, the major bioactive form of vitamin A, acts in a paracrine or autocrine hormone, impacting cellular regulation, growth, and function. Although unusual, deficiencies are usually associated with vision deficiencies (e.g., night blindness), and immune and integumentary issues [30]. However, epidemiologic support has associated higher intake of carotenoid-rich diets with lower CVD risk and low measured serum carotenoids with increased risk of subsequent ischemic event risk [32]. Despite these associations, several clinical trials have thus far failed to provide conclusive evidence that supplementation of vitamin A or provitamin A decreases CVD risk or decreases the risk in those with established heart disease [33]; in contrast, some trials [33–35] have raised concern for a possibly increased risk.

Disagreement between epidemiological associations and clinical trial findings has not been entirely elucidated. The diversity of dietary carotenoids and confounding of a diet rich in carotenoids—rather than carotenoids themselves—have been proposed [36, 37]. Given concerns of potential harms (including lung cancer in smokers or those with asbestos exposure, beyond the scope of this review) in supplementation, routine recommendation for vitamin A or provitamin A is not generally recommended for primary or secondary prevention of CVD [38].

Vitamin D

Vitamin D is predominantly obtained by synthetic processes in the skin by ultraviolet B (UVB) from sunlight, and secondarily from food sources. Once activated from 25(OH)D to 1,25-dihydroxyvitamin D (mostly in the kidneys), the hormone calcitriol plays important homeostatic functions in calcium regulation and acts on numerous different tissues throughout the body including the heart and vascular system, where vitamin D receptors are present [39, 40].

Physiologically, calcitriol has been shown to stop vascular smooth muscle cells from proliferating and have been theorized to contribute to calcium deposition and arterial calcification. Further, low calcitriol serum concentrations cause a homeo-statically regulated increase in parathyroid hor-mone, which has been implicated in increasing both vascular and myocardial calcification. Finally, low calcitriol has been shown to upregu-late pro-inflammatory cytokines (IL-6, TNF-a) and downregulate IL-10, and renin–angiotensin–aldosterone system activation, further supporting its role in heart disease risk. Epidemiological support includes noted associations between country latitude and cardiovascular death rates, seasonality trends and increased incidence of risk in the winter, and decreased rates in higher altitudes of residence, all suggesting the protec-tive role of UVB activation of vitamin D. Serum levels of 25(OH)D have been noted inversely associated with cardiovascular mortality [40, 41]. Additionally, the British Regional Heart Study noted higher risk of ischemic heart disease in men living in more northern locations over time, suggesting more than simple corollary evidence. In this study, while blood levels of vitamin D were not assessed, and smoking rates were noted higher in these locations as well, there was not an association between blood pressure and smok-ing rates, though blood pressure was noted higher in locations further north [42], perhaps explain-ing some of the author's findings as vitamin D deficiency has been associated with increased risk of hypertension [43]. While studies have supported vitamin D supplementation with low-ering C-reactive protein, evidence that supple-mentation has a role in lowering blood pressure has been mixed, especially in healthy individuals [44–46].

Intervention studies regarding CVD and vita-min D supplementation have been limited but generally have not found positive results with supplementation. The Woman's Health Initiative followed post-menopausal women (mean of 7 years) and found no clear association between calcium and vitamin D compared with pla-cebo on cardiovascular outcomes, although this was a secondary endpoint [47]. In addition, the amount supplemented was generally considered low (400 IU daily in two divided doses, with calcium). The ViDA study in New Zealand, in contrast, randomized over 5000 individuals to high-dose monthly (100,000 IU or more) vitamin D and found after over 3 years that compared with placebo, there was no effect on cardiovas-cular outcomes, including in the subgroup analy-sis of individuals with known CVD [48]. Finally, more recently, the VITAL study randomized over 20,000 individuals to 2000 IU daily (see Omega-3 section) and found after a median follow-up of over 5 years, there was similarly no benefit of supplementation on CVD in low-risk individu-als [49]. In both the ViDA and VITAL studies, subgroup analysis similarly failed to show ben-efit in individuals with vitamin D deficiency at randomization.

There still remains incredible interest given the physiological mechanisms and epidemiologi-cal findings, and many trials including higher risk individuals are ongoing. However, currently there is insufficient evidence to recommend vitamin D for primary or secondary prevention of CVD.

Vitamin E

Vitamin E (*tocopherols* and *tocotrienols*) is com-posed of eight isomeric molecules, functions as an important antioxidant, protecting free radical damage to lipid-rich cellular environments such as those found in membranes and lipoproteins, and helps to stabilize membrane structures. Once consumed, vitamin E is transported predomi-nantly by LDL and stored in fat-rich cellular structures throughout the body including the kidney, liver, brain, and heart [50]. Deficiencies of vitamin E are rare and are generally associ-ated with neurologic compromise [31]; however, their role as a potent antioxidant has been theo-rized to be important in cardiovascular protection and chronic disease progression, specifically by preventing oxidative stress and progression of atherosclerosis [51, 52]. Further, vitamin E has a role in decreasing platelet aggregation, thrombosis formation, and monocyte activation [31, 53]. Support for these claims comes from epidemiological studies associating a higher reported intake of vitamin E and lower risk of atherosclerotic heart disease [54, 55]. Because of these associations, in the last 20 years, there has been a tremendous interest in evaluating the effect of vitamin E supplementation for both primary and secondary prevention of heart disease.

While primary prevention studies have had varied methods, generally they have failed to show conclusive evidence that regular supplementation decreases incident myocardial infarction or major adverse cardiac events. For example, while nonsignificant trends have been noted to favor vitamin E supplementation in both the Alpha-Tocopherol Beta-Carotene Cancer Prevention Study and the Woman's Health Study [56], these trends were not supported by the Physicians Health Study (PHI) evaluating healthy men. Further, there was a statistically significant increase in risk of intracranial bleed in men in the PHI who received vitamin E [26].

In individuals with established CVD, vitamin E has been supported by some, but not all clinical trials. An early study in evaluating 52 patients after percutaneous transluminal angioplasty found a nonstatistically significant trend toward less restenosis [57], and the CHAOS trial in 1996 found less composite cardiovascular death and nonfatal MI, though this was driven by decreased nonfatal MI, and there was a trend toward increased total mortality in the intervention arm. In contrast, the HOPE trial (4 years) and HOPE extension trial (median total 7-year follow-up) found no benefit of vitamin E supplementation on major adverse cardiac events, and the extension trial noted an increase in heart failure incidence [58, 59].

Therefore, it remains uncertain if vitamin E supplementation provides cardiovascular benefit in low- or high-risk individuals, and existing evidence refutes supporting routine recommendation for use in individuals. There has been recent suggestion of vitamin E having a role in improving clinical indices noted in non-alcoholic steatohepatitis, thought driven at least in part by

the anti-inflammatory properties of this vitamin [60–62]. However, given some heterogeneity of results in clinical trials, and because of apprehension of safety data balancing benefits and harms (including possibly increased risk of prostate cancer among those taking vitamin E [63]), supplementation recommendations clinically are generally made on a case-by-case basis. This is similarly reflected in the USPSTF review and guidance recommendation for vitamin E supplementation in 2014 [38].

Vitamin K

Vitamin K (in plants, *phylloquinone (K1); menaquinone (K2), and menadione (K3)* ultimately derived from K1) is an essential substrate for physiologic enzymatic processes including converting glutamyl residues to γ-carboxyglutamyl (Gla) residues. This action is important in bone homeostasis, the blood coagulation cascade, as well as in activating matrix Gla proteins, or MGP. MGP is synthesized in smooth muscle cells, and early investigations in animal studies have found it is an important inhibitor of calcification including in the coronary arteries [64]. Vitamin K has also been recognized as having anti-inflammatory actions and suppresses NF-κB, possibly contributing to its role in preventing vascular calcification. While vitamin K deficiencies are rare, in certain high-risk populations (such as those with kidney disease), and in those taking vitamin K antagonist medications, there is epidemiological association with markers of low vitamin K levels and increased cardiovascular mortality and/or vascular calcification [65]. Cohort studies have found circulating phylloquinone levels to not be associated with coronary artery calcification (CAC) progression after over 2 years [66]; in contrast, phylloquinone supplementation in healthy middle aged and older adults was found, after 3 years to decrease progression in CAC in a subgroup analysis of those adherent to treatment, but not stop new CAC formation [67]. K2 has been also subject of research interest, as it has a longer half-life, is considered more potent, and is the major storage form of vitamin K in humans [68]. K2 intake has been shown to decrease arterial stiffness [69], and while cohort studies have found that higher dietary consumption has been associated with lower cardiovascular mortality and aortic calcifications [70, 71], a large meta-analysis only found trends in lower risk of heart disease and serum markers of vitamin K intake [72]. More recently, a meta-analysis of US-based studies similarly failed to find differences in cardiovascular outcomes [73].

Several investigational studies are ongoing; there are no current randomized controlled trials (RCTs) evaluating vitamin K intake showing benefit for supplementation and cardiovascular outcomes. As noted above, several markers of cardiovascular health have shown promise (such as CAC), and thus, these studies will likely provide valuable insight; however, currently there is uncertain benefit of supplementation.

Elemental Mineral Nutrient Supplements

Elemental minerals are essential, meaning they must be obtained from dietary sources as they are not able to be synthesized by the body, and operate as cofactors in multiple crucial physiological processes. Many minerals exhibit a U-shaped curve as it pertains to their relationship with disease, which mirror the homeostatic tendency of the body to require a specific range for optimal function. Adequate dietary intake appears to be linked inversely with CVD while use of supplements especially when internal levels are adequate may increase risk of CVD events and mortality. With this information, the best approach that can be recommended is to gain adequate nutrient intake from dietary sources and supplements if a deficiency is present. Supplementation outside of the need to optimize diet can promote inappropriate use and the perpetuation of poor nutrition as well as potentially increasing the risk of adverse health outcomes. Perturbations of these tightly regulated systems due to dietary inadequacy have widespread consequences, with dysregulation of mineral homeostasis seeming to be one of the

underlying physiological abnormalities contributing to the development of CVD.

Zinc

Zinc is an essential mineral that supports normal growth and development via several cellular processes including protein synthesis, DNA synthesis, cellular division, and cellular metabolism [74]. It also serves as a catalyst and more specifically a cofactor in hundreds of enzymatic reactions and plays a role in immune function, skin integrity, and wound healing as well as the olfactory system with proper taste and smell. Supplemental forms of zinc include zinc acetate, zinc gluconate, and zinc sulfate with the percentage of elemental zinc varying by form. Research is not yet sufficient to provide clarity on the absorption, bioavailability, and tolerance of these forms [75].

Zinc is absorbed by transcellular processes where the highest transport velocity rate occurs in the jejunum of the small intestines. Zinc absorption appears to occur with a level of saturability and dynamic efficiency where transport velocity increases as zinc availability decreases. Zinc concentrations in the blood are tightly regulated where levels can remain fairly stable at both low and high levels of zinc functional stores. Of note, the body requires daily zinc intake as there are no specialized zinc storage systems in the body as observed with other minerals like calcium.

Oxidative stress and inflammation are understood to be key underlying mechanisms in the pathophysiology of CVD, particularly atherosclerosis [76]. Studies have shown an inverse relationship between zinc deficiency and cellular oxidative stress [77, 78], where zinc deficiency increases the production of reactive oxidative species [76]. Zinc also serves to regulate key modulators, such as NF-κB, in inflammatory response pathways, where zinc deficiency has been shown to increase the activation of NF-κB and affect the production of cytokines [79]. Though the exact function of zinc ions in normal cardiac physiology remains unknown, zinc status changes, particularly zinc deficiency, have been reportedly linked to various CVDs [76], including hypertension [80], myocardial infarction [81], atrial fibrillation, and congestive heart failure as well as metabolic syndrome [82]. Studies have implicated zinc deficiency in the development of atherosclerosis and subsequent complications of heart disease including MI and stroke [76]. Evidence from epidemiologic studies suggests that the progression of atherosclerosis is modified by many nutritional factors including zinc. However, this relationship has not been confirmed in randomized clinical trials assessing the role of zinc in primary prevention. Some studies have also shown association between higher intake of zinc and CVD [83], which may be attributed to high meat consumption in Westernized diets. Many RCTs have typically used combination supplements that include zinc but do not provide zinc supplementation solely. Current evidence is not sufficient to support the use of supplementation in primary prevention [84].

Magnesium

Following calcium, sodium, and potassium, magnesium is the fourth most common mineral in the human body [85]. Magnesium is an essential nutrient and is abundant and naturally occurring in many foods. It is crucial to vital processes occurring in the body such as those involved with muscle and nerve function, apoptosis [86], regulation of blood glucose levels, blood pressure [87], and bone formation as well as DNA and protein synthesis [88]. Magnesium, like many other minerals, serves as a cofactor in hundreds of enzymatic reactions, especially those involved with cellular metabolism (i.e., oxidative phosphorylation and glycolysis [87]). In supplemental forms, magnesium is available as magnesium aspartate, magnesium chloride, magnesium citrate, magnesium lactate, and magnesium oxide. Some studies suggest that magnesium is better absorbed and bioavailable in the aspartate, chloride, citrate, and lactate forms compared to oxide and sulfate forms. It has also been found

that zinc consumed at abnormally high doses (142 mg/day) may decrease magnesium absorption [89]. Vitamin D has been linked to improved magnesium absorption [74].

Once consumed, magnesium is efficiently absorbed mainly in the jejunum and ileum [90] and in smaller amounts in the colon [91]. Similar to zinc and calcium, magnesium absorption is inversely related to the magnesium availability in the diet, where the less magnesium is consumed, the more is absorbed. Magnesium absorption is facilitated via both unsaturable passive transport and unsaturable active transport mechanisms. As it relates to the heart, magnesium contributes to normal cardiovascular function by playing a role in the transport of calcium and potassium across cell membranes and thus crucial to the maintenance of normal sinus rhythm [92].

In cardiac physiology, magnesium plays a key role in modulation neuronal excitation, intracardiac conduction, and myocardial contraction [93] and helps to maintain electrical, metabolic, and vascular homeostasis [94]. Magnesium depletion has significant effects on cardiovascular function [95] as well as neuromuscular function and has been associated with CVD [94] risk factors including hypertension [95], diabetes, dyslipidemia, atherosclerosis, and metabolic syndrome [96] and ultimately even CVD [97]. This correlation between hypomagnesemia and CVD is also observed in CKD patients where CVD mortality is higher [98]. Evidence from a variety of studies including epidemiological studies, RCTs, and meta-analyses have suggested an inverse relationship between magnesium intake and CVD. Higher dietary magnesium intake was associated with both lower CV risk factors and CVD-related mortality [99]. Magnesium supplementation has been associated with favorable effects on CVD risk factors, including improvement in arterial stiffness, endothelial function [99], overall blood pressure [100], insulin resistance [101], and metabolic syndrome, but more studies are needed to elucidate the role of supplementation in primary prevention [102]. In one meta-analysis, a 100-mg increment in magnesium intake was associated with 5% risk reduction in hypertension [103]. Evidence of the differential impact of one form compared to another has not been evaluated as yet in the research.

Manganese

Manganese is a naturally occurring, abundant, and essential trace element. It operates as a cofactor for many enzymatic reactions involved with enzymes arginase, pyruvate carboxylase, glutamine synthetase, and manganese superoxide dismutase. It facilitates the metabolism of cholesterol, some amino acids, and glucose. It is also involved in bone formation and antioxidant activity such as reactive oxygen species scavenging [104] and plays a role in homeostasis and the clotting cascade (along with vitamin K) [105]. In supplemental forms, manganese is available in differing formulations (bisglycinate chelate, glycinate chelate, aspartate, gluconate, picolate, citrate, chloride, and sulfate). No current research defines the absorption, bioavailability, and tolerance of these different forms; however, iron status appears to affect manganese absorption [106].

A small percentage of manganese is absorbed in the small intestines via a known active transport system and a lesser known nonsaturable passive mechanism, thought to be facilitated by diffusion when intake is high. Most of the manganese found in the body is present in the bones (25–40%), with the remaining amounts stored in the liver, pancreas, kidney, and brain. Stable manganese concentrations are maintained in the body via a balance of absorption and excretion [74].

Though research is limited, prospective studies have identified manganese deficiency as a likely risk factor for ischemic heart disease including coronary artery disease [107]. In a prospective study, urine manganese had a negative association [108] with systolic and diastolic blood pressure highlighting cardiovascular association with low levels of manganese. Research on the effect of manganese on heart disease has also looked at the interplay between manganese and magnesium. Manganese and magnesium appear to have interchangeable functions where they can occupy activation sites in proteins requiring either Mg or Mn with similar efficiency. Some animal studies have suggested that manganese supplementation can worsen magnesium deficiency and contribute to higher morality [109]. Manganese can also become toxic in high quantities and lead to a manganism, which causes a Parkinson-like illness [110]. Studies of occupation-related manganese exposure reveal that manganese toxicity leads to abnormal ECGs (sinus tachycardia, sinus bradycardia, and arrhythmias), hypertension, and hypotension [111]. There are no clinical trials investigating the impact of manganese on cardiovascular health.

Calcium

Calcium is one of the most abundant elements in the human body, with 99% being stored in the skeleton [74] and teeth and smaller amounts found inside the cells, in blood and tissues such as the muscle. In addition to its role in bone health, it is involved with several cellular and tissue functions including muscle contraction, particularly vasoconstriction and vasodilation, intracellular signaling, nerve transmission, and hormonal secretion. In supplementation, calcium exists in two main forms: calcium carbonate and calcium citrate. Calcium carbonate is more widely available and inexpensive but requires stomach acid to become bioavailable. In contrast, calcium citrate is readily absorbed and optimal for individuals with malabsorptive conditions [112].

Once consumed, calcium is absorbed via active and passive transport in the small intestines [74]. More specifically, the efficiency of calcium is dynamic where absorption increases as the intake level decreases. At low-to-moderate levels, active transport occurs and requires the presence of vitamin D. At high intake levels, passive transport occurs primarily. This dynamic efficiency is a feature of the mechanism that allows tight regulation of calcium in the body where significant changes in intake do not lead to significant changes in concentration unless in severely abnormal states [89] that have been long standing.

Calcium is integral to a healthy cardiovascular system, particularly with its involvement in cardiac muscle function. However, calcium supplementation has been on the rise and evidence from prospective studies [113], RCTs [114], and meta-analyses [115] suggests that calcium supplement intake is associated with an increased risk of CVD events and mortality [116]. Though concerns have been [116] raised with other studies [117] showing some conflicting evidence, the most recent meta-analysis [118] continues to support a concern that calcium supplementation may increase CVD risk. Adverse effects of calcium supplementation seem to occur when total body calcium is already adequate. A recent review suggests that in spite of the widespread use of general supplements, there appears to be no evidence of significant benefit [19]. There have also been studies showing a potential benefit of calcium supplement intake on glucose metabolism [119] on lipid levels [120], where calcium binds to fatty acids leading to decreased absorption in the intestines. The current consensus summarized from a recent review [116] appears to be that a more evidence-based approach is needed and to approach Ca supplementation with caution as the overall body of evidence is not yet fully clear. This has not been shown with dietary intake of calcium in observational studies. High dietary calcium intake (including food sources and supplements) has been associated with lower risk of CVD [121, 122]. The overall recommendation is that use of calcium supplements outside of deficiency should be avoided with the encouragement of dietary intake of calcium. The benefit of the use of calcium and vitamin D supplementation remains conflicting and thus unclear.

Phosphorus

Phosphorus is an abundant mineral of critical importance found naturally in combination with oxygen as phosphate. It is integral to energy production as a component of ATP and is a key element in the formation of cellular membranes, nucleic acids, bone, and teeth [74]. Phosphorus is vital to other processes including maintaining

proper pH and phosphorylation, a step in the catalytic activation of proteins. Phosphorus can be obtained in the diet through the consumption of a variety of whole foods and dietary supplementation in single and combination formulations, which include MVI. Phosphate additives are also largely present in processed foods. In supplementation, phosphorus is available in the form phosphate salts (dipotassium phosphate or disodium phosphate) and phospholipids (phosphatidylcholine and phosphatidylserine). Simultaneous intake of calcium carbonate and antacids can bind to phosphorus and prevent its absorption [123].

Once consumed, most phosphorus absorption occurs in the jejunum by passive concentration-dependent processes though some is also absorbed via active transport and the efficiency of absorption appears to be unaffected by intake levels. Phosphorus is present in food in the form of phosphates and phosphate esters. Phosphate is also stored in the form of phytic acid; however, this form requires the presence of the enzyme phytase, which is not produced in the human intestines. In the body, phosphorus is primarily found in hydroxyapatite (85%), the main component of bone and teeth, and to a much lesser degree in soft tissue (15%).

Many robust studies have outlined an association with higher serum phosphorus concentrations and CVD as well as CVD mortality in the CKD and ESRD populations [124, 125], prompting the development of phosphate binders to reduce phosphorus serum levels. The mechanism underlying this includes disordered mineral metabolism associated with impaired kidney function promoting vascular calcification, arterial stiffness, cardiomyocyte hypertrophy, atherosclerosis, and other pathophysiological processes that impair and damage the cardiovascular system [122, 125, 126]. In the general population, the same association is observed with even mild elevations in serum phosphorus, even at the higher end of the normal range [127–131]. Excess dietary phosphorus intake has been commonly observed in the Westernized population and can lead to perturbations in phosphorus homeostasis. Because of the increasing consumption of processed foods in the American diet, high consumption of dietary phosphorus has increasingly become a topic of interest and concern [131]. It has been suggested that daily intake of phosphorus exceeding 800 mg may have adverse effects [132–134]. Phosphorus restriction has been recommended as a strategy to decrease adverse outcomes in the general population.

Potassium

Potassium is one of the most important minerals found in the body as it serves as one of the main intracellular cations. It is involved in many crucial cellular processes including nerve transmission, muscle contraction, vascular tone, and regulation of intracellular and extracellular fluid volume [74]. Potassium can be obtained from dietary sources via a wide variety of whole foods and dietary supplementation. Forms of potassium supplementation include potassium chloride (the most commonly used), potassium citrate, phosphate aspartate bicarbonate, and gluconate.

Once consumed, potassium is absorbed in the small intestines via passive diffusion and concentrated in the intracellular and extracellular compartments to create a gradient that drives many cellular processes. In a cardiac cell, as in other cells, this gradient is characterized by a high level of potassium inside the cell compared to outside of the cell, up to 30 times higher in the intracellular space than the extracellular space. Enzymatic processes, including sodium–potassium (Na+/K+) ATPase transporter, are responsible for maintaining this gradient. Other cellular ions such as Ca and Na have higher concentrations outside of the cell. In this state, the cell is polarized as it holds a more negative charge inside the cell relative to the outside of the cell. In this state, it is inactive until it depolarizes resulting in the phases 0–4 of the action potential: the rapid upstroke, repolarization, plateau, the late repolarization, and diastole [135]. Subsequently, the action potential facilitates the cellular processes of nerve transmission and muscle contraction.

A low potassium diet has been associated with increased blood pressure, increased risk of stroke, and increased risk of chronic kidney disease. Potassium deficiency serves to induce sodium reabsorption and decrease sodium urinary excretion and decrease vasodilation [136–138]. One of the benefits derived from potassium intake is its effect on blood pressure where high dietary potassium intake has been associated with decreased blood pressure and subsequently lower risk of stroke and coronary heart disease. Potassium supplementation has been used to offset the impact of high sodium consumption. A 2013 systematic review found that high potassium intake was associated with a statistically significant decrease in blood pressure in patients with and without hypertension [137]. A 2011 meta-analysis observed a 21% lower risk of stroke with a 1.64-g higher intake of potassium [138]. Potassium intake was not associated with risk of coronary heart disease or risk factors associated with it such as blood lipid concentrations [138].

Selenium

Selenium is an essential mineral that is found naturally in many foods. It is an integral component of special proteins called selenoproteins that play an important role in thyroid function as cofactors for thyroid hormone deiodinases, reproduction, DNA synthesis, immune function, redox signaling, oxidoreductions, and antioxidant activity [74, 139]. Selenium has also been identified as playing a role in cell cycle progression and cell growth and in cancer prevention via the promotion of cell arrest and induced cell death (apoptosis) [140, 141]. Selenium can be obtained from dietary sources via a wide variety of whole foods and dietary supplementation. In supplementary forms, selenium is available as selenomethionine, selenium-enriched yeast, sodium selenite, and sodium selenite.

Selenium exists in inorganic (selenate and selenite) and organic forms (selenomethionine and selenocysteine) and is present in human tissues in the organic forms. Selenomethionine and selenocysteine are also the dietary forms of selenium, with selenomethionine being the most prominent. Selenate and selenite are not dietary forms and are used to fortify foods and in dietary supplements. Both selenomethionine and selenocysteine are well absorbed in the GI tract. These four forms of selenium can be ingested and converted to metabolites such as selenide, which can operate as a precursor for other reactions in the cell, or methylselenol, which is involved in regulation of the cell cycle. Selenium stores in the body include the skeleton and the liver.

Historically, selenium deficiency has been most associated with a juvenile cardiomyopathy called Keshan disease that is endemic to countries such as China and Eastern Siberia [142, 143]. Though this is a specific disease, the underlying pathology of increased oxidative stress related to Se deficiency has been observed in the development of CVD in the general population [144]. The specific pathophysiology appears to be related to the impaired function of selenoproteins such as glutathione peroxidase, thioredoxin reductases, and methionine sulfoxide reducated B1, which have been specifically linked to cardiovascular stress [145]. Mechanisms supporting the positive impact of selenium on cardiovascular health include increased antioxidant activity, reduced apoptosis, and reduced alteration of inflammatory response pathways. The trend of adverse CVD risk factors and CVD and its association with inadequate mineral levels continues to be observed with respect to selenium. However, high selenium exposure in the setting of adequate selenium intake may be associated with increased risks of Type 2 diabetes, lipid levels, and blood pressure as well as adverse cardiometabolic outcomes, though most studies have been cross-sectional and thus do not prove causation. Currently, there is no conclusive evidence to conclude that use of selenium supplements will prevent CVD in nondeficient populations [144–148]. This is a needed area of research as the use of selenium-enriched foods, supplements, and even fertilizers has notably increased in recent years due to increased marketing and consumer interest in selenium's antioxidant capabilities.

Copper

Copper is an essential mineral found naturally in some foods. It acts as a cofactor for many enzymes known collectively as cuproenzymes, which play an important role as oxidases in the reduction of molecular oxygen. These enzymes include diamine oxidase (inactivates the histamine released in allergic reactions), monoamine oxidase (plays essential role in the degradation of serotonin and metabolism of catecholamines and dopamine), ferroxidases (plays a role in iron transport via ferrous iron oxidation), dopamine, β-monooxygenase (converts dopamine to norepinephrine), and copper/zinc superoxide dismutase (plays a role in antioxidant activity). The activity of these enzymes has been shown to decrease with copper deficiency. Copper also plays an important role in angiogenesis, immune system function, . regulation of gene expression, neurotransmitter homeostasis, and pigmentation [149]. Copper can be obtained from dietary sources via a wide variety of whole foods and dietary supplementation. In supplementation, copper exists as cupric oxide, cupric sulfate, copper amino acid chelates, and copper gluconate [74].

Copper is primarily absorbed in the small intestines via saturable-mediated and non-saturable-mediated processes and as well as energy-dependent transport via Menkes P-type ATPase. Copper absorption is very dependent on dietary intake and can vary from 20% to 50% depending on the milligrams of copper ingested. It is mainly bound by ceruloplasmin and transported through the body for use and storage in cells and specific tissues. Two-thirds of the copper in the body is stored in the skeleton and muscle with the remaining third stored in the liver where 35% of copper is absorbed in the portal vein and delivered to the liver for uptake in the liver cells [74].

Cuproenzymes, such as superoxide dismutase and lysyl oxidase, are crucial for the physiological responses of cardiovascular cells. The expression of cuproenzymes by cardiac cells is tightly regulated and facilitate angiogenesis, cell growth, cell migration, and wound repair [150]. Deficiency in this mineral leads to decreased activities of these enzymes leading to pathological mechanism (peroxidation, glycation, and nitration), resulting in the loss of cell matrix in the heart and blood vessels as well as antioxidant damage [151–153]. Copper, like many other minerals, has a dual nature where levels that are too high or too low are pro-oxidant and are associated with disease while sufficient levels allow for normal antioxidant activity and are associated with prevention of disease. In prospective studies, high serum copper and ceruloplasmin levels have been associated with CVD similar to low serum copper levels [151, 154, 155]. The only randomized trial looking specifically at copper supplement use found the data to be inconsistent where there was both improvement and worsening of metabolic markers [156].

Chromium

Chromium is a trace mineral known to be involved in glucose regulation although a comprehensive understanding of the role it plays in human physiology remains to be elucidated in the research. In addition to playing a role in glucose regulation by potentiating the action of insulin, it also appears to be involved with the metabolism of fats, carbohydrates, and proteins. Chromium can be obtained from dietary sources as well as dietary supplementation. Chromium is widely used as a supplement and is present in single and combination formulations. It is available as chromium chloride, chromium nicotinate, chromium picolinate, high-chromium yeast, and chromium citrate [74]. Clarity on which of these supplemental forms is best to take is limited due to a lack of research.

Chromium exists in two forms: the dietary form, which is trivalent chromium [74] (chromium III), and the form that exists in the environment, hexavalent (chromium VI), which is carcinogenic. The current understanding is that chromium is absorbed in the small intestines via passive diffusion mechanisms and then transported by the protein, transferrin, to various tissues. Chromium absorption is found to be quite low in the body, ranging from 0.5% to 2.5% [74, 157]. Research has suggested that absorption may be potentiated by exercise. In the body, chromium stores include the liver, spleen, and bone.

The impact of chromium on CVD has been studied within the last two decades but data remain limited. Studies from the 1970s revealed that chromium was indeed and essential nutrient that played a role in glucose metabolism, particularly with insulin, and lipid metabolism [158]. The epidemiological evidence on chromium intake and CVD is limited but suggests an inverse relationship between deficient chromium levels [159] and risk of myocardial infarction [160]. Chromium deficiency has been associated with hyperglycemia, hyperinsulinemia, insulin resistance, and hypertension, which are all abnormal physiological states that contribute to type 2 diabetes and metabolic syndrome. In regard to supplementation, some studies have suggested that chromium supplementation improves insulin and glucose control [161–163]. There remains a need for further research to better understand whether chromium supplementation results in cardiovascular benefit.

Macronutrient Supplement Compounds

Macronutrients have also been increasingly evaluated on their role in cardiovascular health. These compounds—usually taken whole or in combination with other supplements—have a variety of impacts in homeostatic function, including muscle and myocardial function. Over the last several decades, several compounds have been evaluated including CoA Q10, garlic, pmega-3 fatty acid oils, resveratrol, red rice yeast, Ginkgo biloba, and curcumin. In general, compared with vitamin and elemental supplementation, relatively less is understand about the use of these as supplements. While some studies have shown promise, the complex interplay for much of these compound's actions remains yet to be elucidated.

CoQ10

CoA Q10 (CoQ10) is the only known endogenous lipid-soluble antioxidant in humans and is found in high concentrations in the bilipid membranes. Its two primary roles are protecting cellular membranes from lipid peroxidation by reactive oxygen species and as a carrier in the electron transport chain [164]. CoQ10 is, unsurprisingly, found in high concentrations in metabolically active tissues such as the heart, liver, kidneys, and nervous system [165]. The evidence supporting its role in cardiovascular health is mounting, both due to its antioxidant effects and its role in energy production. The role of inflammation on CVD is well known, and understanding the effects of CoQ10 on the heart is important given the worldwide burden of CVD.

Endothelial dysfunction, often caused by reactive oxygen species (ROS), is found early on in the development of CVD [165]. A meta-analysis of RCTs looking at CoQ10 supplementation's effects on the vascular flow patterns related to endothelial dysfunction showed that when given oral supplementation of CoQ10, there was an improvement of the flow-mediated dilation of the peripheral arteries indicating improvement of the endothelial dysfunction and the possible therapeutic benefits to the early supplementation of CoQ10 [166]. This relationship is thought to be mediated by the antioxidant effects of CoQ10 and could play a role in both primary and secondary prevention of CVD [167]. Other studies have shown that CoQ10 supplementation reduces inflammatory markers. A case-control study looking at CVD and the interplay of reactive oxygen species and CoQ10 showed that cases who had had a recent coronary stent placed had higher levels of oxidative markers and lower levels of CoQ10 compared to controls who did not have CVD [168–171]. The long-term effects of CoQ10 supplementation were studied in a RCT among elderly adults who were given CoQ10 and selenium supplementation for 4 years. The individuals in the treatment arm had a statistically significant reduction in mortality that continued to be seen even 8 years after the supplementation had been ceased. Reperfusion injury plays a large part in the long-term consequences of ischemic heart disease. Due to CoQ10's mechanism of action both as an antioxidant and as part of the mitochondrial energy machinery, it plays a valuable role in mitigating the effects of ischemic injury during and immediately after myocardial infarctions. Higher levels of CoQ10 have been connected with lower oxidative stress, less myocardial necrosis and apoptosis, improved cardiac functioning, and increased energy available directly following a myocardial infarction. A study looking at the correlations of endogenous levels of CoQ10 in the blood and the long-term effects of ischemic injury and left ventricular function showed that patients with lower levels of CoQ10 had worse outcomes than individuals with higher levels of CoQ10 6 months after the event [172]. Due to the time it takes to build up CoQ10 levels in the blood via oral supplementation, acute use after an MI is often too little too late so the therapeutic benefits are seen best when used earlier on in the course of the disease. While the beneficial effects of CoQ10 are seen in the early stages of CAD, a meta-analysis of CoQ10 supplementation showed that in heart-failure patients CoQ10 lead to decreased mortality and improvements in exercise capacity indicating that it has uses even in secondary prevention [173].

There is insufficient evidence to support CoQ10 has any effect on hyperlipidemia or blood pressure, although preliminary studies suggest it may play a role in mitigating the effects of hyperlipidemia on development of atherosclerosis and coronary artery disease [174].

Anecdotal evidence suggests that some people have resolution of statin-induced myopathy with supplementation of CoQ10; however, the evidence supporting this has been mixed. One meta-analysis [175] did show CoQ10 to be beneficial in the muscle weakness, cramps, and fatigue though not in regards to muscle pain, while another meta-analysis [176] found no benefit with CoQ10 supplementation in regards to statin-induced myopathy. The studies were generally small with significant heterogeneity making conclusions difficult to assess between trials.

Garlic

Garlic (*Allium sativum*) has many claims to health including decreasing lipids, blood pressure, and an antiplatelet effect leading to a risk reduction of CVD. Allicin, the pungent chemical that gives garlic its strong flavor, has not been shown to be absorbed in the gut and is therefore unlikely responsible for the lauded health effects of this plant. However, *S*-allyl-L-cysteine (SAC), a water-soluble organosulfide, found in the aged garlic formulations, has high bioavailability and is thought to be partially responsible for the many bioactive effects of garlic. Due to the many different chemicals in garlic, depending on the formulation, it can lead to either no health effects if the primary components are the more volatile chemicals such as allicin, or to significant improvements in blood pressure and lipid profiles in formulations containing the more water-soluble SAC components [177].

In a double-blind placebo-controlled trial, researchers found that the use of aged garlic extract led to a statistically significant drop in blood pressure among participants with uncontrolled hypertension. A meta-analysis of 20 RCTs showed that garlic supplements lowered both diastolic and systolic blood pressure [178].

Not only has garlic been shown to reduce blood pressure, it also can lead to a small but significant reduction in lipid levels. A meta-analysis looking at clinical trials that used aged black garlic, garlic oil, and garlic supplements showed that) garlic supplementation led to a significant decrease in total cholesterol and LDL levels while increasing HDL levels [179].

While not as supported as the lipid- and blood-pressure-lowering effects of garlic, preliminary studies have shown garlic supplementation has an effect on inhibiting platelet aggregation [180] which could prove to be another beneficial way that garlic is cardioprotective. While there is insufficient evidence on the role garlic plays during acute myocardial infarctions, animal studies have shown that it protects myocytes from hypoxic injury by inducing autophagy instead of necrosis [181]. Further studies are needed to determine how this could lead to a beneficial effect in humans.

Fish Oil

Societies with high amounts of fish in their diets have been shown to have lower rates of CVD, raising interest in the use of fish oil supplementation in the prevention of CVD. Fish contains high levels of polyunsatuated fatty acids (PUFA) with a double bond in the third carbon position, more commonly known as the omega-3 fatty acids. The two primary omega-3 FAs are eicosapentaenoic acid (EPA) and docosahexaenoic acid (DHA). The PUFAs have been shown to have multiple cardioprotective mechanisms including lowering of cholesterol and triglycerides, antiarrhythmic and anti-inflammatory properties [182–185]. Studies have shown that supplementation of 2–4 g/day leads to a decrease in total cholesterol levels in dose dependent manner with or without the use of statin medications [186, 187]. Bioactive derivatives of the omega-3 FAs have been shown to decrease sudden cardiac death and episodes of ventricular tachycardia in patients with recent myocardial infarctions [185] making a case for its use in secondary prevention. While the data are mixed on the use of omega-3 FA for primary prevention [188–190], recent studies looking at formulations containing only EPA have shown a clear decrease in the incidence of primary myocardial infarctions in patients with significant risk factors for CVD [191]. Additionally, bioactive compounds derived from omega-3 have potent anti-inflammatory properties and are integral to the modulation of the immune system and down-regulation of acute phase reactants. Given the role inflammation plays in CVD, this ability may play a role in the primary prevention of CVD. Thus, there is great interest in further understanding the role of EPA supplementation in average and low-risk individuals.

There have been a number of large cohort studies looking at the effects of fish oil on cardiovascular health which are worth noting. One of the difficulties with the use of supplements is the unregulated industry, especially amongst the over-the-counter (OTC) formulations. The JELIS trial, which followed 18,645 Japanese patients and used just the EPA PUFA, and the REDUCE-IT trial, which followed 8179 cardiac patients and gave them icosapent ethyl which is a highly purified stable form of EPA, both showed improvements in cardiovascular outcomes with the use of EPA [176]. However, the VITAL trial, which used a fish oil supplement that combined the EPA and DHA [176], showed no significant cardiovascular benefits. The differences in the trials demonstrate how the specific components of the supplements can change the outcomes; almost all OTC fish oils are a combination of the EPA and DHA PUFA. Because of this, the current recommendations for the use of nonprescription (OTC) fish oil supplementation are class III (no benefit) for primary and secondary prevention of CVD [176].

Resveratrol

Resveratrol (RES) is a potent antioxidant found in the skin of red grapes and is a direct scavenger of hydroxyl ($\bullet OH$) and superoxide ($O_2\bullet^-$) radicals. Given the moderate consumption of red wine among the French, it is thought to be one of the chemicals that explains the "French Paradox," the observation that low levels of CVD has been noted among French individuals despite a diet rich in saturated fats. Clinical trials in patients with CVD have shown that supplementation with RES leads to a decrease in platelet aggregation, improved flow mediated dilation, and left ventricular function in patients with recent MI making a case for its use as a nutraceutical [192]. However, questions about bioavailability with oral supplementation, its ability to inhibit CYP3A4, and the lack of significant clinical evidence on the effects of RES on cardiac health bring into question the efficacy of RES supplementation for primary and secondary prevention of CVD. Further questions

on whether it is RES alone rather than a combination of multiple chemicals in red grapes that explain the "French Paradox" remain.

Red Rice Yeast

Red Yeast Rice (RYR) has been used in Chinese medicine as a lipid lowering cardioprotective supplement for decades. Some formulations of RYR contain high levels of a compound called monocolin K, which is chemically identical to lovastatin. RYR has been shown to lower LDL-C comparable to moderate-dose statin medications, especially in patients who have side effects from or prefer not to take statins [193, 194]. RYR has been shown to reduce cardiovascular mortality in patients with diabetes and hypertension in various clinical trials [195, 196]. One of the concerns that has been brought up by the FDA is the unregulated industry and the amount of monocolin K found in various OTC supplements and concerns over its safety profile given its similarities to prescription medications [193, 194, 196, 197]. Specific safety concerns are due to the metabolite citrinin. Animal studies have shown nephrotoxic effects and renal cancer associated with the chronic use of citrinin. Certain RYR supplements have been found to have concentrations of citrinin over the levels recommended safe [195]. While studies have clearly shown that RYR with high levels of monocolin K does have similar cardioprotective effects of the statins in both lipid-lowering activity and secondary prevention of cardiac mortality, it can be challenging to know what percentage of monocolin K a particular supplement may have.

Ginkgo Biloba

One of the most commonly used herbal remedies in the USA and Europe, Ginkgo biloba is taken with a goal of stabilizing atherosclerotic plaque and improving blood flow [198]. Ginkgo biloba has been shown to have anticoagulation properties by direct inhibition of thrombin. Evidence supports that it may decrease early plaque formation in the coronary arteries and stabilizes existing plaque in CVD patients by downregulating inflammatory markers leading to a decrease in LDL-C oxidation and subsequent foam cell formation [199–201]. While clinical trials are lacking in showing an effect on reduction in morbidity and mortality from cardiovascular events, the reduction and stabilization of plaque do indicate that it may be a useful tool in the prevention and management of CVD.

Curcumin

Curcumin, the active ingredient in turmeric, has long been used in Eastern medicine as a powerful anti-inflammatory agent. Due to its long history of use, recent studies have sought to understand more of what curcumin does in the body. Its primary role in cardiovascular health has to do with its potent anti-inflammatory and antioxidant effects [202]. Curcumin lowers vascular inflammation leading to decreased levels of TNF-a, IL-6, IL-1, and other inflammatory markers, which may help to reduce macrovascular complications, especially among diabetics. In addition

to the anti-inflammatory effects, meta-analyses of RCTs showed that daily use of curcumin reduced LDL-C and total cholesterol levels in adults with metabolic syndrome further decreasing cardiovascular risk. Curcumin also has been shown to have antiplatelet and anticoagulant properties, though no trials have been done to show this has a direct effect on cardiac morbidity and mortality [203–205]. Overall, curcumin has been shown to be safe and effective in clinical trials [202], and thus ongoing trials may provide further evidence to support this compound. As it stands, further research is needed to understand its direct effects on cardiovascular health.

Conclusion

Dietary supplements, vitamins, and minerals are a multibillion-dollar industry that makes all sorts of claims about health benefits. While the use of supplements has been found to confer benefit as evidenced by rigorous studies showing mortality benefit such as CoQ10 and congestive heart failure, others, such as fish oil, have epidemiological support but thus far have failed to show significance of benefit when studied in a systematic way. Table 1.1 outlines an overview

Table 1.1 Summary of supplement dietary sources, common formations, and summary for CVD benefit

Nutrient	Dietary source	Supplement forms	Summary evidence
Multivitamins	Varied—whole grains, plant sources (legumes, green leafy vegetables, fruits, nuts); some animal sources (meat, such as pork, fish, beef)	MVI—multivitamins (varied)	Dietary intake in foods rich in these vitamins has epidemiological support for CVD benefit. Interventional studies have failed to find consistent benefit for CVD risk
B Vitamins	Varied—whole grains, plant sources (legumes, green leafy vegetables, fruits, nuts); some animal sources (meat, such as pork, fish, beef)	B1—thiamine B3—niacin B5—pantothenic acid B6—pyroxidine B9—folate/folic acid B12—cyanocobalamin	Supplements of some may lower surrogate markers of CVD risk; supplements have not consistently been found to confer benefit. Diet intake in foods rich in these vitamins have epidemiological support for CVD benefit
Vitamin C	Varied fruit sources—citrus, potatoes, tomatoes; varied vegetable sources including potato, broccoli, Brussels sprouts, bell pepper	L-ascorbic acid	Diets rich in vitamin C have inverse associations with incident heart disease; supplement use in isolation has not been found to confer CVD risk benefit

Table 1.1   (continued)

Nutrient	Dietary source	Supplement forms	Summary evidence
Vitamin A	Animal derived especially liver; some fish oils; dairy products; vegetable sources include green leafy vegetables, tomatoes, potatoes (especially swell potato)	Retinol, retinal, and retinyl esters; carotenoid compounds or provitamin A compounds (α-carotene, β-carotene, and β-cryptoxanthin)	Carotenoid-rich diets have been found to have a lower cardiovascular disease risk; interventional studies have not found consistent benefit and in some populations (e.g., smokers) may confer harm
Vitamin D	Fatty fish, fish oils; dairy in particular cheese; egg yolks, mushrooms; fortified foods such as milk, certain fortified cereals	25-Hydroxyvitamin D-calcidiol; 1,25-hydroxyvitamin D-calciferol	Epidemiologic support for CVD risk and vitamin D exposure (sun); interventional studies have failed to find consistent CVD risk benefit
Vitamin E	Varied—plant sources (green leafy vegetables, seeds, nuts); some vegetable oils (canola, corn, soybean); some fruits (kiwi, tomato)	Tocopherols; tocotrienols	Largely mixed evidence; large intervention trials have not found benefit and possible harm (intracranial bleeds, heart failure exacerbations)
Vitamin K	Varied—Plant sources (green leafy vegetables); some vegetable oils; some fruits (blueberries, grapes, pomegranate)	K1—Phylloquinone K2—menaquinone K3—menadione, derived from K1	Early studies suggest possible benefit of K1 and K2; interventional studies are ongoing
Zinc	Whole grains, cashews, sesame seeds, pumpkin seeds, almonds, chickpeas, legumes, poultry, beef, lamb, oysters, and shrimp	Zinc acetate; zinc gluconate Zinc sulfate	Though zinc deficiency has been implicated in the development of atherosclerosis, current evidence does not supplementation in primary prevention
Magnesium	Green leafy vegetables, legumes, nuts, seeds, whole grains	Magnesium aspartate; magnesium chloride; magnesium citrate; magnesium lactate; magnesium oxide	Magnesium supplementation has been associated with favorable effects in individuals with CVD risk factors though more research is needed to elucidate its benefit in primary prevention
Manganese	Plant sources (whole grains, nuts, legumes, leafy vegetables, coffee, tea, spices such as black pepper) and animals sources (mollusks)	Manganese bisglycinate chelate; manganese glycinate chelate; manganese aspartate; manganese gluconate; manganese picolate; manganese citrate; manganese chloride; manganese sulfate	Manganese is known more for its potential for toxicity. Some prospective studies have identified an inverse relationship between manganese levels and blood pressure; however, no clinical trials have investigated the impact of manganese on CVD
Calcium	Plant sources such as Chinese cabbage, kale, and broccoli; dairy sources such as milk, yogurt, and cheese; grains when consumed frequently in adequate amounts	Calcium carbonate; calcium citrate	Studies have provided conflicting evidence on the benefit or adverse effects of calcium supplementation. More studies have suggested an increased risk of CVD and CVD mortality. Per most recent guidelines, calcium supplementation is not recommended

(continued)

Table 1.1 (continued)

Nutrient	Dietary source	Supplement forms	Summary evidence
Phosphorus	Plant sources (nuts, legumes, vegetables and grains) and animal sources (dairy products, meats and poultry, fish and eggs); processed foods contain phosphate additives such as phosphoric acid, sodium phosphate, and sodium polyphosphate	Phosphate salts (dipotassium phosphate or disodium phosphate) phospholipids (phosphatidylcholine and phosphatidylserine)	Excess phosphorus intake is a concern, particularly with the dietary patent of westernized cultures. Increased intake of phosphorus has been associated impaired cardiac and renal function. The overall recommendation is to decrease phosphorus intake in the diet
Potassium	Plant sources (legumes, green leafy vegetables, fruits, and nuts) and animal sources (meat, poultry, fish, milk, and yogurt)	Potassium chloride, potassium citrate, potassium phosphate, potassium aspartate, potassium bicarbonate, and potassium gluconate	Dietary intake associated with decreased CVD risk and mortality while supplementation has consistently been found to decrease blood pressure
Selenium	Plant sources (whole grains, fruits, vegetables, nuts, especially Brazil nuts) and animal sources (seafood, meat, and dairy)	Selenomethionine; selenium-enriched yeast; sdium selenite; sodium selenite	Currently, there is no conclusive evidence to conclude that use of selenium supplements will prevent CVD in nondeficient populations
Copper	Plant sources (seeds, nuts, grains, chocolate) and animal sources (shellfish and organ meats)	Cupric oxide; cupric sulfate; copper amino acid chelates; copper gluconate	Both high and low serum copper and ceruloplasmin levels have been associated with CVD in less robust studies. There are no clinical trials demonstrating conclusive evidence on the impact of copper supplementation on CVD health
Chromium	Whole grains, some fruits (apples, bananas, oranges, and grapes), some vegetables (green beans, potatoes, broccoli, garlic, and basil), and meats (beef, turkey, chicken)	Chromium chloride chromium nicotinate; chromium picolinate; high-chromium yeast, chromium citrate	There remains a need for further research to better understand whether chromium supplementation results in cardiovascular benefit
CoQ10	N/a	N/a	Cardioprotective against morbidity and mortality from ischemic heart disease
Garlic	N/a	Aged garlic formulations	Significant decrease in blood pressure and small but significant decreases in LDL-C levels
Fish oil	N/a	N/a	Mixed evidence for cardioprotective benefits. EPA-only formulations show cardioprotective benefits. EPA/DHA OTC formulations do not show evidence of cardioprotective benefits
Resveratrol	Grapes and red wine	N/a	Limited evidence on cardioprotective benefits as a nutraceutical
Red yeast rice	N/a	N/a	Lowers LDL-C similar to statins. Concerns over heterogeneity of active ingredients in supplements
Gingko biloba	N/a	N/a	Anti-inflammatory effects may lead to stabilization and reduction of plaque
Curcumin	Turmeric	N/a	Potent anti-inflammatory agent decreases vascular inflammation and LDL-C levels

and summary of the key findings thus far for the compounds reviewed in this chapter. As many of these confer considerable expense to patients, it is imperative that clinicians are critical of existing evidence, and judicious with recommendation of supplement use. Overwhelmingly, it is consistently safe to recommend the consumption of varied, whole foods that are rich in dietary macronutrients, such as garlic and fish compared to isolated preparations such as garlic extract and fish oil. Ideally, the consumption of these foods is recommended as part of a nutrient-rich plant-predominant dietary pattern as outlined in the Healthy US-Style Dietary Pattern that is referenced in the 2020–2025 Dietary Guidelines for Americans. A perfect example of this is the use of green tea: while there are some concerns over the safety of green tea extract [206], there is consensus in regard to the significant benefits of drinking green tea [207]. The more one can get beneficial compounds such as PUFAs, polyphenols, antioxidants, vitamins, and minerals through regular dietary consumption, over the use of supplements formulation, generally, the better for health-related outcomes.

References

1. Bailey RL, Gahche JJ, Miller PE, Thomas PR, Dwyer JT. Why US adults use dietary supplements. JAMA Intern Med. 2013;173(5):355–61. https://doi.org/10.1001/jamainternmed.2013.2299.
2. Law MR, Morris JK. By how much does fruit and vegetable consumption reduce the risk of ischaemic heart disease? Eur J Clin Nutr. 1998;52(8):549–56. https://doi.org/10.1038/sj.ejcn.1600603.
3. Fortmann SP, Burda BU, Senger CA, Lin JS, Whitlock EP. Vitamin and mineral supplements in the primary prevention of cardiovascular disease and cancer: an updated systematic evidence review for the U.S. preventive services task force. Ann Intern Med. 2013;159(12):824–34. https://doi.org/10.7326/0003-4819-159-12-201312170-00729.
4. Bleys J, Miller ER, Pastor-Barriuso R, Appel LJ, Guallar E. Vitamin-mineral supplementation and the progression of atherosclerosis: a meta-analysis of randomized controlled trials. Am J Clin Nutr. 2006;84(4):880–7. https://doi.org/10.1093/ajcn/84.4.880.
5. Hercberg S, Galan P, Preziosi P, et al. The SU.VI. MAX study: a randomized, placebo-controlled trial of the health effects of antioxidant vitamins and minerals. Arch Intern Med. 2004;164(21):2335–42. https://doi.org/10.1001/archinte.164.21.2335.
6. Gaziano JM, Sesso HD, Christen WG, et al. Multivitamins in the prevention of cancer in men: the physicians' health study II randomized controlled trial. J Am Med Assoc. 2012;308(18):1871–80. https://doi.org/10.1001/jama.2012.14641.
7. Christen WG, Cook NR, Van Denburgh M, Zaharris E, Albert CM, Manson JAE. Effect of combined treatment with folic acid, vitamin B6, and vitamin B12 on plasma biomarkers of inflammation and endothelial dysfunction in women. J Am Heart Assoc. 2018;7(11); https://doi.org/10.1161/JAHA.117.008517.
8. Hosseini B, Saedisomeolia A, Skilton MR. Association between micronutrients intake/status and carotid intima media thickness: a systematic review. J Acad Nutr Diet. 2017;117(1):69–82. https://doi.org/10.1016/j.jand.2016.09.031.
9. Huo Y, Li J, Qin X, et al. Efficacy of folic acid therapy in primary prevention of stroke among adults with hypertension in China: the CSPPT randomized clinical trial. J Am Med Assoc. 2015;313(13):1325–35. https://doi.org/10.1001/jama.2015.2274.
10. Davey Smith G, Ebrahim S. Folate supplementation and cardiovascular disease. Lancet. 2005;366(9498):1679–81. https://doi.org/10.1016/S0140-6736(05)67676-3.
11. Dinicolantonio JJ, Niazi AK, Lavie CJ, O'Keefe JH, Ventura HO. Thiamine supplementation for the treatment of heart failure: a review of the literature. Congest Heart Fail. 2013;19(4):214–22. https://doi.org/10.1111/chf.12037.
12. DiNicolantonio JJ, Lavie CJ, Niazi AK, O'Keefe JH, Hu T. Effects of thiamine on cardiac function in patients with systolic heart failure: systematic review and metaanalysis of randomized, double-blind, placebo-controlled trials. Ochsner J. 2013;13(4):495–9. Accessed 31 Aug 2020. /pmc/articles/PMC3865826/?report=abstract
13. Chen YQ, Zhao SP, Zhao YH. Efficacy and tolerability of coenzyme a vs pantethine for the treatment of patients with hyperlipidemia: a randomized, double-blind, multicenter study. J Clin Lipidol. 2015;9(5):692–7. https://doi.org/10.1016/j.jacl.2015.07.003.
14. Lloyd-Jones DM. Niacin and HDL cholesterol - time to face facts. N Engl J Med. 2014;371(3):271–3. https://doi.org/10.1056/NEJMe1406410.
15. Stamler J. Clofibrate and niacin in coronary heart disease. J Am Med Assoc. 1975;231(4):360–81. https://doi.org/10.1001/jama.1975.03240160024021.
16. Prineas RJ, Friedewald W. Fifteen year mortality in coronary drug project patients: long-term benefit with niacin. J Am Coll Cardiol. 1986;8(6):1245–55. https://doi.org/10.1016/S0735-1097(86)80293-5.
17. Burton E, Lewin G, O'Connell H, Petrich M, Boyle E, Hill KD. Can community care workers deliver a falls prevention exercise program? A feasibility

study. Clin Interv Aging. 2018;13:485–95. https://doi.org/10.2147/CIA.S162728.

18. D'Alonzo KT, Smith BA, Dicker LH. Outcomes of a culturally tailored partially randomized patient preference controlled trial to increase physical activity among low-income immigrant Latinas. J Transcult Nurs. Published online July 27. 2017; https://doi.org/10.1177/1043659617723073.

19. Ingles DP, Cruz Rodriguez JB, Garcia H. Supplemental vitamins and minerals for cardiovascular disease prevention and treatment. Curr Cardiol Rep. 2020;22(4):1–8. https://doi.org/10.1007/s11886-020-1270-1.

20. Knekt P, Ritz J, Pereira MA, et al. Antioxidant vitamins and coronary heart disease risk: a pooled analysis of 9 cohorts. Am J Clin Nutr. 2004;80(6):1508–20. https://doi.org/10.1093/ajcn/80.6.1508.

21. Frei B, England L, Ames BN. Ascorbate is an outstanding antioxidant in human blood plasma (oxidant stress/lipid peroxidation/protein Thiols/a-Tocopherol). Proc Nati Acad Sci USA. 1989;86:6377–81. PMID is 2762330.

22. Honarbakhsh S, Schachter M. Vitamins and cardiovascular disease. Br J Nutr. 2009;101(8):1113–31. https://doi.org/10.1017/S000711450809123X.

23. Li Y, Schellhorn HE. New developments and novel therapeutic perspectives for vitamin C. J Nutr. 2007;137(10):2171–84. https://doi.org/10.1093/jn/137.10.2171.

24. Osganian SK, Stampfer MJ, Rimm E, et al. Vitamin C and risk of coronary heart disease in women. J Am Coll Cardiol. 2003;42(2):246–52. https://doi.org/10.1016/S0735-1097(03)00575-8.

25. Sesso HD, Christen WG, Bubes V, et al. Multivitamins in the prevention of cardiovascular disease in men: the physicians' health study II randomized controlled trial. J Am Med Assoc. 2012;308(17):1751–60. https://doi.org/10.1001/jama.2012.14805.

26. Sesso HD, Buring JE, Christen WG, et al. Vitamins E and C in the prevention of cardiovascular disease in men: the physicians' health study II randomized controlled trial. J Am Med Assoc. 2008;300(18):2123–33. https://doi.org/10.1001/jama.2008.600.

27. Cook NR, Albert CM, Gaziano JM, et al. A randomized factorial trial of vitamins C and E and beta carotene in the secondary prevention of cardiovascular events in women: results from the women's antioxidant cardiovascular study. Arch Intern Med. 2007;167(15):1610–8. https://doi.org/10.1001/archinte.167.15.1610.

28. Salonen JT, Nyyssönen K, Salonen R, et al. Antioxidant supplementation in atherosclerosis prevention (ASAP) study: a randomized trial of the effect of vitamins E and C on 3-year progression of carotid atherosclerosis. J Intern Med. 2000;248(5):377–86. https://doi.org/10.1046/j.1365-2796.2000.00752.x.

29. Al-Khudairy L, Flowers N, Wheelhouse R, et al. Vitamin C supplementation for the primary prevention of cardiovascular disease. Cochrane Database Syst Rev. 2017;(3): https://doi.org/10.1002/14651858.CD011114.pub2.

30. Coates PM, Betz JM, Blackman MR, et al. Encyclopedia of dietary supplements. 2nd ed. Informa Healthcare. New York, NY; 2010.

31. Dietary reference intakes for Vitamin C, Vitamin E, Selenium, and Carotenoids. National Academies Press; 2000. https://doi.org/10.17226/9810.

32. Voutilainen S, Nurmi T, Mursu J, Rissanen TH. Carotenoids and cardiovascular health. Am J Clin Nutr. 2006;83(6):1265–71. https://doi.org/10.1093/ajcn/83.6.1265.

33. Rapola JM, Virtamo J, Ripatti S, et al. Randomised trial of α-tocopherol and β-carotene supplements on incidence of major coronary events in men with previous myocardial infarction. Lancet. 1997;349(9067):1715–20. https://doi.org/10.1016/S0140-6736(97)01234-8.

34. Greenberg ER. Mortality associated with low plasma concentration of beta carotene and the effect of oral supplementation. J Am Med Assoc. 1996;275(9):699. https://doi.org/10.1001/jama.1996.03530330043027.

35. Omenn GS, Goodman GE, Thornquist MD, et al. Effects of a combination of beta carotene and vitamin A on lung cancer and cardiovascular disease. N Engl J Med. 1996;334(18):1150–5. https://doi.org/10.1056/NEJM199605023341802.

36. Lichtenstein AH. Nutrient supplements and cardiovascular disease: a heartbreaking story. J Lipid Res. 2009;50(SUPPL):S429. https://doi.org/10.1194/jlr.R800027-JLR200.

37. Tavani A, La Vecchia C. β-Carotene and risk of coronary heart disease. A review of observational and intervention studies. Biomed Pharmacother. 1999;53(9):409–16. https://doi.org/10.1016/S0753-3322(99)80120-6.

38. Moyer VA. Vitamin, mineral, and multivitamin supplements for the primary prevention of cardiovascular disease and cancer: U.S. preventive services task force recommendation statement. Ann Intern Med. 2014;160(8):558–64. https://doi.org/10.7326/M14-0198.

39. Holick MF, Vitamin D. Deficiency. N Engl J Med. 2007;357(3):266–81. https://doi.org/10.1056/NEJMra070553.

40. Zittermann A, Schleithoff SS, Koerfer R. Putting cardiovascular disease and vitamin D insufficiency into perspective. Br J Nutr. 2005;94(4):483–92. https://doi.org/10.1079/bjn20051544.

41. Khaw KT, Luben R, Wareham N. Serum 25-hydroxyvitamin D, mortality, and incident cardiovascular disease, respiratory disease, cancers, and fractures: a 13-y prospective population study. Am J Clin Nutr. 2014;100(5):1361–70. https://doi.org/10.3945/ajcn.114.086413.

42. Shaper AG, Pocock SJ, Walker M, Cohen NM, Wale CJ, Thomson AG. British regional heart study: cardiovascular risk factors in middle-aged men in 24 towns. Br Med J (Clin Res Ed). 1981;283(6285):179–86. https://doi.org/10.1136/bmj.283.6285.179.

43. Wang L, Ma J, Manson JE, Buring JE, Gaziano JM, Sesso HD. A prospective study of plasma vitamin

D metabolites, vitamin D receptor gene polymorphisms, and risk of hypertension in men. Eur J Nutr. 2013;52(7):1771–9. https://doi.org/10.1007/s00394-012-0480-8.

44. Pfeifer M, Begerow B, Minne HW, et al. Vitamin D status, trunk muscle strength, body sway, falls, and fractures among 237 postmenopausal women with osteoporosis. Exp Clin Endocrinol Diabetes. 2001;109(2):87–92. https://doi.org/10.1055/s-2001-14831.

45. Zhang D, Cheng C, Wang Y, et al. Effect of vitamin D on blood pressure and hypertension in the general population: an update meta-analysis of cohort studies and randomized controlled trials. Prev Chronic Dis. 2020;17:190307. https://doi.org/10.5888/pcd17.190307.

46. Timms PM, Mannan N, Hitman GA, et al. Circulating MMP9, vitamin D and variation in the TIMP-1 response with VDR genotype: mechanisms for inflammatory damage in chronic disorders? QJM. 2002;95(12):787–96. https://doi.org/10.1093/qjmed/95.12.787.

47. LaCroix AZ, Kotchen J, Anderson G, et al. Calcium plus vitamin D supplementation and mortality in postmenopausal women: the women's health initiative calcium-vitamin D randomized controlled trial. J Gerontol A Biol Sci Med Sci. 2009;64(5):559–67. https://doi.org/10.1093/gerona/glp006.

48. Scragg R, Stewart AW, Waayer D, et al. Effect of monthly high-dose vitamin D supplementation on cardiovascular disease in the vitamin D assessment study: a randomized clinical trial. JAMA Cardiol. 2017;2(6):608–16. https://doi.org/10.1001/jamacardio.2017.0175.

49. Manson JE, Cook NR, Lee I-M, et al. Vitamin D supplements and prevention of cancer and cardiovascular disease. N Engl J Med. 2019;380(1):33–44. https://doi.org/10.1056/NEJMoa1809944.

50. Wang X, Quinn PJ. Vitamin E and its function in membranes. Prog Lipid Res. 1999;38(4):309–36. https://doi.org/10.1016/S0163-7827(99)00008-9.

51. Berliner JA, Navab M, Fogelman AM, et al. Atherosclerosis: basic mechanisms. Circulation. 1995;91(9):2488–96. https://doi.org/10.1161/01.CIR.91.9.2488.

52. Witztum JL. The oxidation hypothesis of atherosclerosis. Lancet. 1994;344(8925):793–5. https://doi.org/10.1016/S0140-6736(94)92346-9.

53. Glynn RJ, Ridker PM, Goldhaber SZ, Zee RYL, Buring JE. Effects of random allocation to vitamin E supplementation on the occurrence of venous thromboembolism: report from the women's health study. Circulation. 2007;116(13):1497–503. https://doi.org/10.1161/CIRCULATIONAHA.107.716407.

54. Stampfer MJ, Hennekens CH, Manson JE, Colditz GA, Rosner B, Willett WC. Vitamin E consumption and the risk of coronary disease in women. N Engl J Med. 1993;328(20):1444–9. https://doi.org/10.1056/NEJM199305203282003.

55. Rimm EB, Stampfer MJ, Ascherio A, Giovannucci E, Colditz GA, Willett WC. Vitamin E consumption and

the risk of coronary heart disease in men. N Engl J Med. 1993;328(20):1450–6. https://doi.org/10.1056/NEJM199305203282004.

56. Lee IM, Cook NR, Gaziano JM, et al. Vitamin E in the primary prevention of cardiovascular disease and cancer. The women's health study: a randomized controlled trial. J Am Med Assoc. 2005;294(1):56–65. https://doi.org/10.1001/jama.294.1.56.

57. Demaio SJ, King SB, Lembo NJ, et al. Vitamin E supplementation, plasma lipids and incidence of restenosis after percutaneous transluminal coronary angioplasty (PTCA). https://doi.org/10.1080/07315724.1992.10718198.

58. Lonn E. Effects of long-term Vitamin E supplementation on cardiovascular events and Cancer. JAMA. 2005;293(11):1338. https://doi.org/10.1001/jama.293.11.1338.

59. Yusuf S. Vitamin E supplementation and cardiovascular events in high-risk patients. N Engl J Med. 2000;342(3):154–60. https://doi.org/10.1056/NEJM200001203420302.

60. Pacana T, Sanyal AJ. Vitamin E and nonalcoholic fatty liver disease. Curr Opin Clin Nutr Metab Care. 2012;15(6):641–8. https://doi.org/10.1097/MCO.0b013e328357f747.

61. Sanyal AJ, Chalasani N, Kowdley KV, et al. Pioglitazone, Vitamin E, or placebo for nonalcoholic Steatohepatitis. N Engl J Med. 2010;362(18):1675–85. https://doi.org/10.1056/NEJMoa0907929.

62. Thendiono E. IDDF2018-ABS-0025 the effect of vitamin e (mixed tocotrienol) on the liver stiffness measurement measured by transient elastography (FIBROSCAN) among nafld patients. Gut. 2018;67:A89.2–A90. https://doi.org/10.1136/gutjnl-2018-iddfabstracts.189.

63. Klein EA, Thompson IM, Tangen CM, et al. Vitamin E and the risk of prostate cancer: the selenium and vitamin E cancer prevention trial (SELECT). J Am Med Assoc. 2011;306(14):1549–56. https://doi.org/10.1001/jama.2011.1437.

64. Luo G, Ducy P, McKee MD, et al. Spontaneous calcification of arteries and cartilage in mice lacking matrix GLA protein. Nature. 1997;386(6620):78–81. https://doi.org/10.1038/386078a0.

65. Tsugawa N. Cardiovascular diseases and fat soluble Vitamins: Vitamin D and Vitamin K. J Nutr Sci Vitaminol (Tokyo). 2015;61:S170–2.

66. Shea MK, Booth SL, Miller ME, et al. Association between circulating vitamin K1 and coronary calcium progression in community-dwelling adults: the multi-ethnic study of atherosclerosis. Am J Clin Nutr. 2013;98(1):197–208. https://doi.org/10.3945/ajcn.112.056101.

67. Shea MK, O'Donnell CJ, Hoffmann U, et al. Vitamin K supplementation and progression of coronary artery calcium in older men and women. Am J Clin Nutr. 2009;89(6):1799–807. https://doi.org/10.3945/ajcn.2008.27338.

68. van Ballegooijen AJ, Beulens JW. The role of Vitamin K status in cardiovascular health: evidence from observational and clinical studies. Curr Nutr Rep. 2017;6(3):197–205. https://doi.org/10.1007/s13668-017-0208-8.

69. Knapen MH, Braam LA, Drummen NE, Bekers O, Hoeks APG, Vermeer C. Menaquinone-7 supplementation improves arterial stiffness in healthy postmenopausal women a double-blind randomised clinical trial. Thromb Haemost. 2015;113. https://doi.org/10.1160/TH14-08-0675.

70. Geleijnse JM, Vermeer C, Grobbee DE, et al. Dietary intake of menaquinone is associated with a reduced risk of coronary heart disease: the Rotterdam study. J Nutr. 2004;134(11):3100–5. https://doi.org/10.1093/jn/134.11.3100.

71. Gast GCM, de Roos NM, Sluijs I, et al. A high menaquinone intake reduces the incidence of coronary heart disease. Nutr Metab Cardiovasc Dis. 2009;19(7):504–10. https://doi.org/10.1016/j.numecd.2008.10.004.

72. Zhang S, Guo L, Bu C. Vitamin K status and cardiovascular events or mortality: a meta-analysis. Eur J Prev Cardiol. 2019;26(5):549–53. https://doi.org/10.1177/2047487318808066.

73. Shea MK, Barger K, Booth SL, et al. Vitamin K status, cardiovascular disease, and all-cause mortality: a participant-level meta-analysis of 3 US cohorts. Am J Clin Nutr. 2020;111(6):1170–7. https://doi.org/10.1093/ajcn/nqaa082.

74. Institute of Medicine. Dietary reference intakes: the essential guide to nutrient requirements; 2006. https://doi.org/10.17226/11537.

75. Office of Dietary Supplements. Zinc - health professional fact sheet. Accessed 31 Aug 2020. https://ods.od.nih.gov/factsheets/Zinc-HealthProfessional/

76. Choi S, Liu X, Pan Z. Zinc deficiency and cellular oxidative stress: prognostic implications in cardiovascular diseases. Acta Pharmacol Sin. 2018;39:1120–32. https://doi.org/10.1038/aps.2018.25.

77. Prasad AS. Zinc is an antioxidant and anti-inflammatory agent: its role in human health. Front Nutr. 2014;1. https://doi.org/10.3389/fnut.2014.00014.

78. Eide DJ. The oxidative stress of zinc deficiency. Metallomics. 2011;3(11):1124–9. https://doi.org/10.1039/c1mt00064k.

79. Bonaventura P, Benedetti G, Albarède F, Miossec P. Zinc and its role in immunity and inflammation. Autoimmun Rev. 2015;14(4):277–85. https://doi.org/10.1016/j.autrev.2014.11.008.

80. Yao J, Hu P, Zhang D. Associations between copper and zinc and risk of hypertension in US adults. Biol Trace Elem Res. 2018;186(2):346–53. https://doi.org/10.1007/s12011-018-1320-3.

81. Choi S, Liu X, Pan Z. Zinc deficiency and cellular oxidative stress: prognostic implications in cardiovascular diseases review-article. Acta Pharmacol Sin. 2018;39(7):1120–32. https://doi.org/10.1038/aps.2018.25.

82. Miao X, Sun W, Fu Y, Miao L, Cai L. Zinc homeostasis in the metabolic syndrome and diabetes. Front Med China. 2013;7(1):31–52. https://doi.org/10.1007/s11684-013-0251-9.

83. Milton AH, Vashum KP, McEvoy M, et al. Prospective study of dietary zinc intake and risk of cardiovascular disease in women. Nutrients. 2018;10(1). https://doi.org/10.3390/nu10010038.

84. Schwingshackl L, Boeing H, Stelmach-Mardas M, et al. Dietary supplements and risk of cause-specific death, cardiovascular disease, and cancer: a systematic review and meta-analysis of primary prevention trials. Adv Nutr. 2017;8(1):27–39. https://doi.org/10.3945/an.116.013516.

85. Schwalfenberg GK, Genuis SJ. The importance of magnesium in clinical healthcare. Scientifica (Cairo). 2017. https://doi.org/10.1155/2017/4179326.

86. Muñoz-Castañeda JR, Pendón-Ruiz De Mier M V., Rodríguez M, Rodríguez-Ortiz ME Magnesium replacement to protect cardiovascular and kidney damage? Lack of prospective clinical trials. Int J Mol Sci. 2018;19(3). https://doi.org/10.3390/ijms19030664.

87. Dietary reference intakes for Calcium, Phosphorus, Magnesium, Vitamin D, and Fluoride. National Academies Press; 1997. https://doi.org/10.17226/5776.

88. de Baaij JHF, Hoenderop JGJ, Bindels RJM. Magnesium in man: implications for health and disease. Physiol Rev. 2015;95:1–46. https://doi.org/10.1152/physrev.00012.2014.-Mag.

89. Spencer H, Norris C, Williams D. Inhibitory effects of zinc on magnesium balance and magnesium absorption in man. J Am Coll Nutr. 1994;13(5):479–84. https://doi.org/10.1080/07315724.1994.10718438.

90. Kiela PR, Ghishan FK. Physiology of intestinal absorption and secretion. Best Pract Res Clin Gastroenterol. 2016;30(2):145–59. https://doi.org/10.1016/j.bpg.2016.02.007.

91. Swaminathan R. Magnesium metabolism and its disorders. Clin Biochem Rev. 2003;24(2):47–66. Accessed 31 Aug 2020. http://www.ncbi.nlm.nih.gov/pubmed/18568054

92. Ross AC, Caballero BH, Cousins RJ, Tucker KL, Ziegler TR. *Modern nutrition in health and disease.* 11th ed. Wolters Kluwer Health Adis (ESP); 2012. Accessed 31 Aug 2020. https://jhu.pure.elsevier.com/en/publications/modern-nutrition-in-health-and-disease-eleventh-edition

93. Tangvoraphonkchai K, Davenport A. Magnesium and cardiovascular disease. Adv Chronic Kidney Dis. 2018;25(3):251–60. https://doi.org/10.1053/j.ackd.2018.02.010.

94. Severino P, Netti L, Mariani MV, et al. Prevention of cardiovascular disease: screening for magnesium deficiency. Cardiol Res Pract. 2019; https://doi.org/10.1155/2019/4874921.

95. Gums JG. Magnesium in cardiovascular and other disorders. Am J Heal Pharm. 2004;61(15):1569–76. https://doi.org/10.1093/ajhp/61.15.1569.

96. Shechter M. Magnesium and cardiovascular system. Magnes Res. 2010;23(2):60–72. https://doi.org/10.1684/mrh.2010.0202.

97. Larsson SC, Burgess S, Michaëlsson K. Serum magnesium levels and risk of coronary artery disease: Mendelian randomisation study. BMC Med. 2018;16(1). https://doi.org/10.1186/s12916-018-1065-z.

98. Massy ZA, Drüeke TB. Magnesium and cardiovascular complications of chronic kidney disease. Nat Rev Nephrol. 2015;11(7):432–42. https://doi.org/10.1038/nrneph.2015.74.

99. Rosique-Esteban N, Guasch-Ferré M, Hernández-Alonso P, Salas-Salvadó J. Dietary magnesium and cardiovascular disease: a review with emphasis in epidemiological studies. Nutrients. 2018;10(2). https://doi.org/10.3390/nu10020168.

100. Dibaba DT, Xun P, Song Y, Rosanoff A, Shechter M, He K. The effect of magnesium supplementation on blood pressure in individuals with insulin resistance, prediabetes, or noncommunicable chronic diseases: a meta-analysis of randomized controlled trials. Am J Clin Nutr. 2017;106(3):921–9. https://doi.org/10.3945/ajcn.117.155291.

101. Verma H, Garg R. Effect of magnesium supplementation on type 2 diabetes associated cardiovascular risk factors: a systematic review and meta-analysis. J Hum Nutr Diet. 2017;30(5):621–33. https://doi.org/10.1111/jhn.12454.

102. Dinicolantonio JJ, Liu J, O'keefe JH. Magnesium for the prevention and treatment of cardiovascular disease. Open Hear. 2018;5:775. https://doi.org/10.1136/openhrt-2018-000775.

103. Han H, Fang X, Wei X, et al. Dose-response relationship between dietary magnesium intake, serum magnesium concentration and risk of hypertension: a systematic review and meta-analysis of prospective cohort studies. Nutr J. 2017;16(1). https://doi.org/10.1186/s12937-017-0247-4.

104. Li L, Yang X. The essential element manganese, oxidative stress, and metabolic diseases: links and interactions. Oxidative Med Cell Longev. 2018. https://doi.org/10.1155/2018/7580707.

105. Aschner JL, Aschner M. Nutritional aspects of manganese homeostasis. Mol Asp Med. 2005;26(4–5 SPEC. ISS):353–62. https://doi.org/10.1016/j.mam.2005.07.003.

106. Finley JW, Davis CD. Manganese deficiency and toxicity: are high or low dietary amounts of manganese cause for concern? Biofactors. 1999;10(1):15–24. https://doi.org/10.1002/biof.5520100102.

107. Mahalle N, Garg MK, Naik SS, Kulkarni MV. Association of dietary factors with severity of coronary artery disease. Clin Nutr ESPEN. 2016;15:75–9. https://doi.org/10.1016/j.clnesp.2016.06.004.

108. Wu C, Woo JG, Zhang N. Association between urinary manganese and blood pressure: Results from National Health and Nutrition Examination Survey (NHANES), 2011-2014. PLoS One.

2017;12(11):2011–4. https://doi.org/10.1371/journal.pone.0188145.

109. Miller KB, Caton JS, Schafer DM, Smith DJ, Finley JW. High dietary manganese lowers heart magnesium pigs fed a low-magnesium diet. J Nutr. 2000;130(8):2032–5. https://doi.org/10.1093/jn/130.8.2032.

110. O'Neal SL, Zheng W. Manganese toxicity upon overexposure: a decade in review. Curr Environ Health Rep. 2015;2(3):315–28. https://doi.org/10.1007/s40572-015-0056-x.

111. Jiang Y, Zheng W. Cardiovascular toxicities upon manganese exposure. Cardiovasc Toxicol. 2005;5(4):345–54. https://doi.org/10.1385/CT:5:4:345.

112. Office of Dietary Supplements. Calcium - Health Professional Fact Sheet. Published March 26, 2020. Accessed 31 Aug 2020. https://ods.od.nih.gov/factsheets/Calcium-HealthProfessional/

113. Bolland MJ, Grey A, Reid IR. Calcium supplements and cardiovascular risk: 5 years on. Ther Adv Drug Saf. 2013;4(5):199–210. https://doi.org/10.1177/2042098613499790.

114. Bolland MJ, Barber PA, Doughty RN, et al. Vascular events in healthy older women receiving calcium supplementation: randomised controlled trial. BMJ. 2008;336(7638):262–6. https://doi.org/10.1136/bmj.39440.525752.BE.

115. Bolland MJ, Avenell A, Baron JA, et al. Effect of calcium supplements on risk of myocardial infarction and cardiovascular events: meta-analysis. BMJ. 2010;341(7767):289. https://doi.org/10.1136/bmj.c3691.

116. Tankeu AT, Ndip Agbor V, Noubiap JJ. Calcium supplementation and cardiovascular risk: a rising concern. J Clin Hypertens. 2017;19(6):640–6. https://doi.org/10.1111/jch.13010.

117. Shin CS, Kim KM. Calcium, is it better to have less? - Global health perspectives. J Cell Biochem. 2015;116(8):1513–21. https://doi.org/10.1002/jcb.25119.

118. Yang C, Shi X, Xia H, et al. The evidence and controversy between dietary calcium intake and calcium supplementation and the risk of cardiovascular disease: a systematic review and meta-analysis of cohort studies and randomized controlled trials. J Am Coll Nutr. 2020;39(4):352–70. https://doi.org/10.1080/07315724.2019.1649219.

119. Asemi Z, Foroozanfard F, Hashemi T, Bahmani F, Jamilian M, Esmaillzadeh A. Calcium plus vitamin D supplementation affects glucose metabolism and lipid concentrations in overweight and obese vitamin D deficient women with polycystic ovary syndrome. Clin Nutr. 2015;34(4):586–92. https://doi.org/10.1016/j.clnu.2014.09.015.

120. Reid IR, Mason B, Horne A, et al. Effects of calcium supplementation on serum lipid concentrations in normal older women: a randomized controlled trial. Am J Med. 2002;112(5):343–7. https://doi.org/10.1016/S0002-9343(01)01138-X.

121. Umesawa M, Iso H, Date C, et al. Dietary intake of calcium in relation to mortality from cardiovascular disease: the JACC study. Stroke. 2006;37(1):20–6. https://doi.org/10.1161/01.STR. 0000195155.21143.38.

122. Kong SH, Kim JH, Hong AR, Cho NH, Shin CS. Dietary calcium intake and risk of cardiovascular disease, stroke, and fracture in a population with low calcium intake. Am J Clin Nutr. 2017;106(1):27–34. https://doi.org/10.3945/ajcn.116.148171.

123. Heaney RP, Nordin BEC. Calcium effects on phosphorus absorption: implications for the prevention and co-therapy of osteoporosis. J Am Coll Nutr. 2002;21(3):239–44. https://doi.org/10.1080/073157 24.2002.10719216.

124. Palmer SC, Hayen A, Macaskill P, et al. Serum levels of phosphorus, parathyroid hormone, and calcium and risks of death and cardiovascular disease in individuals with chronic kidney disease a systematic review and meta-analysis. J Am Med Assoc. 2011;305(11):1119–27. https://doi.org/10.1001/ jama.2011.308.

125. Menon MC, Ix JH. Dietary phosphorus, serum phosphorus, and cardiovascular disease. Ann N Y Acad Sci. 2013;1301(1):21–6. https://doi.org/10.1111/ nyas.12283.

126. Kendrick J, Chonchol M. The role of phosphorus in the development and progression of vascular calcification. Am J Kidney Dis. 2011;58(5):826–34. https://doi.org/10.1053/j.ajkd.2011.07.020.

127. Gutiérrez OM. The connection between dietary phosphorus, cardiovascular disease, and mortality: where we stand and what we need to know. Adv Nutr. 2013;4(6):723–9. https://doi.org/10.3945/ an.113.004812.

128. Bai W, Li J, Liu J. Serum phosphorus, cardiovascular and all-cause mortality in the general population: a meta-analysis. Clin Chim Acta. 2016;461:76–82. https://doi.org/10.1016/j.cca.2016.07.020.

129. Chang AR, Lazo M, Appel LJ, Gutiérrez OM, Grams ME. High dietary phosphorus intake is associated with all-cause mortality: results from NHANES III1-3. Am J Clin Nutr. 2014;99(2):320–7. https:// doi.org/10.3945/ajcn.113.073148.

130. Uribarri J, Calvo MS. Introduction to *dietary phosphorus excess and health*. Ann N Y Acad Sci. 2013;1301(1):iii–iv. https://doi.org/10.1111/ nyas.12302.

131. Wang J, Wang F, Dong S, Zeng Q, Zhang L. Levels of serum phosphorus and cardiovascular surrogate markers: a population-based cross-sectional study. J Atheroscler Thromb. 2016;23(1):95–104. https:// doi.org/10.5551/jat.31153.

132. Shimada M, Shutto-Uchita Y, Yamabe H. Lack of awareness of dietary sources of phosphorus is a clinical concern. In Vivo (Brooklyn). 2019;33(1):11–6. https://doi.org/10.21873/invivo.11432.

133. Uribarri J, Calvo MS. Dietary phosphorus excess: a risk factor in chronic bone, kidney, and cardiovascu-

lar disease? Adv Nutr. 2013;4(5):542–4. https://doi. org/10.3945/an.113.004234.

134. Savica V, Duro G, Bellingheri G, Monroy A. Between the utility and hazards of phosphorus through the centuries. G Ital Nefrol. 2016;33(Suppl 66):33.S66.31.

135. Larry Jameson J, Fauci AS, Kasper DL, Hauser SL, Longo DL, Loscalzo J, editors. Harrison's principles of internal medicine. 20th ed. McGraw-Hill Medical. Accessed 31 Aug 2020. https://accessmedicine. mhmedical.com/book.aspx?bookID=2129

136. Weaver CM. Potassium and health. Adv Nutr. 2013;4(3):368S. https://doi.org/10.3945/an.112. 003533.

137. Ellison DH, Terker AS. Why your mother was right: how potassium intake reduces blood pressure. Trans Am Clin Climatol Assoc. 2015;126:46–55. Accessed August 31, 2020. /pmc/articles/ PMC4530669/?report=abstract

138. Aburto NJ, Hanson S, Gutierrez H, Hooper L, Elliott P, Cappuccio FP. Effect of increased potassium intake on cardiovascular risk factors and disease: systematic review and meta-analyses. BMJ. 2013;346(7903). https://doi.org/10.1136/bmj.f1378.

139. Lu J, Holmgren A. Selenoproteins. J Biol Chem. 2009;284(2):723–7. https://doi.org/10.1074/jbc. R800045200.

140. Huawei Z. Selenium as an essential micronutrient: roles in cell cycle and apoptosis. Molecules. 2009;14(3):1263–78. https://doi.org/10.3390/molecules14031263.

141. Zeng H, Wu M, Botnen JH. Methylselenol, a selenium metabolite, induces cell cycle arrest in G1 phase and apoptosis via the extracellular-regulated-and other cancer signaling kinase 112 pathway genes 1-3. J Nutr. 2009;139:1613–8. https://doi. org/10.3945/jn.109.110320.

142. Chen J. *An original discovery:* selenium deficiency and Keshan disease (an endemic heart disease). Asia Pac J Clin Nutr. 2012;21(3):320–326.144.

143. Navarro-Alarcon M, Cabrera-Vique C. Selenium in food and the human body: a review. Sci Total Environ. 2008;400(1–3):115–41. https://doi. org/10.1016/j.scitotenv.2008.06.024.

144. Benstoem C, Goetzenich A, Kraemer S, et al. Selenium and its supplementation in cardiovascular disease—what do we know? Nutrients. 2015;7(5):3094–118. https://doi.org/10.3390/nu 7053094.

145. Tanguy S, Grauzam S, de Leiris J, Boucher F. Impact of dietary selenium intake on cardiac health: experimental approaches and human studies. Mol Nutr Food Res. 2012;56(7):1106–21. https:// doi.org/10.1002/mnfr.201100766.

146. Zhang X, Liu C, Guo J, Song Y. Selenium status and cardiovascular diseases: meta-analysis of prospective observational studies and randomized controlled trials. Eur J Clin Nutr. 2016;70(2):162–9. https://doi. org/10.1038/ejcn.2015.78.

147. Stranges S, Navas-Acien A, Rayman MP, Guallar E. Selenium status and cardiometabolic health: state of the evidence. Nutr Metab Cardiovasc Dis. 2010;20(10):754–60. https://doi.org/10.1016/j.numecd.2010.10.001.

148. Gharipour M, Sadeghi M, Behmanesh M, Salehi M, Nezafati P, Gharipour A. Selenium homeostasis and clustering of cardiovascular risk factors: a systematic review. Acta Biomed. 2017;88(3):263–70. https://doi.org/10.23750/abm.v%vi%i.5701.

149. Office of Dietary Supplements. Copper - health professional fact sheet. Published July 2020. Accessed 31 Aug 2020. https://ods.od.nih.gov/factsheets/Copper-HealthProfessional/.

150. Fukai T, Ushio-Fukai M, Kaplan JH. Copper transporters and copper chaperones: roles in cardiovascular physiology and disease. Am J Physiol Cell Physiol. 2018;315(2):C186–201. https://doi.org/10.1152/ajpcell.00132.2018.

151. Klevay LM. Cardiovascular disease from copper deficiency - a history. J Nutr. 2000;130. American Institute of Nutrition. https://doi.org/10.1093/jn/130.2.489s.

152. Fukai T, Ushio-Fukai M. Superoxide dismutases: role in redox signaling, vascular function, and diseases. Antioxid Redox Signal. 2011;15(6):1583–606. https://doi.org/10.1089/ars.2011.3999.

153. Saari JT. Copper deficiency and cardiovascular disease: role of peroxidation, glycation, and nitration. Can J Physiol Pharmacol. 2000;78(10):848–55. https://doi.org/10.1139/cjpp-78-10-848.

154. Ford ES. Serum copper concentration and coronary heart disease among US adults. Am J Epidemiol. 2000;151(12):1182–8. https://doi.org/10.1093/oxfordjournals.aje.a010168.

155. Reunanen A, Knekt P, Marniemi J, Mäki J, Maatela J, Aromaa A. Serum calcium, magnesium, copper and zinc and risk of cardiovascular death. Eur J Clin Nutr. 1996;50(7):431–7. Accessed 31Aug 2020. https://europepmc.org/article/med/8862478

156. Disilvestro RA, Joseph EL, Zhang W, Raimo AE, Kim YM. A randomized trial of copper supplementation effects on blood copper enzyme activities and parameters related to cardiovascular health. Metabolism. 2012;61(9):1242–6. https://doi.org/10.1016/j.metabol.2012.02.002.

157. Vincent JB, Edwards KC. The absorption and transport of chromium in the body. In: The nutritional biochemistry of chromium (III). Elsevier; 2019. p. 129–74. https://doi.org/10.1016/b978-0-444-64121-2.00004-0.

158. Cefalu WT, Hu FB. Role of chromium in human health and in diabetes. Diabetes Care. 2004;27(11):2741–51.

159. Rajpathak S, Rimm EB, Li T, et al. Lower toenail chromium in men with diabetes and cardiovascular disease compared with healthy men. Diabetes Care. 2004;27(9):2211–6. https://doi.org/10.2337/diacare.27.9.2211.

160. Hummel M, Standl E, Schnell O. Chromium in metabolic and cardiovascular disease. Horm Metab Res. 2007;39:743–51. https://doi.org/10.1055/s--2007-985847.

161. A scientific review: the role of chromium in insulin resistance - PubMed. Diabetes Educ. 2004;Suppl:2–14. Accessed 31 Aug 2020. https://pubmed.ncbi.nlm.nih.gov/15208835/.

162. Bai J, Xun P, Morris S, Jacobs DR, Liu K, He K. Chromium exposure and incidence of metabolic syndrome among American young adults over a 23-year follow-up: the CARDIA trace element study. Sci Rep. 2015;5: https://doi.org/10.1038/srep15606.

163. Ngala RA, Awe MA, Nsiah P. The effects of plasma chromium on lipid profile, glucose metabolism and cardiovascular risk in type 2 diabetes mellitus. A case - control study. PLoS One. 2018;13(7): https://doi.org/10.1371/journal.pone.0197977.

164. Ernster L, Dallner G. Biochemical, physiological and medical aspects of ubiquinone function. BBA - Mol Basis Dis. 1995;1271(1):195–204. https://doi.org/10.1016/0925-4439(95)00028-3.

165. Sohal RS, Kamzalov S, Sumien N, et al. Effect of coenzyme Q10 intake on endogenous coenzyme Q content, mitochondrial electron transport chain, antioxidative defenses, and life span of mice. Free Radic Biol Med. 2006;40(3):480–7. https://doi.org/10.1016/j.freeradbiomed.2005.08.037.

166. Gutiérrez E, Flammer AJ, Lerman LO, Elízaga J, Lerman A, Francisco FA. Endothelial dysfunction over the course of coronary artery disease. Eur Heart J. 2013;34(41):3175. https://doi.org/10.1093/eurheartj/eht351.

167. Gao L, Mao Q, Cao J, Wang Y, Zhou X, Fan L. Effects of coenzyme Q10 on vascular endothelial function in humans: a meta-analysis of randomized controlled trials. Atherosclerosis. 2012;221(2):311–6. https://doi.org/10.1016/j.atherosclerosis.2011.10.027.

168. Huo J, Xu Z, Hosoe K, et al. Coenzyme Q10 prevents senescence and dysfunction caused by oxidative stress in vascular endothelial cells. Oxidative Med Cell Longev. 2018; https://doi.org/10.1155/2018/3181759.

169. Alehagen U, Aaseth J, Johansson P. Reduced cardiovascular mortality 10 years after supplementation with selenium and coenzyme q10 for four years: follow-up results of a prospective randomized double-blind placebo-controlled trial in elderly citizens. PLoS One. 2015;10(12): https://doi.org/10.1371/journal.pone.0141641.

170. Lee BJ, Lin YC, Huang YC, Ko YW, Hsia S, Lin PT. The relationship between coenzyme Q10, oxidative stress, and antioxidant enzymes activities and coronary artery disease. Sci World J. 2012; https://doi.org/10.1100/2012/792756.

171. Jorat MV, Tabrizi R, Kolahdooz F, et al. The effects of coenzyme Q10 supplementation on biomarkers of inflammation and oxidative stress in among coronary artery disease: a systematic review and meta-analysis of randomized controlled trials. Inflammopharma-

cology. 2019;27(2):233–48. https://doi.org/10.1007/s10787-019-00572-x.

172. Huang CH, Kuo CL, Huang CS, et al. High plasma coenzyme Q10 concentration is correlated with good left ventricular performance after primary angioplasty in patients with acute myocardial infarction. Med (United States). 2016;95(31): https://doi.org/10.1097/MD.0000000000004501.

173. Lei L, Liu Y. Efficacy of coenzyme Q10 in patients with cardiac failure: a meta-analysis of clinical trials. BMC Cardiovasc Disord. 2017;17(1):196. https://doi.org/10.1186/s12872-017-0628-9.

174. Zhang X, Liu H, Hao Y, et al. Coenzyme Q10 protects against hyperlipidemia-induced cardiac damage in apolipoprotein E-deficient mice. Lipids Health Dis. 2018;17(1): https://doi.org/10.1186/s12944-018-0928-9.

175. Qu H, Guo M, Chai H, Wang W-T, Zhu-Ye G, Da-Zhuo S. Effects of coenzyme Q10 on statin-induced myopathy: an updated meta-analysis of randomized controlled trials. https://doi.org/10.1161/JAHA.118.009835.

176. Kennedy C, Köller Y, Surkova E. Effect of coenzyme Q10 on statin-associated myalgia and adherence to statin therapy: a systematic review and meta-analysis. Atherosclerosis. 2020;299:1–8. https://doi.org/10.1016/j.atherosclerosis.2020.03.006.

177. Amagase H. Clarifying the real bioactive constituents of garlic. J Nutr. 2006;136:716S–25S. https://doi.org/10.1093/jn/136.3.716s. American Institute of Nutrition

178. Ried K, Travica N, Sali A. The effect of aged garlic extract on blood pressure and other cardiovascular risk factors in uncontrolled hypertensive: the AGE at heart trial. Integr Blood Press Control. 2016;9:9–21. https://doi.org/10.2147/IBPC.S93335.

179. Ried K. Garlic lowers blood pressure in hypertensive individuals, regulates serum cholesterol, and stimulates immunity: an updated meta-analysis and review. J Nutr. 2016;146(2):389S–96S. https://doi.org/10.3945/jn.114.202192.

180. Sun YE, Wang W, Qin J. Anti-hyperlipidemia of garlic by reducing the level of total cholesterol and low-density lipoprotein. Med (United States). 2018;97(18): https://doi.org/10.1097/MD.0000000000010255.

181. Bordia A, Verma SK, Srivastava KC. Effect of garlic on platelet aggregation in humans: a study in healthy subjects and patients with coronary artery disease. Prostaglandins Leukot Essent Fat Acids. 1996;55(3):201–5. https://doi.org/10.1016/S0952-3278(96)90099-X.

182. Adkins Y, Kelley DS. Mechanisms underlying the cardioprotective effects of omega-3 polyunsaturated fatty acids. J Nutr Biochem. 2010;21(9):781–92. https://doi.org/10.1016/j.jnutbio.2009.12.004.

183. Mozaffarian D, Wu JHY. Omega-3 fatty acids and cardiovascular disease: effects on risk factors, molecular pathways, and clinical events. J Am Coll Cardiol. 2011;58(20):2047–67. https://doi.org/10.1016/j.jacc.2011.06.063.

184. Rees K, Hartley L, Flowers N, et al. "Mediterranean" dietary pattern for the primary prevention of cardiovascular disease. Cochrane Database Syst Rev. 2013;(8): https://doi.org/10.1002/14651858.CD009825.pub2.

185. Schrepf R, Limmert T, Weber PC, Theisen K, Sellmayer A. Immediate effects of n-3 fatty acid infusion on the induction of sustained ventricular tachycardia. Lancet. 2004;363(9419):1441–2. https://doi.org/10.1016/S0140-6736(04)16105-9.

186. Maki KC, Orloff DG, Nicholls SJ, et al. A highly bioavailable omega-3 free fatty acid formulation improves the cardiovascular risk profile in high-risk, statin-treated patients with residual hypertriglyceridemia (the ESPRIT trial). Clin Ther. 2013;35(9): https://doi.org/10.1016/j.clinthera.2013.07.420.

187. Backes J, Anzalone D, Hilleman D, Catini J. The clinical relevance of omega-3 fatty acids in the management of hypertriglyceridemia. Lipids Health Dis. 2016;15(1):1–12. https://doi.org/10.1186/s12944-016-0286-4.

188. AbuMweis S, Jew S, Tayyem R, Agraib L. Eicosapentaenoic acid and docosahexaenoic acid containing supplements modulate risk factors for cardiovascular disease: a meta-analysis of randomised placebo-control human clinical trials. J Hum Nutr Diet. 2018;31(1):67–84. https://doi.org/10.1111/jhn.12493.

189. Abdelhamid AS, Brown TJ, Brainard JS, et al. Omega-3 fatty acids for the primary and secondary prevention of cardiovascular disease. Cochrane Database Syst Rev. 2018;2018(7): https://doi.org/10.1002/14651858.CD003177.pub3.

190. Marchioli R. Dietary supplementation with N-3 polyunsaturated fatty acids and vitamin E after myocardial infarction: results of the GISSI-Prevenzione trial. Lancet. 1999;354(9177):447–55. https://doi.org/10.1016/S0140-6736(99)07072-5.

191. Manson JE, Cook NR, Lee I-M, et al. Marine n−3 fatty acids and prevention of cardiovascular disease and Cancer. N Engl J Med. 2019;380(1):23–32. https://doi.org/10.1056/NEJMoa1811403.

192. Magyar K, Halmosi R, Palfi A, et al. Cardioprotection by resveratrol: a human clinical trial in patients with stable coronary artery disease. Clin Hemorheol Microcirc. 2012;50(3):179–87. https://doi.org/10.3233/CH-2011-1424.

193. Moriarty PM, Roth EM, Karns A, et al. Effects of Xuezhikang in patients with dyslipidemia: a multicenter, randomized, placebo-controlled study. J Clin Lipidol. 2014;8(6):568–75. https://doi.org/10.1016/j.jacl.2014.09.002.

194. Red Yeast Rice | NCCIH. Published July 2013. Accessed 31 Aug 2020. https://www.nccih.nih.gov/health/red-yeast-rice

195. Ye P, Lu ZL, Du BM, et al. Effect of xuezhikang on cardiovascular events and mortality in elderly patients with a history of myocardial infarction: a

subgroup analysis of elderly subjects from the China Coronary Secondary Prevention Study. J Am Geriatr Soc. 2007;55(7):1015–22. https://doi.org/10.1111/j.1532-5415.2007.01230.x.

196. Zhao S, Lu Z, Du B, et al. Xuezhikang, an extract of Cholestin, reduces cardiovascular events in type 2 diabetes patients with coronary heart disease: subgroup analysis of patients with type 2 diabetes from China coronary secondary prevention study (CCSPS). J Cardiovasc Pharmacol. 2007;49(2):81–4. https://doi.org/10.1097/FJC.0b013e31802d3a58.

197. Gerards MC, Terlou RJ, Yu H, Koks CHW, Gerdes VEA. Traditional Chinese lipid-lowering agent red yeast rice results in significant LDL reduction but safety is uncertain - a systematic review and meta-analysis. Atherosclerosis. 2015;240(2): 415–23. https://doi.org/10.1016/j.atherosclerosis.2015.04.004.

198. Heinonen T, Gaus W. Cross matching observations on toxicological and clinical data for the assessment of tolerability and safety of Ginkgo biloba leaf extract. Toxicology. 2015;327:95–115. https://doi.org/10.1016/j.tox.2014.10.013.

199. Chen TR, Wei LH, Guan XQ, et al. Biflavones from Ginkgo biloba as inhibitors of human thrombin. Bioorg Chem. 2019;92: https://doi.org/10.1016/j.bioorg.2019.103199.

200. Rodríguez M, Ringstad L, Schäfer P, et al. Reduction of atherosclerotic nanoplaque formation and size by Ginkgo biloba (EGb 761) in cardiovascular high-risk patients. Atherosclerosis. 2007;192(2):438–44. https://doi.org/10.1016/j.atherosclerosis.2007.02.021.

201. Feng Z, Yang X, Zhang L, et al. Ginkgolide B ameliorates oxidized low-density lipoprotein-induced endothelial dysfunction via modulating Lectin-like ox-LDL-receptor-1 and NADPH oxidase 4 expression and inflammatory cascades. Phytother Res. 2018;32(12):2417–27. https://doi.org/10.1002/ptr.6177.

202. Kim Y, Clifton P. Curcumin, cardiometabolic health and dementia. Int J Environ Res Public Health. 2018;15(10): https://doi.org/10.3390/ijerph15102093.

203. Yuan F, Dong H, Gong J, et al. A systematic review and meta-analysis of randomized controlled trials on the effects of turmeric and curcuminoids on blood lipids in adults with metabolic diseases. Adv Nutr. 2019;10(5):791–802. https://doi.org/10.1093/advances/nmz021.

204. Qin S, Huang L, Gong J, et al. Efficacy and safety of turmeric and curcumin in lowering blood lipid levels in patients with cardiovascular risk factors: a meta-analysis of randomized controlled trials. Nutr J. 2017;16(1):68. https://doi.org/10.1186/s12937-017-0293-y.

205. Keihanian F, Saeidinia A, Bagheri RK, Johnston TP, Sahebkar A. Curcumin, hemostasis, thrombosis, and coagulation. J Cell Physiol. 2018;233(6):4497–511. https://doi.org/10.1002/jcp.26249.

206. Oketch-Rabah HA, Roe AL, Rider CV, et al. United States Pharmacopeia (USP) comprehensive review of the hepatotoxicity of green tea extracts. Toxicol Rep. 2020;7:386–402. https://doi.org/10.1016/j.toxrep.2020.02.008.

207. Hartley L, Flowers N, Holmes J, et al. Green and black tea for the primary prevention of cardiovascular disease. Cochrane Database Syst Rev. 2013;2013(6): https://doi.org/10.1002/14651858.CD009934.pub2.

Impact of Nutrition on Biomarkers of Cardiovascular Health

2

Cameron K. Ormiston, Rebecca Ocher, and Pam R. Taub

Introduction

The role of nutrition and lifestyle as effective strategies to decrease diabetes and cardiovascular disease risk is becoming increasingly important as over one-third of Americans are prediabetic and more than 60% of Americans eat more than the daily recommended amount of sodium, added sugar, and saturated fats [1, 2]. Although a wide variety of diet and lifestyle treatment options are available to patients, clinical dietary counseling often fails to meet patient needs and provide sufficient guidance and feedback on progress [3]. One way to understand the impact of diet is through biomarkers, which serve as noninvasive, cost-effective, and diverse tools for physicians to quantify a patient's responses to nutritional therapy. While there are several methods of monitoring a patient's response to nutritional therapy, biomarkers are preferred due to their low cost, greater accessibility, and avail-

ability of rapid testing. The biomarkers discussed in this chapter were selected based on their clinical relevance and strength of literature available. This chapter will focus on how biomarkers can be used to assess the impact of diet and lifestyle changes on cardiovascular health (Fig. 2.1).

BMI/Body Composition

Obesity, defined by a BMI of greater than 30 kg/m^2, is a well-known risk factor for dyslipidemia, hypertension, diabetes, cardiometabolic syndrome, CVD, and cancer. However, extending beyond a pure weight-based assessment, new evidence sheds light on the importance of body fat distribution and body composition in overall health [4, 5]. Numerous tools are available to clinicians to quantify body composition. For example, dual energy absorptiometry (DEXA) scans are used to analyze body composition and are an important diagnostic tool for osteopenia and osteoporosis. Further, DEXA scans have been utilized to assess fat mass normalized by height squared (FMI), which is advantageous over BMI in that the value is independent of lean muscle mass, and FMI may be used as a predictor for cardiovascular health [6]. DEXA scans have been used in clinical research and in special populations such as athletes [7]. However, current guidelines suggest that the clinical utility of DEXA scans in metabolic syndrome evaluation requires further research [8].

C. K. Ormiston · P. R. Taub (✉)
Division of Cardiovascular Medicine, Department of Medicine, University of California San Diego, San Diego, CA, USA
e-mail: cormisto@ucsd.edu; ptaub@health.ucsd.edu

R. Ocher
Department of Medicine, University of California, Los Angeles, Los Angeles, CA, USA

© Springer Nature Switzerland AG 2021
M. J. Wilkinson et al. (eds.), *Prevention and Treatment of Cardiovascular Disease*, Contemporary Cardiology, https://doi.org/10.1007/978-3-030-78177-4_2

Achieving Balance

The Benefits and Risks of each Food Group

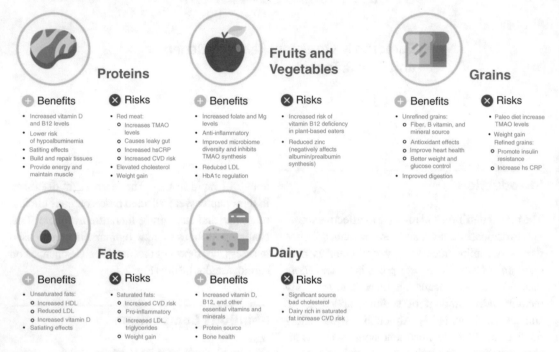

Fig. 2.1 The effects of each major food group on cardiovascular biomarkers reviewed in this chapter

An even less invasive measurement of body composition is the waist-to-hip ratio, measured simply by circumference. An increased waist-to-hip ratio shows a significant association with risk of myocardial infarction, as well as coronary artery disease, and T2D [9], [10]. In fact, waist-to-hip ratio shows both a graded and a significant association with myocardial infarction, especially in comparison to BMI, across ethnic groups [11]. The population-attributable risks of MI for waist-to-hip ratio in the top two quintiles of INTERHEART study participants was 24.3% compared with only 7.7% for the top two quintiles of BMI [9]. The importance of waist-to-hip ratio and waist circumference in predicting cardiometabolic risk has been increasingly recognized in the literature, and qualitative descriptors known as "pear" body shaped and "apple" body have been applied to describe patients with more weight around the hips and more weight around the waist, respectively [12, 13]. Furthermore, there

is evidence to suggest that even in women with normal weight, central obesity is associated with increased risk of mortality, similar to mortality in women with elevated BMI with central obesity [14]. These findings underscore the importance of assessing not only BMI as a risk factor for future cardiovascular disease, but also central obesity.

Studies have shown when body composition is modified with modalities such as high intensity exercise and diet, there is a reduction in body fat, waist circumference and increase in muscle mass. For example, patients with a history of myocardial infarction ($n = 90$) who performed high intensity exercise lost 4 pounds more of body fat, gained 1.5 pounds more of muscle, and reduced their waist circumference by 2.54 cm more than those who solely performed moderate exercise [15]. In addition, the Mediterranean diet (MD) in particular can be useful in reducing weight circumference, as demonstrated in a meta-analysis by Kastorini et al. [16].

Blood Pressure

Numerous large-scale studies have provided strong and consistent evidence that both systolic (SBP) and diastolic (DBP) blood pressures are positively associated with cardiovascular disease outcomes [17]. These findings are consistent across genders, various age groups, racial and ethnic groups, and across different countries. Not only is elevated blood pressure an overall predictor for cardiovascular outcomes, systolic and diastolic values are helpful in differentiating risk for patients and may act as a marker to assess risk of cardiometabolic syndrome [17]. While hypertension significantly affects the heart, it has multi-organ effects and is a risk factor for kidney disease and stroke [18].

Vegetarians have been shown to have lower blood pressure than those who eat omnivorous diets. In a meta-analysis of 258 studies, vegetarian diets were found to reduce SBP ~5–7 mm Hg and DBP by ~2–5 mm Hg, which is equivalent to the effect of losing 2.5 lbs [19]. Mirroring these findings , the MD decreases both SBP (-2.35 mm Hg) and DBP (-1.58 mm Hg) blood pressure [16]. Conversely, salty foods increase risk of hypertension: increasing SBP by 4.58 mm Hg and DBP by 2.25 mm Hg per 1000 mg of sodium [20]. Alarmingly, the risk of hypertension for participants in the upper third and fourth quartile (>3819 mg/day) is more than 4x higher compared to those in the lower two quartiles ($P < 0.01$).

Exercise also plays a crucial role in managing hypertension. Endurance training, dynamic resistance training and isometric training lower both SBP and DBP [21]. A systematic review and meta-analysis by Cornelissen and Smart in 2013 found that blood pressure reductions after low-intensity endurance exercise were smaller than blood pressure reductions after moderate- or high-intensity training [21]. (Low-intensity exercise training was defined by <55% of heart rate maximum or < 40% of heart rate reserve) [21]. Surprisingly, this same meta-analysis found that the groups exercising >210 min a week had the smallest reductions in blood pressure, possibly due to the fact that more exercise was performed at a lower intensity [21]. There are many different effective options for exercise to reduce blood pressure, but it may be worthwhile to consider prescribing a supervised facility-based exercise program for patients new to exercise, as this does yield the highest adherence [21].

Total Cholesterol

Total cholesterol, a commonly performed measure, is the sum of LDL cholesterol, VLDL cholesterol, HDL cholesterol, intermediate-density lipoprotein (IDL) cholesterol and cholesterol associated with lipoprotein(a) (Lp(a)). Cholesterol is a requirement for physiological function—it is an essential structural component of cell membranes and acts as a precursor for steroid hormones produced by the body. While the liver's synthesis of cholesterol is largely determined by genetic factors and feedback mechanisms, the remainder of cholesterol is obtained through dietary intake. Foods such as dairy products, eggs, meat, and poultry are significant sources of cholesterol in the diet. Though reducing such animal product intake seems intuitive to lower total cholesterol in patients with hyperlipidemia, dietary cholesterol has little effect on cardiovascular disease risk [22]. In fact, the relationship between dietary cholesterol and cardiovascular disease is different in a given individual; studies demonstrate that the fractional absorption rate of dietary cholesterol is variable, ranging from 20% to 80% [22].

According to US population studies, an optimal total cholesterol level in an adult is <150 mg/dL [23]. It is important to note, however, that there is a large difference in cardiovascular mortality rates for a given total cholesterol value [24]. Total serum cholesterol may be tracked longitudinally as a way to assess both risk for cardiovascular disease and nutrition status, alongside other clinically significant values, discussed below.

Low-Density Lipoproteins (LDL)

While total cholesterol is an important value to track over time and is a predictor of cardiovascular risk, LDL is colloquially termed "bad cholesterol" and is the main target of lipid lowering therapies such as statins. LDL is particularly utilized clinically as epidemiologic data demonstrates a positive and consistent relationship between LDL concentration and cardiovascular mortality and cardiovascular events. There is also substantial data to support the effort of lowering LDL, as reduction decreases patients' cardiovascular risk across a wide spectrum of patients, including those with known cardiovascular disease.

LDL is known to play a key role in the pathophysiology of atherosclerosis. Portions of blood vessels that are susceptible to atherosclerosis retain lipoproteins like LDL, and it is this retention that is an initial and key step in the formation of atherosclerotic plaques in the arteries. The mechanism of plaque formation is well understood, and the evidence for LDL's key role in atherosclerotic formation is corroborated by the understanding of Familial Hypercholesterolemia, an inherited disease associated with severely elevated LDL levels and premature atherosclerotic cardiovascular disease [25].

While LDL is the target of pharmacotherapy, diet plays a vital role in LDL reduction. The MD, which contains large amounts of plant sterols and nuts, lowers LDL, as compared to a low-fat controlled diet [26]. Meta-analyses of vegetarian diets corroborate that vegetarian diets not only lower total cholesterol, but LDL as well [27]. Further, nuts such as almonds, hazelnuts, and walnuts have been linked with a decrease in LDL and C-reactive protein, an acute phase reactant discussed later in this chapter. Additionally, viscous fiber has been shown to reduce LDL by trapping bile salts and preventing reuptake in the GI tract, as well as interfering with cholesterol being absorbed into cells [26].

Target LDL is based on multiple factors, but US population studies suggest that LDL <100 mg/dL manifests in low levels of atherosclerotic cardiovascular disease and patients with an LDL >190 mg/dL have a high risk of atherosclerotic cardiovascular disease [23]. LDL is an important value in the clinical assessment of risk for heart disease, and clinicians target therapies based on changes in LDL, which acts as a useful biomarker. Pharmacologic therapies used to lower LDL include statins, ezetimibe, bile acid sequestrants, and PCSK9 inhibitors [23].

High-Density Lipoproteins (HDL)

Opposite of LDL, HDL is often introduced to patients as the "good cholesterol." And unlike LDL, there is a known inverse relationship between HDL and the risk for cardiovascular events [28]. HDL is a scavenger of cholesterol—it assists in facilitating the return of cholesterol from the blood vessels back to the liver for eventual elimination. Furthermore, HDL prevents oxidation of LDL to limit LDL's role in the generation of atherosclerotic plaque and prevents secretion of the vasoconstrictor endothelin [29].

HDL values <40 mg/dL are considered an independent risk factor for cardiovascular disease [30]. Although low HDL is correlated with cardiovascular disease, raising HDL by pharmacologic interventions has not been consistently shown to have significant clinical benefit [31]. Some diets, such as the MD, have been shown to increase HDL levels, but the maximum threshold of improvement appears to be as low as 12%. Importantly, saturated fats and, to a lesser extent, unsaturated fatty acids have been shown to increase HDL [32]. Moderate alcohol consumption, specifically wine, is positively associated with higher levels of HDL [33, 34]. Conversely, diets high in carbohydrates and low in fats have been associated with low HDL [35]. There is preliminary evidence that aerobic exercise improves the anti-inflammatory and anti-oxidative properties of HDL, but the lack of consistent findings in this regard warrants more studies to determine the importance of exercise on HDL values and function [31].

Non-HDL Cholesterol

The sum of LDL and VLDL values is termed non-HDL cholesterol , which is more atherogenic than LDL or VLDL alone [23]. Therefore, non-HDL more accurately assesses atherogenic lipids and CV risk than LDL, especially in patients with hypertriglyceridemia. In patients with high triglycerides, such as patients with metabolic syndrome and Type II Diabetes, LDL is less accurately estimated by means of the Friedewald equation [23, 25]. Due to the limitations of the Friedewald equation, other ways of estimating LDL have been developed such as the Martin-Hopkins equation, which is a novel method to estimate LDL by using an adjustable factor of triglycerides to VLDL ratio [36]. Given that there are atherogenic lipids beyond LDL, some evidence suggests non-HDL cholesterol values could be more predictive of cardiovascular risk than LDL [37, 38]. In a recent 10-year risk cohort study, both LDL and non-HDL cholesterol values above 160 mg/dL were independently associated with a 50–80% increased relative risk of mortality [39].

In addition to underscoring the importance of non-HDL cholesterol as a marker of atherogenicity, the 2018 cholesterol management guidelines also underscore apolipoprotein B (apoB), the major apolipoprotein embedded in LDL and VLDL, as a stronger indicator of atherogenicity than LDL [23]. Another atherogenic biomarker similar in clinical utility and risk assessment to apoB is LDL particle number [40]. Both apoB and LDL particle number have been shown to be stronger cardiovascular disease risk factors than LDL cholesterol, but apoB has been the preferable particle for guideline adoption given lower cost, standardization, and scalability [40].

Triglycerides

Meta-analyses have demonstrated that both elevated fasting and non-fasting triglycerides are associated with increased risk of coronary artery disease [41]. The Women's Health Study further corroborated the strong association between raised triglycerides and coronary artery disease, as well as risk of myocardial infarction and all-cause mortality [42, 43]. In addition to cardiovascular risk, a triglyceride level > 150 mg/dL is a significant risk factor for metabolic syndrome, a cluster of pathological processes related to insulin resistance and elevated free fatty acids [44]. Additionally, elevated triglyceride concentrations (>885 mg/dL) are associated with risk of pancreatitis [45].

While these correlations between hypertriglyceridemia and risk for cardiovascular disease have been well studied, there is a need to further evaluate the clinical significance of lowering triglycerides by pharmacotherapy [45]. However, triglycerides are highly affected by diet and lifestyle. The MD, high in MUFA, PUFA and dietary fiber, can be particularly helpful in lowering triglycerides [44]. Many studies have shown that high intake of carbohydrates (greater than 60% of caloric intake) is associated with a rise in triglycerides [44]. In addition, high alcohol consumption is associated with elevated triglycerides, but low and moderate alcohol intake are associated with lower triglycerides; this is likely dependent on the type of alcohol consumed [46].

There are several classes of pharmacologic agents, such as fibrates, that reduce triglyceride levels, but both weight loss and moderate intensity exercise, such as brisk walking and social dancing, have been identified as key interventions to reduce triglyceride levels [47]. Additionally, dietary supplementation of ω-3 acid ethyl esters can be considered as an additional therapy for hypertriglyceridemia with a very minimal side effect profile [48]. Icospaent ethyl, a prescription highly purified eicosapentaenoic acid, has been shown to lower triglycerides and reduce the risk of ischemic cardiac events [49].

Lipoprotein(a)

Lp(a) is a well-known risk factor for coronary disease that is highly heritable; elevated levels are associated with atherosclerosis development and incidence of cardiovascular events [50]. Specifically, elevated Lp(a) levels have been associated with both coronary disease and calcific aortic valve disease. Lp(a) is distinguished from LDL by the presence of apolipoprotein (a), which likely mediates proinflammatory and prothrombotic effects of the protein [51]. While Lp(a) is a modified LDL particle, Lp(a) levels are independent of LDL levels [25]. There is significant evidence to support the use of Lp(a) as a risk factor for CVD, and there are randomized trials ongoing that are targeting Lp(a) [52, 53]. It is important to note that treatment with niacin can reduce Lp(a) up to 20–30% but has not been associated with improved outcomes [25]. Interestingly, monoclonal antibodies to PCSK9 may lower Lp(a) by 30% and have been associated with improved outcomes in large clinical trials such as FOURIER and ODESSEY [25, 54, 55]. Additionally, there are new pharmacologic approaches in phase III clinical trials that target Lp(a) lowering and it will be important to assess if lowering Lp (a) translates to decreased CV events [53]. There are little data available to support the influence of dietary choices on lowering Lp(a), but several studies suggest that low-fat diets may result in an increase in Lp(a) [56].

Hs-CRP

C-reactive protein (CRP), produced by the liver, is a marker of systemic inflammation [57]. High-sensitivity C-reactive protein (hs-CRP) is a higher sensitivity test that can detect lower grades of inflammation than a standard CRP test [57]. While numerous pathologic processes ranging from infection to autoimmune disease can elevate hs-CRP levels, it can also be used as a global assessment of cardiovascular risk. Given that many processes can lead to systemic inflammation, hs-CRP elevations may be transient in response to infection and should be repeated when these confounding processes are quiescent. Meta-analysis conducted by Li et al. suggests hs-CRP can stratify cardiovascular risk and all-cause mortality risk in the general population [57]. Further, data from the Women's Health

Study suggests hs-CRP predicts cardiovascular events even in groups that have no other apparent markers of cardiovascular disease [58]. An hs-CRP <2.0 mg/L is often considered the threshold for low risk and a value of >2.0 mg/L is considered the threshold for higher risk [59].

Provided that inflammation plays a key role in the pathophysiology of atherosclerotic formation, the correlation between hs-CRP and cardiovascular disease is not surprising. Even in patients with low levels of atherogenic biomarkers such as non-HDL cholesterol and apoB, a discordantly elevated hs-CRP level resulted in a 30–60% greater relative risk of developing ASCVD compared to patients with low hs-CRP [59]. While many cardiovascular risk factors such as smoking, diabetes, and hypertension can increase the inflammatory response and, thereby, hs-CRP, an anti-inflammatory diet may be helpful in reducing systemic inflammation and could help improve cardiovascular outcomes. Anti-inflammatory diets are the subject of many studies currently, but it has been well established that ω-3 fatty acids are anti-inflammatory, and ω-6 fatty acids tend to be pro-inflammatory. ω-3 fatty acids may be found in walnuts, canola oil, and soybean oil, and fish such as salmon, halibut, and mackerel. Conversely, ω-6 acids are found in corn and sunflower oils. It is generally recommended that protein in an anti-inflammatory diet be plant-based with small amounts of fish and lean meats. Further, the phytonutrients found in soy-based proteins have been demonstrated to have anti-inflammatory properties [60]. While a comprehensive anti-inflammatory diet is beyond the scope of this text, the Mediterranean and other plant-based diets have been identified as general guidelines with anti-inflammatory properties.

TMAO and the Gut Microbiome
(Fig. 2.2)

Trimethylamine N-oxide is a gut microbiota-dependent biomarker derived from L-carnitine, choline, and betaine. TMAO levels reflect a pro-atherogenic milieu in the gut microbi-

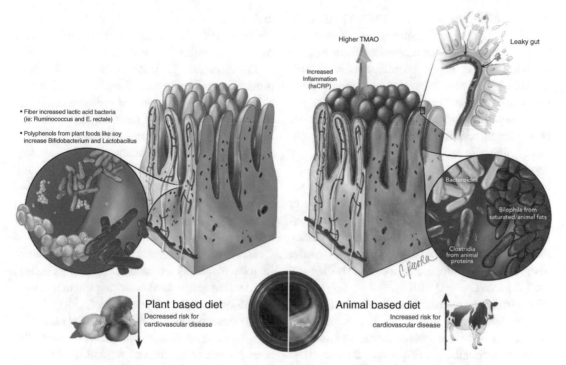

Fig. 2.2 The impacts of a plant-based diet vs. animal-based diet on TMAO levels, the gut microbiome, and the risk of coronary arterial plaque buildup. (Printed with permission from ©*Christina Pecora*)

ome and is associated with poor CV outcomes [61]. The normal range for serum TMAO is 0.5–5 µmol/L. TMAO is felt to play a role in cardiovascular disease and enhancing CV risk. A study on adults undergoing elective diagnostic cardiac catheterization found that participants who had a major cardiac event ≤3 years of catheterization had higher baseline TMAO levels compared to those who did not experience a cardiac event (5.0 µM vs. 3.5 µM; $P < 0.001$). Furthermore, elevated levels of TMAO were associated with a significant risk of mortality (hazard ratio (HR): 3.37; $P < 0.001$) and non-fatal myocardial infarction/stroke (HR: 2.135; $P < 0.001$) [61].

Foods rich in phosphatidylcholine (beef, eggs, and pork) get converted into trimethylamine and then TMAO. Increased choline levels induce greater gut microbial activity and, subsequently higher levels of TMAO. The KarMeN study, which monitored plasma TMAO levels in healthy adults after eating red meat, found a positive correlation ($r = 0.25$) between red meat consumption and choline levels. Additionally, participants

with TMAO levels >3.98 µmol/L ate more than the daily recommended amount of red meat per day [62].

Conversely, plant-based diets can decrease TMAO levels by promoting more diverse and stable microbiota. This is due to greater intake of fiber, polyphenols, and beneficial bacteria. For example, Klimenko et al. found plant-based diets greatly improve microbiome diversity [63]. Long-term fruit and vegetable consumption also improved local microbial diversity ($p < 0.05$). Moreover, reduced meat and greater fruit/vegetable consumption can be cardioprotective and inhibit TMAO production. In Koeth et al.'s study on L-carnitine metabolism, omnivores produced >20× more plasma TMAO than vegans despite consuming the same amount of L-carnitine ($p = 0.001$) [64].

The MD has also shown to promote gut diversity and reduce TMAO levels. De Filippis et al. examined the relationship between MD adherence and gut microbiota, observing significantly lower urinary TMAO levels in plant-based eaters vs. omnivores ($p < 0.0001$) and MD adherence having a negative correlation with TMAO levels [65]. Also, 25% of plasma metabolites are different between vegetarians and omnivores, further showing how diet can change the gut microbiome [66].

Although advertised as anti-inflammatory, the paleo diet may adversely interact with our gut microbiota and increase TMAO levels. Genoni et al. found serum TMAO levels were significantly higher in strict paleo diet eaters (<1 daily serving of grains/dairy) compared to those who eat a healthy balanced diet (9.53 μmol/L vs. 3.93 μmol/L, $P < 0.01$). This is possibly due to the lack of fiber in paleo diets [67]. In comparing the Atkins diet and Ornish diet after 4 weeks, Park et al. found the Atkins diet had higher TMAO levels compared to the Ornish diet: 3.3 vs. 1.8 μmol/L, $p = 0.01$ [68].

Additionally, Verdam et al. showed microbiome diversity is linked to inflammation in individuals who are obese. Compared to non-obese participants, participants who are obese exhibited lower *Bacteroidetes:Firmicutes* ratios ($p = 0.007$) and higher levels of *Proteobacteria*, inflammatory bacteria positively associated with BMI and CRP ($p = 0.0005$). Klimenko et al. also showed an inverse relationship between gut diversity and BMI ($p < 0.05$) [63]. This suggests obesity-induced loss of microbiota diversity results in greater inflammation [69]. Other studies, however, show an opposite relationship between obesity and *Bacteroidetes:Firmicutes* ratios, indicating further research is needed on the specific interactions between our gut microbiota and lifestyle [70, 71].

Albumin and Prealbumin

Albumin and prealbumin give important information into a patient's protein and calorie intake. Albumin, the most abundant serum protein, is a moderate indicator of malnutrition, with the normal range being 3.5–5.2 g/dL. As a negative acute-phase protein, its serum concentration and production is downregulated during inflammation [72]. Although prealbumin is also a negative acute-phase protein, its shorter half-life (~2 days)

makes it a more sensitive indicator of acute malnutrition and protein-calorie consumption compared to albumin. Prealbumin's reference range is 15–35 mg/dL [73]. As negative acute-phase proteins, prealbumin and albumin have high sensitivities to inflammation and additional steps are required to determine if reduced levels are malnutrition- or inflammation-induced.

Prealbumin and malnutrition risk are inversely related, where hypoalbuminemia (<3.5 g/dL) and/or hypoprealbuminemia (<15 mg/dL) indicate higher malnutrition risk. This is because visceral protein synthesis is not prioritized by the liver and is only made in sufficiently nourished states. Consequently, inadequate nutritional intake inhibits synthesis of albumin and prealbumin, and subsequently lowers each protein's levels. Additionally, Saka et al. ($n = 97$, 55 malnourished) observed prealbumin levels increased by 20% and risk of malnutrition decreased by 12% after 1 week of nutritional support, highlighting prealbumin's sensitivity to dietary changes [74].

Maintaining healthy nutritional intake is also integral in predicting morbidity and mortality. A study on admitted patients with acute coronary syndrome and lower prealbumin levels showed their risk of a major in-hospital cardiac event was more than 3× the risk of patients with normal prealbumin levels: 20.8 vs 6.1% [75]. Also, Lourenço et al. found the risk of heart failure death doubled in patients with discharge prealbumin levels ≤15 mg/dL, citing an imbalance protein-energy demands [76].

There are concerns, however, on albumin's reliability in monitoring nutritional status. For example, Lee et al. showed patients did not exhibit abnormal albumin levels until they reached extreme starvation: <12 BMI or > 6 weeks of starvation [77]. And while a meta-analysis found the risk ratio for a CVD event per 1 g/dL decrease in plasma albumin was 1.96 (95% CI, 1.43–2.68), this was likely due to inflammation and not malnutrition [78]. Additionally, another study ($n = 262$) showed 80% of geriatric patients had low albumin levels despite receiving adequate nutrition [79]. Additional steps beyond albumin testing should therefore be taken to accurately determine a patient's nutritional status.

Magnesium

Magnesium plays a dual role as a marker of nutritional status and cardiovascular health due to its interactions with CRP and serum plasma. Hypomagnesemia (<1.4 mg/dL) is linked to such conditions as hypertension, arrhythmia, diabetes, and CHD [80]. Magnesium deficiency is so prevalent, in fact, that over 10% of hospitalized patients exhibit hypomagnesaemia [81]. Also, thiazide and loop diuretics have been shown to induce moderate reductions in magnesium concentration, but usually at or close to the normal range [82]. The normal range of serum magnesium is 1.46–2.68 mg/dL and 4.2–6.8 mg/dL for RBC magnesium [80, 83].

Magnesium is often acquired through green vegetables, meat, and dietary supplements. Global trends in diet have contributed to declining magnesium intakes through increased consumption of soda and processed foods, which increase bodily phosphorus levels and thus the required daily magnesium intake. Additionally, the Framingham Heart Study ($n = 2695$) showed hypomagnesemia can increase the risk of connective tissue inflammation and aortic calcification due to a surplus of intracellular calcium. It was found that a 50-mg/day magnesium intake (by diet and supplements) was linked to 22% lower coronary artery calcification (CAC) ($p < 0.001$) and 12% lower abdominal aortic calcification (AAC) ($p = 0.07$). Further, the risk of having CAC was 58% lower ($p < 0.001$) and any AAC was 34% lower ($p = 0.01$) in those with the highest magnesium intake compared to those with the lowest magnesium intake [84]. This is because the deficiency of magnesium allows calcium ions to dominate the binding sites of cardiac and smooth muscle cells, resulting in intracellular calcium buildup. Salaminia et al. showed magnesium supplementation plays a role in cardiac arrhythmia risk, with magnesium supplements decreasing ventricular and supraventricular arrhythmias compared to placebo (OR = 0.32;

$p < 0.001$ and OR = 0.42; $p < 0.001$, respectively) [85]. Moreover, each 100 mg/day increase of dietary magnesium has been linked to a 22% reduction in HF risk [86].

Magnesium intake is often higher in those eating a plant-based diet, as indicated by Koebnick et al.'s prospective study of 108 pregnant women. Women eating a plant-based diet (ovo-lacto vegetarian or low meat) had significantly higher magnesium intakes compared to women on the Western (control) diet: 508 ± 14 mg/day for ovo-lacto vegetarians ($P < 0.001$) 504 ± 11 mg/day for low-meat eaters ($P < 0.001$) vs. 412 ± 9 mg/day for the control diet. While serum magnesium levels were similar across groups, RBC magnesium levels were higher in the low-meat group than the control group ($P = 0.058$) [87]. The MD has also exhibited moderate success in ensuring sufficient magnesium intake, with 66.9% of participants in the MEAL study ($n = 1838$) meeting the daily recommended intake (~200–522 mg/day) [88].

Numerous magnesium diagnostic tests are currently available. Although using RBC magnesium is sometimes preferable given RBC's higher magnesium content, its utility and reliability has yet to be established [83, 89]. A 24-h urine analysis has also shown to be unreliable due to variability of renal magnesium reabsorption and excretion [90, 91]. Additionally, current serum magnesium guidelines have come under scrutiny for being insufficient in ascertaining a patient's status [92]. As such, the combined use of 24 h urine, serum, and dietary magnesium tests is suggested to gain the most complete picture of a patient's magnesium status.

HbA$_{1c}$ and Fasting Glucose

Normal range for fasting blood glucose is 70–99 mg/dL, with hyperglycemia resulting in risk of diabetes and hypoglycemia leading to acute neurological changes. HbA1$_c$ is a quantitative measure of average blood glucose of the past 2–3 months and is critical for diagnosing and monitoring diabetes and determining cardiovascular mortality. The ideal range for non-diabetics is <5.7% and ≤ 7.0% for patients with T2D [93, 94].

Plant-based diets have shown to be successful in regulating blood glucose levels and reducing insulin resistance [95]. A meta-analysis found that T2D patients eating a plant-based diet reduced their HbA_{1c} levels by 3.9% ($P = 0.001$) but had a nonsignificant 6.49 mg/dL decrease ($P = 0.301$) in fasting blood glucose levels [96]. Further, a randomized, 10-week study on eight men with untreated T2D showed diets composed of high-protein and low-carbohydrate foods can potentially improve blood glucose and HbA_{1c} levels, exhibiting an average glucose of 126 mg/dL and 7.6 ± 0.3 HbA_{1c} in the diet group vs. 198 mg/dL glucose and 9.8 ± 0.5 HbA_{1c} in the control group [97]. The MD has also shown potential, reducing blood glucose levels by 3.89 mg/dL in a meta-analysis ($n = 534,906$) [16]. Intermittent fasting (500–600 cal/day for 2 nonconsecutive days/week), an increasingly popular eating pattern, can also slightly decrease HbA_{1c} levels in patients with T2D. In a 12-month randomized noninferiority trial, HbA_{1c} lowered by 0.3% but did not show as much of an improvement compared to the continuous restriction diet group (1200–1500 cal/day), which showed a 0.5% reduction [98].

Vitamin D

Vitamin D is a prohormone produced by the kidneys to regulate serum calcium concentration levels and immunological processes. As an essential vitamin it must be acquired externally. The greatest natural source of vitamin D, besides sunlight, is animal products such as dairy, fatty fish (salmon, tuna, etc), and some red meat and cruciferous vegetables. As we transition into a more indoors-oriented society, with 62% of respondents in the Indoor Generation Report ($n = 16,000$) spending 15–24 h indoors per day, vitamin D supplementation is becoming increasingly important [99]. The most clinically relevant form of serum vitamin D is 25(OH)D and the reference range is 50 nmol/L to 125 nmol/L.

Since the majority of vitamin D rich foods are derived from animal sources and vitamin D fortified foods are not common, vegans and vegetarians may be at a greater risk of vitamin D deficiency. In fact, the EPIC Oxford Study ($n = 226$ omnivores, 231 vegetarians, 232 vegans) found male vegans, vegetarians, and omnivores ate 0.88 μg/day, 1.56 μg/day, and 3.39 μg/day, respectively. Women had similar results: 0.88 μg/day, 1.51 μg/day, and 3.32 μg/day [100].

In terms of supplementation, Barger-Lux et al. ($n = 116$) found supplementing with the recommended vitamin D3 intake of 10 μg/day (400 IU/day), the equivalent of 10 large eggs or 3 oz. of salmon, raises 25(OH)D by 11 nmol/L [101]. The issue therefore becomes the efficacy and sustainability of acquiring vitamin D from food sources, a concern also brought up in the Adventist Health-2 study, since salmon is expensive and eating ten eggs a day introduces numerous other health risks, namely hypercholesterolemia. Also, as the EPIC Oxford study showed, neither omnivores nor vegetarians/vegans are meeting their recommended daily vitamin D intake, meaning all eating groups have to augment their diet with vitamin D3 supplements to fulfill the recommended dietary intake.

Additionally, vitamin D may possess anti-inflammatory effects against cancer and diabetes, with several meta-analyses indicating vitamin D supplementation lowers cancer mortality rates [102]. In fact, a double-blinded randomized study on vitamin D supplementation and prostate cancer risk ($n = 250$) found 58% of patients in the supplement group vs 49% in the placebo group had a ≥ 50% reduction of prostate-specific antigens (PSA) and a HR of 0.67 ($P = 0.04$) [103]. Also, Mousa et al. ($n = 1270$) found patients with T2D and taking vitamin D supplements had lower levels of CRP (standardized mean difference (SMD) −0.23; $P = 0.002$), tumor necrosis factor α (SMD −0.49; $P = 0.005$), erythrocyte sedimentation rate (SMD −0.47; $P = 0.03$), and higher levels of leptin (SMD 0.42; $P = 0.03$) compared to control groups, highlighting how vitamin D supplementation can mediate chronic inflammation in T2D patients [104]. Further, the Health Professionals Follow-up Study ($n = 18,225$ men) found those with 25(OH)D deficiencies were 2× more likely to develop myocardial infarction than those who had healthy 25(OH)D concentrations (relative risk, 2.42; $P < 0.001$) [105].

The nationwide, randomized, placebo-controlled VITAL Study ($n = 25,871$) shows further research is required, however, with vitamin D3 supplementation showing no significant effects on cardiovascular health and cancer risk. For example, the HR between the vitamin D supplementation and placebo group was 0.96 ($P = 0.47$) and incidence of a major cardiovascular event had a hazard ratio of 0.97 ($P = 0.69$) [102]. Michos et al. parallel these findings, suggesting diet and sunlight should be prioritized over supplements for optimizing vitamin D levels [106]. The authors also found calcium supplements can increase one's risk of myocardial infarction and stroke, indicating dietary calcium and physical activity are safer methods of calcium intake.

Vitamin B12 and Folate

While the plant-based diet dramatically improves cardiovascular health, there are limitations of implementing this diet–primarily risks of essential vitamin deficiencies. Vitamin B12, the largest and most complex essential vitamin, is primarily sourced from animal products and is a critical enzyme cofactor involved in the oxidation of odd-numbered fatty acid chains. Additionally, it is neuroprotective and converts homocysteine into nontoxic molecules. B12 deficiency not only leads to neurological damage but also a buildup of homocysteine, which promotes arterial plaque buildup, increasing the risk of atherothrombosis [107, 108]. Folate is another essential vitamin and is critical for the biosynthesis of nucleotide bases involved in amino acid synthesis and metabolism. Folate in its natural form is commonly found and consumed in spinach, nuts, beans, and other leafy green vegetables. In its synthetic form, folic acid, folate can be found in fortified foods such as bread and cereals.

While meats are rich in B12, folate is primarily found in plant-based foods. It therefore comes as no surprise that vegetarians and vegans may have B12 deficiencies since their diets lack the only natural source of B12: meat. Rauma et al.'s analysis of serum B12 concentrations and dietary intakes of living food diet vegans, who follow a strict raw food diet, and omnivores, it was found vegans have significantly ($P < 0.001$) lower average B12 serum concentrations (193 pmol/L) as opposed to omnivores (311 pmol/L). Additionally, the serum concentrations in participants who supplemented their diets with B12 rich foods, such as seaweed, had levels twice as high compared to those who did not supplement, having an average B12 concentration of 221 pmol/L vs 105 pmol/L ($P = 0.025$). It should be noted, however, that this study population is part of a very strict subset of vegans and their B12 levels could be drastically different from average vegans due to dietary differences [109]. In a study on B12 supplementation in 50 vegetarians with B12 deficiency (<150 pmol/L), supplementation was shown to be crucial for vegans in keeping healthy B12 concentrations. By supplementing with 500 µg/day, participants exhibited significant improvements in B12 serum concentration (from 134 ± 125.6 to 379 ± 206.2 pmol/L, $p < 0.0001$) and reductions in plasma homocysteine levels (from 16.7 ± 11 to 11.3 ± 6 µmol/L, $p < 0.01$) [110].

In the EPIC-Oxford study ($n = 689$: 226 omnivores, 231 vegetarians, and 232 vegans), 52% of vegans, 7% of vegetarians, and 1 omnivore were B12 deficient (<118 pmol/L). Consequently, average serum B12 concentrations in vegans were the lowest (122 pmol/L), with vegetarians coming second (182 pmol/L), and omnivores with the average highest concentration (281 pmol/L) ($P < 0.001$). This is, of course, due to plant-based diets lacking natural sources of B12. Also, of the vegans and vegetarians that were not using B12 supplements, 95% and 31% of vegans and vegetarians were failing to meet the recommended daily intake (1.5 µg/day), mirroring the trends found in Rauma et al. Conversely, folate concentrations were highest in vegans (37.5 nmol/L) and lowest in omnivores (20.0 nmol/L), indicating an inverse relationship between folate and B12 ($P < 0.001$) [111]. Schupbach et al.'s study ($n = 206$, 100 omnivores, 53 vegans, 53 vegetarians) corroborates these findings, with 58% of omnivores being deficient in folate (<15 nmol/L, $p < 0.05$) [112].

The MD, a diet rich in fruits, vegetables, and lean meats (fish, poultry, etc.), can mediate B12 deficiency in vegans. In the KIDMED study ($n = 3166$, 6- to 24-yr-olds), none of the participants were found to have B12 deficiencies however 14.3% of 6- to 14-yr-olds ($P = 0.021$) and 25.5% of 15- to 24-yr-olds ($P = 0.002$) were deficient in folate [113]. This is likely due to a lack of MD adherence and greater average consumption of sweet drinks and processed foods found in younger adults [114]. Fortified foods rich in folate and other essential vitamins such as ready-to-eat cereals, however, have been shown to decrease folate deficiency risk ($p < 0.001$) in MD eaters ($n = 3534$) [115]. Also, Planells et al. ($n = 384$) showed the MD provided enough B12 (89.1% had acceptable levels) but was moderately successful in mediating folate deficiency (57.6% acceptable) [116]. In a study on the MD and pregnant women ($n = 72$), however, 70.8% were B12 deficient and none were folate deficient, indicating pregnant women may be a vulnerable population to B12 deficiency [117].

Conclusion

The role and use of biomarkers and lifestyle changes to monitor and treat cardiovascular health and nutrition are of increasing interest among health providers and patients. In this chapter, we reviewed the potential of biomarkers to monitor the impact of lifestyle changes. We also presented data on how plant-based diets and minimal red meat consumption can have positive effects on biomarkers like triglycerides, TMAO, and cholesterol.

While the biomarkers reviewed in this chapter are the most clinically relevant and useful measures for detecting the impact of diets and nutritional therapy, the list of possible biomarkers that could contribute to clinical nutrition is continually evolving.

References

1. CDC. Prediabetes - your chance to prevent type 2 diabetes. In: Centers for Disease Control and Prevention. 2020. https://www.cdc.gov/diabetes/basics/prediabetes.html. Accessed 26 Feb 2020.
2. Meghan M, Slining BMP. Trends in intakes and sources of solid fats and added sugars among US children and adolescents: 1994–2010. Pediatr Obes. 2013;8:307.
3. Phillips K, Wood F, Spanou C, Kinnersley P, Simpson SA, Butler CC, PRE-EMPT Team. Counselling patients about behaviour change: the challenge of talking about diet. Br J Gen Pract. 2012;62:e13–21.
4. Poirier P, Després J-P. Waist circumference, visceral obesity, and cardiovascular risk. J Cardiopulm Rehab. 2003;23:161–9.
5. Fox KR, Hillsdon M. Physical activity and obesity. Obes Rev. 2007;8 Suppl 1:115–21.
6. Lang P-O, Trivalle C, Vogel T, Proust J, Papazyan J-P, Dramé M. Determination of cutoff values for DEXA-based body composition measurements for determining metabolic and cardiovascular health. Biores Open Access. 2015;4:16–25.
7. Shepherd J, Ng B, Sommer M, Heymsfield SB. Body composition by DXA. Bone. 2017;104:101.
8. American Heart Association, National Heart, Lung, and Blood Institue, Grundy SM, Cleeman JI, Daniels SR, Donato KA, Eckel RH, Franklin BA, Gordon DJ, Krauss RM, Savage PJ, Smith SC Jr, Spertus JA, Costa F. Diagnosis and management of the metabolic syndrome. An American Heart Association/National Heart, Lung, and Blood Institute Scientific Statement. Executive summary. Cardiol Rev. 2005;13: 322–7.
9. Iqbal R, Anand S, Ounpuu S, Islam S, Zhang X, Rangarajan S, Chifamba J, Al-Hinai A, Keltai M, Yusuf S, INTERHEART Study Investigators. Dietary patterns and the risk of acute myocardial infarction in 52 countries: results of the INTERHEART study. Circulation. 2008;118:1929–37.
10. Emdin CA, Khera AV, Natarajan P, Klarin D, Zekavat SM, Hsiao AJ, Kathiresan S. Genetic association of waist-to-hip ratio with cardiometabolic traits, type 2 diabetes, and coronary heart disease. JAMA. 2017;317:626–34.
11. Yusuf S, Hawken S, Ounpuu S, Bautista L, Franzosi MG, Commerford P, Lang CC, Rumboldt Z, Onen CL, Lisheng L, Tanomsup S, Wangai P Jr, Razak F, Sharma AM, Anand SS, INTERHEART Study Investigators. Obesity and the risk of myocardial infarction in 27,000 participants from 52 countries: a case-control study. Lancet. 2005;366:1640–9.
12. Wang S, Liu Y, Li F, Jia H, Liu L, Xue F. A novel quantitative body shape score for detecting association between obesity and hypertension in China. BMC Public Health. 2015;15. https://doi.org/10.1186/s12889-014-1334-5.

13. Jingyuan F, Hofker M, Wijmenga C. Apple or pear: size and shape matter. Cell Metab. 2015;21:507–8.

14. Sun Y, Liu B, Snetselaar LG, Wallace RB, Caan BJ, Rohan TE, Neuhouser ML, Shadyab AH, Chlebowski RT, Manson JE, Bao W. Association of normal-weight central obesity with all-cause and cause-specific mortality among postmenopausal women. JAMA Netw Open. 2019;2:e197337.

15. Kuehn BM. Evidence for HIIT benefits in cardiac rehabilitation grow. Circulation. 2019;140:514–5.

16. Kastorini C-M, Milionis HJ, Esposito K, Giugliano D, Goudevenos JA, Panagiotakos DB. The effect of Mediterranean diet on metabolic syndrome and its components: a meta-analysis of 50 studies and 534,906 individuals. J Am Coll Cardiol. 2011;57:1299–313.

17. Vasan RS, Larson MG, Leip EP, Evans JC, O'Donnell CJ, Kannel WB, Levy D. Impact of high-normal blood pressure on the risk of cardiovascular disease. N Engl J Med. 2001;345:1291–7.

18. Kjeldsen SE. Hypertension and cardiovascular risk: general aspects. Pharmacol Res. 2018;129:95–9.

19. Yokoyama Y, Nishimura K, Barnard ND, Takegami M, Watanabe M, Sekikawa A, Okamura T, Miyamoto Y. Vegetarian diets and blood pressure: a meta-analysis. JAMA Intern Med. 2014;174:577–87.

20. Jackson SL, Cogswell ME, Zhao L, Terry AL, Wang C-Y, Wright J, Coleman King SM, Bowman B, Chen T-C, Merritt R, Loria CM. Association between urinary sodium and potassium excretion and blood pressure among adults in the united states: national health and nutrition examination survey, 2014. Circulation. 2018;137:237–46.

21. Cornelissen VA, Smart NA. Exercise training for blood pressure: a systematic review and meta-analysis. J Am Heart Assoc. 2013;2:e004473.

22. McNamara DJ. Dietary cholesterol, heart disease risk and cognitive dissonance. Proc Nutr Soc. 2014;73:161–6.

23. Grundy SM, Stone NJ, Bailey AL, Beam C, Birtcher KK, Blumenthal RS, Braun LT, de Ferranti S, Faiella-Tommasino J, Forman DE, Goldberg R, Heidenreich PA, Hlatky MA, Jones DW, Lloyd-Jones D, Lopez-Pajares N, Ndumele CE, Orringer CE, Peralta CA, Saseen JJ, Smith SC Jr, Sperling L, Virani SS, Yeboah J. 2018 AHA/ACC/AACVPR/AAPA/ABC/ACPM/ADA/AGS/APhA/ASPC/NLA/PCNA guideline on the management of blood cholesterol: a report of the American College of Cardiology/American Heart Association Task Force on Clinical Practice Guidelines. Circulation. 2019;139:e1082–143.

24. Monique Verschuren WM, Jacobs DR, Bloemberg BPM, Kromhout D, Menotti A, Aravanis C, Blackburn H, Buzina R, Dontas AS, Fidanza F, Karvonen MJ, Nedelijković S, Nissinen A, Toshima H. Serum total cholesterol and long-term coronary heart disease mortality in different cultures: twenty-five-year follow-up of the seven countries study. JAMA. 1995;274:131–6.

25. Linton MF, Yancey PG, Davies SS, Gray Jerome W, Linton EF, Song WL, Doran AC, Vickers KC. The role of lipids and lipoproteins in atherosclerosis. MDText.com, Inc; 2019.

26. Jenkins W, MSc AJB, Rd AJP, Caroline Brydson B. The portfolio diet for cardiovascular disease risk reduction: an evidence based approach to lower cholesterol through plant food consumption. Amsterdam: Elsevier; 2019.

27. Wang F, Zheng J, Yang B, Jiang J, Fu Y, Li D. Effects of vegetarian diets on blood lipids: a systematic review and meta-analysis of randomized controlled trials. J Am Heart Assoc. 2015;4:e002408.

28. Rubenfire M, Brook RD. HDL cholesterol and cardiovascular outcomes: what is the evidence? Curr Cardiol Rep. 2013;15:349.

29. Ahn N, Kim K. High-density lipoprotein cholesterol (HDL-C) in cardiovascular disease: effect of exercise training. Integr Med Res. 2016;5:212–5.

30. Barter P. HDL-C: role as a risk modifier. Atheroscler Suppl. 2011;12:267–70.

31. Ruiz-Ramie JJ, Barber JL, Sarzynski MA. Effects of exercise on HDL functionality. Curr Opin Lipidol. 2019;30:16–23.

32. DiNicolantonio JJ, O'Keefe JH. Effects of dietary fats on blood lipids: a review of direct comparison trials. Open Heart. 2018;5:e000871.

33. Nova E, San Mauro-Martín I, Díaz-Prieto LE, Marcos A. Wine and beer within a moderate alcohol intake is associated with higher levels of HDL-c and adiponectin. Nutr Res. 2019;63:42–50.

34. KrálováLesná I, Suchánek P, Stávek P, Poledne R. May alcohol-induced increase of HDL be considered as atheroprotective? Physiol Res. 2010;59:407–13.

35. Lee HA, An H. The effect of high carbohydrate-to-fat intake ratios on hypo-HDL-cholesterolemia risk and HDL-cholesterol levels over a 12-year follow-up. Sci Rep. 2020;10:1–9.

36. Martin SS, Blaha MJ, Elshazly MB, Toth PP, Kwiterovich PO, Blumenthal RS, Jones SR. Comparison of a novel method vs the Friedewald equation for estimating low-density lipoprotein cholesterol levels from the standard lipid profile. JAMA. 2013;310:2061–8.

37. Boekholdt SM, Arsenault BJ, Mora S, Pedersen TR, LaRosa JC, Nestel PJ, Simes RJ, Durrington P, Hitman GA, Welch KMA, DeMicco DA, Zwinderman AH, Clearfield MB, Downs JR, Tonkin AM, Colhoun HM, Gotto AM Jr, Ridker PM, Kastelein JJP. Association of LDL cholesterol, non-HDL cholesterol, and apolipoprotein B levels with risk of cardiovascular events among patients treated with statins: a meta-analysis. JAMA. 2012;307:1302–9.

38. Liu J, Sempos CT, Donahue RP, Dorn J, Trevisan M, Grundy SM. Non-high-density lipoprotein and very-low-density lipoprotein cholesterol and their risk predictive values in coronary heart disease. Am J Cardiol. 2006;98:1363–8.

39. Abdullah SM, Defina LF, Leonard D, Barlow CE, Radford NB, Willis BL, Rohatgi A, McGuire DK, de Lemos JA, Grundy SM, Berry JD, Khera A. Long-term association of low-density lipoprotein choles-

terol with cardiovascular mortality in individuals at low 10-year risk of atherosclerotic cardiovascular disease. Circulation. 2018;138:2315–25.

40. AACC Lipoproteins and Vascular Diseases Division Working Group on Best Practices, Cole TG, Contois JH, Csako G, McConnell JP, Remaley AT, Devaraj S, Hoefner DM, Mallory T, Sethi AA, Warnick GR. Association of apolipoprotein B and nuclear magnetic resonance spectroscopy-derived LDL particle number with outcomes in 25 clinical studies: assessment by the AACC Lipoprotein and Vascular Diseases Division Working Group on Best Practices. Clin Chem. 2013;59:752–70.

41. Hokanson JE, Austin MA. Plasma triglyceride level is a risk factor for cardiovascular disease independent of high-density lipoprotein cholesterol level: a meta-analysis of population-based prospective studies. J Cardiovasc Risk. 1996;3:213–9.

42. Nordestgaard BG, Benn M, Schnohr P, Tybjaerg-Hansen A. Nonfasting triglycerides and risk of myocardial infarction, ischemic heart disease, and death in men and women. JAMA. 2007;298:299–308.

43. Bansal S, Buring JE, Rifai N, Mora S, Sacks FM, Ridker PM. Fasting compared with nonfasting triglycerides and risk of cardiovascular events in women. JAMA. 2007;298:309–16.

44. Miller M, Stone NJ, Ballantyne C, Bittner V, Criqui MH, Ginsberg HN, Goldberg AC, Howard WJ, Jacobson MS, Kris-Etherton PM, Lennie TA, Levi M, Mazzone T, Pennathur S, American Heart Association Clinical Lipidology, Thrombosis, and Prevention Committee of the Council on Nutrition, Physical Activity, and Metabolism, Council on Arteriosclerosis, Thrombosis and Vascular Biology, Council on Cardiovascular Nursing, Council on the Kidney in Cardiovascular Disease. Triglycerides and cardiovascular disease: a scientific statement from the American Heart Association. Circulation. 2011;123:2292–333.

45. Nordestgaard BG, Varbo A. Triglycerides and cardiovascular disease. Lancet. 2014;384:626–35.

46. Klop B, Rego AT, Cabezas MC. Alcohol and plasma triglycerides. Curr Opin Lipidol. 2013. https://doi.org/10.1097/MOL.0b013e3283606845.

47. Jacobson TA, Miller M, Schaefer EJ. Hypertriglyceridemia and cardiovascular risk reduction. Clin Ther. 2007;29:763–77.

48. Handelsman Y, Shapiro MD. Triglycerides, atherosclerosis, and cardiovascular outcome studies: focus on omega-3 fatty acids. Endocr Pract. 2017;23:100–12.

49. Bhatt DL, Steg PG, Miller M, Brinton EA, Jacobson TA, Ketchum SB, Doyle RT Jr, Juliano RA, Jiao L, Granowitz C, Tardif J-C, Ballantyne CM, REDUCE-IT Investigators. Cardiovascular risk reduction with icosapent ethyl for hypertriglyceridemia. N Engl J Med. 2019;380:11–22.

50. Bittner V, Szarek M, Aylward PE, Bhatt DL, Diaz R, Fras Z, Goodman S, Hanotin C, Harrington R, Jukema JW, Loizeau V, Moriarty P, Moryusef A, Pordy R, Roe MT, Sinnaeve P, White HD, Zahger D, Zeiher A, Steg PG, Schwartz G. Lp(a) and cardiovascular outcomes: an analysis from the ODYSSEY OUTCOMES trial. Atheroscler Suppl. 2018;32:24–5.

51. Borrelli MJ, Youssef A, Boffa MB, Koschinsky ML. New frontiers in Lp(a)-targeted therapies. Trends Pharmacol Sci. 2019;40:212–25.

52. Randomized controlled trial of lipid apheresis in patients with elevated lipoprotein(a) - full text view - ClinicalTrials.Gov. https://clinicaltrials.gov/ct2/show/NCT01064934. Accessed 1 Mar 2021.

53. Assessing the impact of lipoprotein (a) lowering with TQJ230 on major cardiovascular events in patients with CVD - full text view - ClinicalTrials.Gov. https://clinicaltrials.gov/ct2/show/NCT04023552. Accessed 1 Mar 2021.

54. Sabatine MS, Giugliano RP, Keech AC, Honarpour N, Wiviott SD, Murphy SA, Kuder JF, Wang H, Liu T, Wasserman SM, Sever PS, Pedersen TR, FOURIER Steering Committee and Investigators. Evolocumab and clinical outcomes in patients with cardiovascular disease. N Engl J Med. 2017;376:1713–22.

55. Schwartz GG, Steg PG, Szarek M, Bhatt DL, Bittner VA, Diaz R, Edelberg JM, Goodman SG, Hanotin C, Harrington RA, Jukema JW, Lecorps G, Mahaffey KW, Moryusef A, Pordy R, Quintero K, Roe MT, Sasiela WJ, Tamby J-F, Tricoci P, White HD, Zeiher AM, ODYSSEY OUTCOMES Committees and Investigators. Alirocumab and cardiovascular outcomes after acute coronary syndrome. N Engl J Med. 2018;379:2097–107.

56. Fitó M, Estruch R, Salas-Salvadó J, Martínez-Gonzalez MA, Arós F, Vila J, Corella D, Díaz O, Sáez G, de la Torre R, Mitjavila M-T, Muñoz MA, Lamuela-Raventós R-M, Ruiz-Gutierrez V, Fiol M, Gómez-Gracia E, Lapetra J, Ros E, Serra-Majem L, Covas M-I, PREDIMED Study Investigators. Effect of the Mediterranean diet on heart failure biomarkers: a randomized sample from the PREDIMED trial. Eur J Heart Fail. 2014;16:543–50.

57. Li Y, Zhong X, Cheng G, Zhao C, Zhang L, Hong Y, Wan Q, He R, Wang Z. Hs-CRP and all-cause, cardiovascular, and cancer mortality risk: a meta-analysis. Atherosclerosis. 2017;259:75–82.

58. Ridker PM, Buring JE, Shih J, Matias M, Hennekens CH. Prospective study of C-reactive protein and the risk of future cardiovascular events among apparently healthy women. Circulation. 1998;98:731–3.

59. Quispe R, Michos ED, Martin SS, Puri R, Toth PP, Al Suwaidi J, Banach M, Virani SS, Blumenthal RS, Jones SR, Elshazly MB. High-sensitivity C-reactive protein discordance with atherogenic lipid measures and incidence of atherosclerotic cardiovascular disease in primary prevention: the ARIC study. J Am Heart Assoc. 2020;9:e013600.

60. Ricker MA, Haas WC. Anti-inflammatory diet in clinical practice: a review. Nutr Clin Pract. 2017;32:318–25.

61. Tang WHW, Wang Z, Levison BS, Koeth RA, Britt EB, Fu X, Wu Y, Hazen SL. Intestinal microbial

metabolism of phosphatidylcholine and cardiovascular risk. N Engl J Med. 2013;368:1575–84.

62. Krüger R, Merz B, Rist MJ, Ferrario PG, Bub A, Kulling SE, Watzl B. Associations of current diet with plasma and urine TMAO in the KarMeN study: direct and indirect contributions. Mol Nutr Food Res. 2017;61. https://doi.org/10.1002/mnfr.201700363.

63. Klimenko NS, Tyakht AV, Popenko AS, Vasiliev AS, Altukhov IA, Ischenko DS, Shashkova TI, Efimova DA, Nikogosov DA, Osipenko DA, Musienko SV, Selezneva KS, Baranova A, Kurilshikov AM, Toshchakov SM, Korzhenkov AA, Samarov NI, Shevchenko MA, Tepliuk AV, Alexeev DG. Microbiome responses to an uncontrolled short-term diet intervention in the frame of the citizen science project. Nutrients. 2018;10. https://doi.org/10.3390/nu10050576.

64. Koeth RA, Lam-Galvez BR, Kirsop J, Wang Z, Levison BS, Gu X, Copeland MF, Bartlett D, Cody DB, Dai HJ, Culley MK, Li XS, Fu X, Wu Y, Li L, DiDonato JA, Tang WHW, Garcia-Garcia JC, Hazen SL. l-Carnitine in omnivorous diets induces an atherogenic gut microbial pathway in humans. J Clin Invest. 2019;129. https://doi.org/10.1172/JCI94601.

65. De Filippis F, Pellegrini N, Vannini L, Jeffery IB, La Storia A, Laghi L, Serrazanetti DI, Di Cagno R, Ferrocino I, Lazzi C, Turroni S, Cocolin L, Brigidi P, Neviani E, Gobbetti M, O'Toole PW, Ercolini D. High-level adherence to a Mediterranean diet beneficially impacts the gut microbiota and associated metabolome. Gut. 2016;65:1812–21.

66. Tomova A, Bukovsky I, Rembert E, Yonas W, Alwarith J, Barnard ND, Kahleova H. The effects of vegetarian and vegan diets on gut microbiota. Front Nutr. 2019;6:47.

67. Genoni A, Christophersen CT, Lo J, Coghlan M, Boyce MC, Bird AR, Lyons-Wall P, Devine A. Long-term Paleolithic diet is associated with lower resistant starch intake, different gut microbiota composition and increased serum TMAO concentrations. Eur J Nutr. 2019. https://doi.org/10.1007/s00394-019-02036-y.

68. Park JE, Miller M, Rhyne J, Wang Z, Hazen SL. Differential effect of short-term popular diets on TMAO and other cardio-metabolic risk markers. Nutr Metab Cardiovasc Dis. 2019;29:513–7.

69. Verdam FJ, Fuentes S, de Jonge C, Zoetendal EG, Erbil R, Greve JW, Buurman WA, de Vos WM, Rensen SS. Human intestinal microbiota composition is associated with local and systemic inflammation in obesity. Obesity. 2013;21:E607–15.

70. Andoh A, Nishida A, Takahashi K, Inatomi O, Imaeda H, Bamba S, Kito K, Sugimoto M, Kobayashi T. Comparison of the gut microbial community between obese and lean peoples using 16S gene sequencing in a Japanese population. J Clin Bio chem Nutr. 2016;59:65–70.

71. Schwiertz A, Taras D, Schäfer K, Beijer S, Bos NA, Donus C, Hardt PD. Microbiota and SCFA in lean and overweight healthy subjects. Obesity. 2010;18:190–5.

72. Jain S, Gautam V, Naseem S. Acute-phase proteins: as diagnostic tool. J Pharm Bioallied Sci. 2011;3:118–27.

73. Kuszajewski ML, Clontz AS. Prealbumin is best for nutritional monitoring. Nursing. 2005;35:70–1.

74. Saka B, Ozturk GB, Uzun S, Erten N, Genc S, Karan MA, Tascioglu C, Kaysi A. Nutritional risk in hospitalized patients: impact of nutritional status on serum prealbumin. Rev Nutr. 2011;24:89–98.

75. Wang W, Wang C-S, Ren D, Li T, Yao H-C, Ma S-J. Low serum prealbumin levels on admission can independently predict in-hospital adverse cardiac events in patients with acute coronary syndrome. Medicine. 2018;97:e11740.

76. Lourenço P, Silva S, Friões F, Alvelos M, Amorim M, Couto M, Torres-Ramalho P, Guimarães JT, Araújo JP, Bettencourt P. Low prealbumin is strongly associated with adverse outcome in heart failure. Heart. 2014;100:1780–5.

77. Lee JL, Oh ES, Lee RW, Finucane TE. Serum albumin and prealbumin in calorically restricted, nondiseased individuals: a systematic review. Am J Med. 2015;128:1023.e1–22.

78. Andreas R, Kirkegaard-KlitboDitte M, Dohlmann TL, Jens L, Sabin CA, Phillips AN, Nordestgaard BG, Shoaib A. Plasma albumin and incident cardiovascular disease. Arterioscler Thromb Vasc Biol. 2020;40:473–82.

79. Kuzuya M, Izawa S, Enoki H, Okada K, Iguchi A. Is serum albumin a good marker for malnutrition in the physically impaired elderly? Clin Nutr. 2007;26:84–90.

80. Gragossian A, Bashir K, Friede R. Hypomagnesemia. In: StatPearls. Treasure Island: StatPearls Publishing; 2020.

81. Ismail Y, Ismail AA, Ismail AAA. The underestimated problem of using serum magnesium measurements to exclude magnesium deficiency in adults; a health warning is needed for "normal" results. Clin Chem Lab Med. 2010;48:323–7.

82. Dørup I, Skajaa K, Clausen T, Kjeldsen K. Reduced concentrations of potassium, magnesium, and sodium-potassium pumps in human skeletal muscle during treatment with diuretics. Br Med J. 1988;296:455–8.

83. Workinger JL, Doyle RP, Bortz J. Challenges in the diagnosis of magnesium status. Nutrients. 2018;10. https://doi.org/10.3390/nu10091202.

84. Hruby A, O'Donnell CJ, Jacques PF, Meigs JB, Hoffmann U, McKeown NM. Magnesium intake is inversely associated with coronary artery calcification: the Framingham Heart Study. JACC Cardiovasc Imaging. 2014;7:59–69.

85. Salaminia S, Sayehmiri F, Angha P, Sayehmiri K, Motedayen M. Evaluating the effect of magnesium supplementation and cardiac arrhythmias after acute coronary syndrome: a systematic review and meta-analysis. BMC Cardiovasc Disord. 2018;18:129.

86. Fang X, Wang K, Han D, He X, Wei J, Zhao L, Imam MU, Ping Z, Li Y, Xu Y, Min J, Wang F. Dietary mag-

nesium intake and the risk of cardiovascular disease, type 2 diabetes, and all-cause mortality: a dose–response meta-analysis of prospective cohort studies. BMC Med. 2016;14:1–13.

87. Koebnick C, Leitzmann R, García AL, Heins UA, Heuer T, Golf S, Katz N, Hoffmann I, Leitzmann C. Long-term effect of a plant-based diet on magnesium status during pregnancy. Eur J Clin Nutr. 2005;59:219–25.

88. Castiglione D, Platania A, Conti A, Falla M, D'Urso M, Marranzano M Dietary micronutrient and mineral intake in the Mediterranean healthy eating, ageing, and lifestyle (MEAL) study. Antioxidants (Basel). 2018;7. https://doi.org/10.3390/antiox7070079.

89. Basso LE, Ubbink JB, Delport R. Erythrocyte magnesium concentration as an index of magnesium status: a perspective from a magnesium supplementation study. Clin Chim Acta. 2000;291:1–8.

90. Joosten MM, Gansevoort RT, Mukamal KJ, van der Harst P, Geleijnse JM, Feskens EJM, Navis G, Bakker SJL, PREVEND Study Group. Urinary and plasma magnesium and risk of ischemic heart disease. Am J Clin Nutr. 2013;97:1299–306.

91. Djurhuus MS, Gram J, Petersen PH, Klitgaard NA, Bollerslev J, Beck-Nielsen H. Biological variation of serum and urinary magnesium in apparently healthy males. Scand J Clin Lab Invest. 1995;55:549–58.

92. Costello RB, Nielsen F. Interpreting magnesium status to enhance clinical care: key indicators. Curr Opin Clin Nutr Metab Care. 2017;20:504–11.

93. Pongudom S, Chinthammitr Y. Determination of normal HbA1C levels in non-diabetic patients with hemoglobin E. Ann Clin Lab Sci. 2019;49:804–9.

94. UpToDate. https://www.uptodate.com/contents/initial-management-of-hyperglycemia-in-adults-with-type-2-diabetes-mellitus. Accessed 10 Feb 2021.

95. Kahleova H, Fleeman R, Hlozkova A, Holubkov R, Barnard ND. A plant-based diet in overweight individuals in a 16-week randomized clinical trial: metabolic benefits of plant protein. Nutr Diabetes. 2018;8:58.

96. Yokoyama Y, Barnard ND, Levin SM, Watanabe M. Vegetarian diets and glycemic control in diabetes: a systematic review and meta-analysis. Cardiovasc Diagn Ther. 2014;4:373–82.

97. Gannon MC, Nuttall FQ. Effect of a high-protein, low-carbohydrate diet on blood glucose control in people with type 2 diabetes. Diabetes. 2004;53:2375–82.

98. Carter S, Clifton PM, Keogh JB. Effect of intermittent compared with continuous energy restricted diet on glycemic control in patients with type 2 diabetes: a randomized noninferiority trial. JAMA Netw Open. 2018;1:e180756.

99. Kelly L. "Indoor generation": a quarter of Americans spend all day inside, survey finds. In: The Washington Times. 2018. https://www.washingtontimes.com/news/2018/may/15/quarter-americans-spend-all-day-inside/. Accessed 29 Feb 2020.

100. Davey GK, Spencer EA, Appleby PN, Allen NE, Knox KH, Key TJ. EPIC-Oxford: lifestyle characteristics and nutrient intakes in a cohort of 33 883 meat-eaters and 31 546 non meat-eaters in the UK. Public Health Nutr. 2003;6:259–69.

101. Barger-Lux MJ, Heaney RP, Dowell S, Chen TC, Holick MF. Vitamin D and its major metabolites: serum levels after graded oral dosing in healthy men. Osteoporos Int. 1998;8:222–30.

102. Manson JE, Cook NR, Lee I-M, Christen W, Bassuk SS, Mora S, Gibson H, Gordon D, Copeland T, D'Agostino D, Friedenberg G, Ridge C, Bubes V, Giovannucci EL, Willett WC, Buring JE, VITAL Research Group. Vitamin D supplements and prevention of cancer and cardiovascular disease. N Engl J Med. 2019;380:33–44.

103. Beer TM, Ryan CW, Venner PM, Petrylak DP, Chatta GS, Ruether JD, Redfern CH, Fehrenbacher L, Saleh MN, Waterhouse DM, Carducci MA, Vicario D, Dreicer R, Higano CS, Ahmann FR, Chi KN, Henner WD, Arroyo A, Clow FW, ASCENT Investigators. Double-blinded randomized study of high-dose calcitriol plus docetaxel compared with placebo plus docetaxel in androgen-independent prostate cancer: a report from the ASCENT Investigators. J Clin Oncol. 2007;25:669–74.

104. Mousa A, Naderpoor N, Teede H, Scragg R, de Courten B. Vitamin D supplementation for improvement of chronic low-grade inflammation in patients with type 2 diabetes: a systematic review and meta-analysis of randomized controlled trials. Nutr Rev. 2018;76:380–94.

105. Giovannucci E, Liu Y, Hollis BW, Rimm EB. 25-hydroxyvitamin D and risk of myocardial infarction in men: a prospective study. Arch Intern Med. 2008;168:1174–80.

106. Michos ED, Cainzos-Achirica M, Heravi AS, Appel LJ. Vitamin D, calcium supplements, and implications for cardiovascular health: JACC focus seminar. J Am Coll Cardiol. 2021;77:437–49.

107. Ganguly P, Alam SF. Role of homocysteine in the development of cardiovascular disease. Nutr J. 2015;14:6.

108. Karger AB, Steffen BT, Nomura SO, Guan W, Garg PK, Szklo M, Budoff MJ, Tsai MY. Association between homocysteine and vascular calcification incidence, prevalence, and progression in the MESA cohort. J Am Heart Assoc. 2020;9:e013934.

109. Rauma AL, Törrönen R, Hänninen O, Mykkänen H. Vitamin B-12 status of long-term adherents of a strict uncooked vegan diet ("living food diet") is compromised. J Nutr. 1995;125:2511–5.

110. Kwok T, Chook P, Qiao M, Tam L, Poon YKP, Ahuja AT, Woo J, Celermajer DS, Woo KS. Vitamin B-12 supplementation improves arterial function in vegetarians with subnormal vitamin B-12 status. J Nutr Health Aging. 2012;16:569–73.

111. Gilsing AMJ, Crowe FL, Lloyd-Wright Z, Sanders TAB, Appleby PN, Allen NE, Key TJ. Serum concentrations of vitamin B12 and folate in British male

omnivores, vegetarians and vegans: results from a cross-sectional analysis of the EPIC-Oxford cohort study. Eur J Clin Nutr. 2010;64:933–9.

112. Schüpbach R, Wegmüller R, Berguerand C, Bui M, Herter-Aeberli I. Micronutrient status and intake in omnivores, vegetarians and vegans in Switzerland. Eur J Nutr. 2017;56:283–93.

113. Serra-Majem L, Ribas L, García A, Pérez-Rodrigo C, Aranceta J. Nutrient adequacy and Mediterranean diet in Spanish school children and adolescents. Eur J Clin Nutr. 2003;57 Suppl 1:S35–9.

114. Serra-Majem L, Ribas L, Ngo J, Aranceta J, Garaulet M, Carazo E, Mataix J, Pérez-Rodrigo C, Quemada M, Tojo R, Vázquez C. Risk of inadequate intakes of vitamins A, B1, B6, C, E, folate, iron and calcium in the Spanish population aged 4 to 18. Int J Vitam Nutr Res. 2001;71:325–31.

115. van den Boom A, Serra-Majem L, Ribas L, Ngo J, Pérez-Rodrigo C, Aranceta J, Fletcher R. The contribution of ready-to-eat cereals to daily nutrient intake and breakfast quality in a Mediterranean setting. J Am Coll Nutr. 2006;25:135–43.

116. Planells E, Sánchez C, Montellano MA, Mataix J, Llopis J. Vitamins B6 and B12 and folate status in an adult Mediterranean population. Eur J Clin Nutr. 2003;57:777–85.

117. Balcı YI, Ergin A, Karabulut A, Polat A, Doğan M, Küçüktaşcı K. Serum vitamin B12 and folate concentrations and the effect of the Mediterranean diet on vulnerable populations. Pediatr Hematol Oncol. 2014;31:62–7.

The Mediterranean Dietary Pattern

3

Jessica K. Bjorklund, Carol F. Kirkpatrick, and Eugenia Gianos

Section 1: Background

The Mediterranean diet (MedDiet) is among the most extensively studied dietary patterns with evidence that high adherence improves atherosclerotic cardiovascular disease (ASCVD) risk factors, reduces cardiovascular (CV) events, and positively impacts a number of other chronic diseases [48]. The origins of the MedDiet can be traced back to ancient Greece where food groups central to the dietary pattern were preferentially consumed as part of a lifestyle that included physical activity, communal gatherings, and sharing of meals, all of which were deemed a core part of the culture. Hippocrates was one of the great supporters of

J. K. Bjorklund
North Shore University Hospital, Manhasset, NY, USA

Zucker School of Medicine, Hempstead, NY, USA
e-mail: JBjorklund@northwell.edu

C. F. Kirkpatrick
Idaho State University Wellness Center, Pocatello, ID, USA
e-mail: carolkirkpatrick@isu.edu

E. Gianos (✉)
Zucker School of Medicine, Hempstead, NY, USA

Cardiovascular Prevention, Northwell Health, New Hyde Park, NY, USA

Western Region, Katz Institute Women's Heart Program, Manhasset, NY, USA

Women's Heart Program, Lenox Hill Hospital, New York, NY, USA
e-mail: EGianos@northwell.edu

the MedDiet for maintenance of health and treatment of disease, and although unconfirmed, he is credited with preaching, "Let food be thy medicine and medicine be thy food." Over the years, the MedDiet has been the primary dietary pattern in various Mediterranean countries, which has evidence to support that it resulted in a decreased risk of disease and mortality. However, the influence of the Western diet has led to the reversal of a number of health benefits in the populations of the Mediterranean region [35].

In order to analyze the impact of the MedDiet, this discussion will consider its overall effect on CV outcomes, dissect how much of those benefits are secondary to improvements in CV risk factors, and explore the direct effects of the dietary pattern on biomarkers and other physiologic effects.

Components of a Mediterranean Diet

The MedDiet is a plant-based, carbohydrate-rich, moderate-fat diet typically consumed by people (or populations) living in olive-growing areas of the Mediterranean region. The typical MedDiet includes an abundance of plant foods, including fruits, vegetables, grains, legumes, nuts, seeds, cereals, whole grains, and potatoes with olive oil being the primary source of fat. Dairy products (primarily cheese and yogurt), fish, poultry, eggs, and wine are typically consumed in low to

© Springer Nature Switzerland AG 2021
M. J. Wilkinson et al. (eds.), *Prevention and Treatment of Cardiovascular Disease*, Contemporary Cardiology, https://doi.org/10.1007/978-3-030-78177-4_3

moderate amounts. Other key principles of the MedDiet are that it is low in processed foods and saturated fat, rich in unsaturated fats (primarily monounsaturated fat from olive oil), and includes only small amounts of red and processed meat [62] (Fig. 3.1).

The Mediterranean Diet Score

Epidemiologic studies have assessed adherence to a MedDiet by determining a Mediterranean

Diet Score (MDS) of study participants. The scoring tool has been used as a dietary exposure variable in epidemiological studies or for directing dietary counseling specific to an individual in clinical care. The MDS was first proposed by Trichopoulou et al. in 1995 and consists of a minimum of eight main food categories: the ratio of monounsaturated fat (from olive oil) to saturated fats, whole grains, vegetables, fruit and nuts, legumes, alcohol, red and processed meat, and milk/dairy products [60]. Multiple validated MDSs exist, varying from 9–14 food category

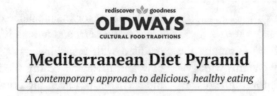

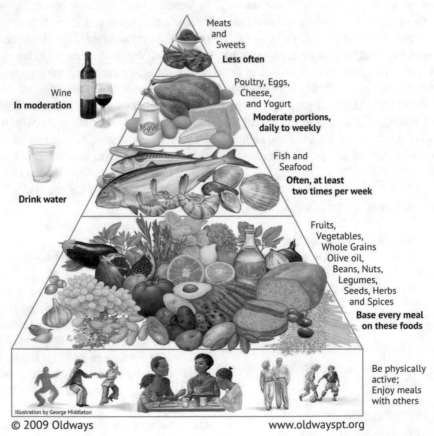

Fig. 3.1 Mediterranean diet pyramid. This is the Oldways Mediterranean Diet Pyramid available at https://oldwayspt.org/traditional-diets/mediterranean-diet

components, and different scoring systems have been used in trials and modified for clinical use [6]. The availability of various MDSs is useful considering time limitations to complete longer assessment tools in some cases; however, this also leads to a lack of consistency in the dietary assessment done in different populations.

Section 2: Evidence for Atherosclerotic Cardiovascular Disease Reduction and Outcomes

The evidence for ASCVD reduction associated with higher adherence to a MedDiet is robust, largely because it transcends human epidemiologic/clinical trials and basic science studies in animals with similar benefits consistently found on a molecular and population level [21]. One of the earliest studies to identify the relationship between the MedDiet and CV health is the Seven Countries Study by Ancel Keys and colleagues in the 1950s. It includes over 50 years of data evaluating cohorts in Finland, Greece, Italy, Japan, Netherlands, the USA, former Yugoslavia, and other countries. This epidemiologic study hypothesized that there was an association between dietary habits, lifestyle, and CV health, and noted that populations in regions bordering the Mediterranean Sea experienced lower morbidity and mortality rates from ASCVD compared to Northern European countries and the USA [31]. Adult life expectancy for populations in the Mediterranean regions was one of the highest in the world with low rates of coronary heart disease (CHD). These findings were attributed to the consumption of what is now known as the MedDiet and propelled future research into this dietary pattern. Although the Seven Countries Study has been criticized for excluding outliers that had both differing dietary patterns and low rates of ASCVD [44], the key findings of the study have consistently been confirmed in more recent epidemiologic studies and randomized controlled trials (RCTs).

Since the Seven Countries Study, epidemiological studies applying the MDS to very large populations have found significant improvements for a variety of health outcomes, including ASCVD, mortality, development of cognitive disorders, and even alterations in genetic makeup. For example, in a United Kingdom cohort (n = 23,902), greater adherence to the MedDiet was associated with a decreased incidence in ASCVD (HR 0.95; 95% CI: 0.92–0.97), ASCVD mortality (HR 0.91; 95% CI: 0.87–0.96), and all-cause mortality (HR 0.95; 95% CI: 0.93–0.98) [58]. In a meta-analysis of nine cohort studies (n = 34,168), the highest MDS was inversely associated with the development of cognitive disorders (RR 0.79; 95% CI: 0.70–0.90) [63]. Furthermore, in a subset of participants in the Nurses' Health Study, longer telomeres were associated with greater adherence to the MedDiet, suggesting that the MedDiet promotes health and longevity [5]. Importantly, the results of epidemiological studies showing health benefits associated with the MedDiet have been supported by RCTs.

Although large RCTs are rare in the field of nutrition science, there have been several examining the health effects of the MedDiet, two of which will be discussed here. The Lyon Diet Heart study was conducted in 605 post-myocardial infarction patients randomized to either a "Mediterranean-style diet " or control (American Heart Association Step 1 Diet) with a 27-month average follow-up for major adverse CV events (MACE) [9]. Participants in the intervention group were advised to eat a diet largely composed of bread, vegetables, fruit, and fish. Participants were instructed to limit meat intake and replace it with poultry, and butter and cream were replaced with canola margarine high in alpha-linolenic acid. Although the study had limitations with respect to quality of data, the results are among the most impressive for the secondary prevention of ASCVD, with a 73% relative risk reduction noted in CV mortality and 70% reduction in overall mortality. Remarkably, these results were consistent at the 5-year follow-up for multiple combinations of MACE. Interestingly, a significant difference was not noted in CV risk factors (i.e., blood pressure (BP), weight, lipid profile) in the MedDiet group compared to the control group suggesting other beneficial effects of the MedDiet.

One of the landmark CV primary prevention trials in nutrition science is the Prevención con DietaMediterránea (PREDIMED) trial, which was conducted in patients with high CV risk, but without established ASCVD. It was a multicenter nutritional intervention study conducted in Spain from 2003–2011, with 7,447 participants randomized to either a MedDiet supplemented with mixed nuts (30 g/d; 15 g walnuts; 7.5 g almonds; 7.5 g hazelnuts), a MedDiet supplemented with extra-virgin olive oil (EVOO; 50 g/d), or a control diet (advice to reduce dietary fat intake) [17]. Total calorie restriction was not advised and physical activity was not promoted as part of the study recommendations. The median follow-up of the trial was 4.8 years with a reduction in MACE found when the two MedDiet arms were compared to the control group. Of note, the reduction in CV events was driven predominantly by a reduced rate of stroke (HR 0.65, 95% CI: 0.44–0.95) with no difference noted in myocardial infarction, CV mortality, or all-cause mortality [17]. The significant reduction in stroke is impressive considering that very few medical or nutritional therapies have been found to have similar outcomes in the primary prevention setting.

The benefits of the MedDiet interventions of the PREDIMED trial have been attributed to the supplementation of either nuts or EVOO. In a prospective analysis of 16,217 participants with type 2 diabetes (T2D), higher nut consumption (consumption of 5 or more servings of total nuts per week [1 serving = 28 g] vs consumption of <1 serving/month), especially tree nuts (almond, walnuts, and hazelnuts), was associated with lower total ASCVD incidence (HR 0.83; 95% CI: 0.71–0.98; P trend = 0.01), CHD incidence (HR 0.80; 95% CI: 0.67–0.96; P trend = 0.005), CVD mortality (HR 0.66; 95% CI: 0.52–0.84; P trend <0.001) and all-cause mortality (HR 0.69; 95% CI: 0.61–0.77; P trend <0.001) [37]. The exact mechanism of benefit remains unknown, but it is thought to be related to the unique nutritional profile of nuts, with components such as unsaturated fatty acids, fiber, vitamins, minerals, and phytochemicals [37]. EVOO is the primary source of fat in the MedDiet. In a prospective cohort of 92,978 US adults, higher olive oil consumption (>0.5

tablespoon/day vs nonconsumers) was associated with 14% lower risk of ASCVD (pooled HR 0.86; 95% CI: 0.79–0.94) and 18% lower risk of CHD (pooled HR 0.82; 95% CI: 0.73–0.91) [26]. The replacement of margarine, butter, mayonnaise, or dairy fat with the equivalent amount of olive oil was also associated with lower risk of ASCVD and CHD [26], but it is important to keep in mind that olive oil was compared to other forms of fat as opposed to nothing at all. The study found no significant associations when olive oil was compared to other plant oils, suggesting that plant-based oils may be a healthier alternative to animal fats [26]. The benefits of olive oil may be derived from the rich polyphenol profile and the antioxidant impact on inflammatory biomarkers and lipids [26].

While the PREDIMED trial found supplementation with either nuts or EVOO to be beneficial, it is difficult to ascertain if the benefit was solely due to the nuts or EVOO after careful examination of the supplemental tables, which show a difference in the amount of vegetables, fruits, legumes, fish, and sofrito sauce consumed by participants in the MedDiet interventions compared to the control group [17]. There are data to suggest that these individual food components may convey health benefits. Additional analysis of the PREDIMED data found that, when examining participants by quintiles of plant-based foods, participants in the highest quintile had the lowest mortality rates suggesting that the health benefits of the MedDiet are associated with the food components similar to other healthy dietary patterns, such as vegan/vegetarian and the Dietary Approaches to Stop Hypertension (DASH) dietary patterns. It is important to note that the PREDIMED investigators faced criticism when it was realized that participants enrolled within a given household were randomized to the same group without accounting for this change in protocol in the analysis of data. Critics argued that this may have not only altered the results of the trial but also puts into question the quality of the remaining data of the trial. Although this was an error on the part of the investigators, an analysis excluding those participants held true to the results of the original analysis and the study remains the strongest level of evidence for a RCT with a dietary intervention to date [17]. In addition to the Lyon Heart Study and the PREDIMED, other RCTs have found that the MedDiet decreases the risk of ASCVD and CVD mortality (Fig. 3.2).

Section 3: Impact on Atherosclerotic Cardiovascular Disease Risk Factors

There is a large body of evidence that has examined the impact of the MedDiet on individual ASCVD risk factors, such as dyslipidemia, T2D, and hypertension, and collectively as part of metabolic syndrome (MetS). Most studies are prospective cohorts with few RCTs. The evidence is conflicting at times, but overall shows a trend toward a positive impact on ASCVD risk factors. The discussion in this section will review key studies, including meta-analyses, which provide the highest level of evidence available, and offer insight into the MedDiet's impact on ASCVD risk factors (Table 3.1).

Table 3.1 Impact of the foods that are part of the Mediterranean diet on ASCVD risk factors

Foods	CVD risk factor effects
Fruits and vegetables	↓ LDL-C, ↓ BP, ↑ glycemic control ↓ oxidative stress
Whole grains vs. refined CHO	↓ LDL-C, ↓ BP, ↑ glycemic control
Vegetable oils vs. solid fat	↓ LDL-C
Dairy products (skim/low-fat vs. full-fat)	↓ BP (↓ LDL-C)
Lean meat, poultry (vs. high-fat)	↓ BP (↓ LDL-C)
Seafood	↓ TG, ↓ BP, ↓ arrhythmia, ↓ inflammation
Legumes, soy	↓ LDL-C, ↓ BP
Nuts, seeds	↓ LDL-C, ↑ HDL-C, ↓ BP, ↓ oxidative stress

From: Flock et al. [20]
BP blood pressure, *CHO* carbohydrate, *CVD* cardiovascular disease, *HDL-C* high-density lipoprotein cholesterol, *LDL-C* low-density lipoprotein cholesterol, *TG* triglycerides

CVD outcomes	No. of studies	Pooled RR [95% CI]	RR and 95%CI	Residual I^2 [%]
Total CVD^x				
Sofi et al 2008 (12)	4	0.91 [0.87, 0.95]		32.6
Sofi et al 2010 (13)	8	0.90 [0.87, 0.93]		35
Sofi et al 2013 (14)	20	0.90 [0.87, 0.92]		38
Martínez-González et al 2014 (15)	16	0.90 [0.86, 0.94]		77.5
Grosso et al 2017 (16)	30	0.71 [0.65, 0.78]		78
Rosato et al 2017 (17)	11	0.81 [0.74, 0.88]		79.9
CVD incidence§				
Grosso et al 2017 (16)	14	0.73 [0.66, 0.80]		36
CVD mortality*				
Grosso et al 2017 (16)	16	0.75 [0.68, 0.83]		75
Coronary heart disease				
Grosso et al 2017 (16)	4	0.72 [0.60, 0.86]		NA
Rosato et al 2017† (17)	11	0.70 [0.62, 0.80]		44.5
Stroke				
Psaltopoulou et al 2013‡ (23)	12	0.71 [0.57, 0.89]		69.1
Grosso et al 2017 (16)	5	0.76 [0.60, 0.96]		52
Rosato et al 2017† (17)	6	0.73 [0.59, 0.91]		46.1
Myocardial infarction				
Grosso et al 2017 (16)	3	0.67 [0.54, 0.83]		NA
Heart failure				
Papadaki et al 2017 (24)	3	0.92 [0.90, 0.95]		0

0.5   0.75   1   1.25
Benefit   Harm

Fig. 3.2 Impact of the Mediterranean diet on CV events. (From: Salas-Salvadó et al. [48])

Effect on Glucose/Insulin Resistance and Risk of T2D

Adhering to the MedDiet lowers the risk of new-onset T2D. Two meta-analyses have shown a 19–23% reduction in the risk of developing T2D in populations with higher adherence to the MedDiet. Schwingshackl et al. conducted a meta-analysis of 1 RCT and 8 prospective cohort studies and Koloverou et al. conducted a meta-analysis of 1 RCT, 9 prospective, and 7 cross-sectional studies, both of which found higher adherence to a MedDiet was associated with a significant reduction in the risk of developing T2D (RR = 0.81; 95% CI: 0.73, 0.90, P < 0.0001, I^2 = 55%; and RR = 0.77; 95% CI: 0.66, 0.89, respectively) [33, 51].

The MedDiet has been shown to improve glycemic control and decrease hemoglobin A1c (HbA1c) in patients with T2D. Two meta-analyses found that individuals with T2D who followed a MedDiet achieved a reduction of HbA1c by 0.30–0.47% compared to individuals with T2D following a control diet (e.g., low-fat, high-carbohydrate, or usual care), and the MedDiet is more effective in improving glycemic control compared to other dietary patterns [15, 27]. A network meta-analysis found that, compared to eight other dietary approaches (low-fat, vegan/vegetarian, high-protein, moderate-carbohydrate, low-carbohydrate, low glycemic index/glycemic load [GI/GL], Paleolithic, and a control diet), the MedDiet was the most effective dietary approach in improving glycemic control in patients with T2D [52]. A narrative review found that, compared to other dietary patterns, the MedDiet has the most evidence for glycemic control and decreased ASCVD risk in patients with T2D [36] and is recommended by several guidelines as an eating plan for the management of T2D [2, 18, 32, 36].

Effect on Lipids

RCTs show a beneficial effect of the MedDiet on lipid profiles, with an increase in high-density lipoprotein cholesterol (HDL-C) and lowering of triglycerides (TGs); however, there is a high degree of inconsistency across studies and the results must be interpreted with caution [48]. For example, in a meta-analysis by Kastorini et al., participants assigned to the MedDiet saw an improvement in HDL-C (1.17 mg/dL; 95% CI: 0.38, 1.96) and TGs (−6.14 mg/dL; 95% CI: −10.35, −1.93), whereas in the meta-analysis by Garcia et al., participants assigned to the MedDiet had improved TGs (−40.7 mg/dL; 95% CI: −0.72, −0.21), but no significant change in HDL-C [24, 28].

A network meta-analysis of 52 RCTs, with an intervention period of ≥12 weeks, compared the effect of the MedDiet and eight other dietary patterns (low-fat, vegan/vegetarian, high-protein, moderate-carbohydrate, low-carbohydrate, low GI/GL, Paleolithic diet, and a control diet) on blood lipids in patients with T2D [41]. The results showed that the moderate-carbohydrate and vegan/vegetarian dietary patterns were most effective at reducing low-density lipoprotein cholesterol (LDL-C) compared to the control diet. The MedDiet was the only dietary pattern that increased HDL-C.

The MedDiet, along with the low-carbohydrate dietary pattern, significantly reduced TG compared with the low-fat and control dietary patterns [36, 41]. Overall, the authors of this network meta-analysis concluded that the MedDiet was the most effective dietary pattern to manage the dyslipidemia associated with diabetes (i.e., increased TG, decreased HDL-C), but cautioned that the findings are limited by low credibility of evidence.

The network meta-analysis discussed above found that the MedDiet was ranked fourth for lowering LDL-C with vegan/vegetarian, low GI/GL, and moderate-carbohydrate dietary patterns ranked higher. Other studies have found a modest LDL-C lowering effect of the MedDiet [12, 46], although, similar to the network meta-analysis results discussed above, some researchers have found vegan/vegetarian dietary patterns are more effective at lowering LDL-C compared to the MedDiet [54].

Effect on Blood Pressure

A limited number of studies have evaluated the influence of the MedDiet specifically on BP; however, patients are more commonly counseled to follow the MedDiet as part of overall primary or secondary prevention strategy that would potentially impact various risk factors [10]. In the PREDIMED study, more than 80% of the 7,447 participants had hypertension. Yet, after 4 years of follow-up, the researchers found that participants assigned to the MedDiet supplemented with either EVOO or mixed nuts had no significant change in systolic BP (SBP) compared to the control group. Both MedDiet groups had a reduction in diastolic BP (DBP), −1.53 mmHg in the EVOO group (95% CI: −2.01, −1.04) and −0.65 mmHg (95% CI: −1.15, −0.15) in the mixed nuts group, compared to the control group [57].

A meta-analysis by Nissensohn et al. identified 6 studies and included more than 7,000 participants who followed either a MedDiet or low-fat dietary pattern and found a positive and significant association between the MedDiet and reduction in BP. However, the authors interpreted the results with caution, finding insufficient evidence to suggest that the MedDiet reduces BP more than the low-fat dietary pattern due to the limited number of studies and their heterogeneity [42]. Furthermore, a systematic review found low- to moderate-quality evidence for beneficial changes in SBP and DBP with the MedDiet for primary prevention [46]. The MedDiet likely has a favorable effect on reducing BP, but the mechanism of benefit is unclear and more studies are needed.

Effect on Weight Loss/Obesity

The MedDiet may be an effective dietary pattern for weight loss in some patient populations. In a meta-analysis of 16 RCTs that included 3,436 participants, Esposito et al. found that, compared to a control diet (e.g., low-fat, high-carbohydrate, or usual care), groups assigned to the MedDiet had a significantly reduced body weight

(−1.75 kg; 95% CI: 0.64, 2.86) and reduced body mass index (0.57 kg/m^2; 95% CI: 0.21, 0.93). Furthermore, larger reductions in body weight were seen when the MedDiet intervention groups were energy restricted (weighted mean difference [WMD]—3.88 kg; 95% CI: −6.54, −1.21), included counseling to increase physical activity (WMD −4.01 kg; 95% CI: −5.79, −2.23), or had follow-up longer than 6 months (WMD −2.69 kg; 95% CI: −3.99, −1.38) [14].

Metabolic Syndrome

MetS is characterized as a group of interrelated risk factors that are metabolic in origin and increase the risk of developing T2D and ASCVD. A patient is diagnosed with MetS if they have at least three of the following five risk factors: increased waist circumference, elevated TGs (≥150 mg/dL or drug treatment for elevated TGs), reduced HDL-C (<40 mg/dL in men and <50 mg/dL in women), elevated BP (≥130 mmHg systolic and/or ≥85 mmHg diastolic or antihypertensive drug treatment), and elevated fasting glucose (FG; ≥100 mg/dL or drug treatment for elevated FG) [1]. In addition to the benefit of the MedDiet on the separate risk factors of MetS discussed previously, numerous studies have shown that the MedDiet is an effective tool for the primary and secondary prevention of MetS [24, 25, 28].

Prevention of MetS with MedDiet

Studies support the use of the MedDiet, along with other lifestyle modifications, for the prevention of MetS. Kesse-Guyot et al. evaluated the association of adherence to the MedDiet with the risk of MetS in a 6-year prospective study that included 3,232 participants and found that higher adherence to the MedDiet was associated with a lower incidence of MetS [30]. A meta-analysis of prospective studies and clinical trials (35 clinical trials, 2 prospective studies, and 13 cross-sectional studies) with a total of 534,906 participants found that adherence to the MedDiet was associated with a reduced risk of MetS (log hazard ratio: −0.69; 95% CI: −1.24, −1.16) [28]. Results from clinical trials in the meta-analysis also revealed the protective role of the MedDiet on components of MetS, such as waist circumference (−0.42 cm; 95% CI: −0.82, −0.02), HDL-C (1.17 mg/dL; 95% CI: 0.38, 1.96), TG (−6.14 mg/dL; 95% CI: −10.35, −1.93), SBP (−2.35 mm Hg; 95% CI: −3.51, −1.18), and DBP (−1.58 mm Hg; 95% CI: −2.02, −1.13), and FG (−3.89 mg/dL; 95% CI: −5.84, −1.95) [28]. Recently, the results of a systematic review was conducted to examine evidence for impact of the MedDiet on *cardiodiabesity*, a new term that describes the interrelationship of obesity, MetS, ASCVD, and T2D [22]. The results of the systematic review indicated that a higher adherence to the MedDiet was inversely related to the incidence of MetS in healthy individuals, although some studies found no association [22].

Treatment of MetS with MedDiet

The MedDiet may be used as a treatment modality for MetS. In a RCT by Esposito et al., 180 patients with MetS were randomized to either a MedDiet (n = 90) or a low-fat control diet (n = 90) (50–60% total daily energy [TDE] carbohydrate; 15–20% TDE protein; <30% TDE fat). At the end of 2 years, only 48% of the participants in the MedDiet group continued to have features of MetS compared to 95% in the control group (*P* < 0.001), suggesting that the MedDiet is a reasonable option to treat MetS. Additionally, individuals in the MedDiet group experienced a significant reduction in body weight, insulin resistance, and inflammatory markers (high sensitivity C-reactive protein [CRP], and interleukin 6 [IL-6], IL-7, and IL-18) compared to the control group [13].

A meta-analysis of 29 intervention trials with 4,133 participants found that the MedDiet had significant beneficial effects on five or six metabolic risk factors: waist circumference (−0.54 cm; 95% CI: −0.77, −0.31), TG (−40.7 mg/dL; 95% CI: −0.72, −0.21), FG (−9 mg/dL; 95% CI:

−0.81, −0.20), SBP (−0.72 mmHg; 95% CI: −1.03, −0.42), and DBP (−0.94 mmHg; 95% CI: −1.45, −0.44). No significant effects on HDL-C were found. It is worth noting that the significant beneficial effects were found in studies conducted in Europe (where the MedDiet may be followed more closely) and perhaps not applicable in other populations. Additionally, the beneficial effects were noted in studies of longer duration, which may be needed to appreciate the benefits of the various nutrients and non-nutrients in the MedDiet and reduction in disease. Lastly, the beneficial effects were also noted in studies that used behavioral change techniques that may make dietary change more durable and are often predictors of improved outcomes in most dietary trials [24].

Although there is inconsistency in the results of studies evaluating the impact of the MedDiet on individual CV risk factors, such as HDL-C, LDL-C, and BP [11] and the effects are likely modest at best, there is evidence to suggest that higher adherence to the MedDiet results in a mortality benefit and decreased incidence of CHD. Although a number of CV risk factors are surrogates for CHD, improved health outcomes associated with the MedDiet are now also believed to be due to independent mechanisms, such as beneficial effects on inflammation, oxidative stress, and endothelial dysfunction, which are some of the key first steps in the pathogenesis of atherosclerosis [48, 59]. The effects of the MedDiet on various biomarkers and processes related to ASCVD are discussed below.

Section 4: Impact on Biomarkers

The exact mechanisms by which the MedDiet exerts its beneficial effects in lowering mortality and the incidence of ASCVD are unknown [59]. Because the improvements of ASCVD risk factors achieved with following the MedDiet are modest, especially given the impact on health outcomes (i.e., decreased CV mortality), other metabolic and molecular effects, including effects on endothelial function, inflammation, oxidative stress, trimethylamine N-oxide (TMAO) production, and genomic stability, may be playing a role . The mechanisms are likely multifactorial and interrelated with benefit derived from a variety of nutrients and non-nutrients.

Inflammation, Oxidative Stress, and Endothelial Dysfunction

Chronic low-grade inflammation is key in the pathogenesis of atherosclerosis, the main cause of ASCVD. The deleterious impact of inflammation is present from the initial to the final phases of atheromatous plaque development, rupture, and thrombus formation. Inflammation is involved in macrophage and T-lymphocyte infiltration, lipid deposition, and vascular wall thickening in response to the release of chemokines and cytokines [50]. Increased expression and activation of CRP, tumor necrosis factor (TNF)-α, and pro-inflammatory cytokines, such as IL-6, at the level of endothelial cells have all be identified in the pathways that lead to the development of atherosclerosis and are independent predictors of ASCVD and T2D [3].

Dietary intake has the ability to modify inflammatory and oxidative stress pathways in the endothelium and, therefore, can impact the prevention, pathogenesis, and even regression of atherosclerosis [43, 49]. The food components of the MedDiet appear to favorably impact these pathways and potentially provide protection. Meanwhile, dietary patterns that are high in sugars, refined starches and grains, red meat, saturated and trans fats, and low in fiber and antioxidants from fruits and vegetables, as well as omega-3 fatty acids from fish/seafood, are thought to activate the innate immune system, which leads to the production of pro-inflammatory cytokines [3]. Continuous production of inflammatory cytokines leads to a chronic low-grade inflammatory state. It has been demonstrated that the MedDiet may play a beneficial role in improving the main risk factors for the development of ASCVD, which may be explained by its anti-inflammatory effects.

Impact on Inflammation

Higher adherence to the MedDiet has been shown to effectively reduce CRP, IL-6, and TNF-α. For example, in the RCT by Esposito et al. discussed previously, patients with MetS randomized to the MedDiet were found to have significantly reduced high sensitivity CRP, IL-6, IL-7, and IL-18 at the end of 2 years, in addition to a 52% decrease in the features of MetS whereas the control group had 5% decrease [13]. The relationship between MedDiet and reduction in inflammatory markers has been demonstrated by other studies, as well. The Nurses' Health Study, the ATTICA Study, and sub-studies from the PREDIMED trial showed an independent association between greater adherence to a MedDiet and reduction in CRP, IL-6, TNF-alpha, intercellular adhesion molecule 1 (ICAM-1), vascular cell adhesion molecule 1, E-selection, fibrinogen, white blood cells, and homocysteine levels [4, 16, 23]. Furthermore, a meta-analysis including 17 RCTs by Schwingshackl et al. also demonstrated that higher adherence to the MedDiet was associated with a greater reduction in IL-6 and CRP compared to the control diet [50]. These studies demonstrate that the MedDiet decreases inflammation and adherence to the MedDiet may be used as part of a lifestyle strategy to reduce the risk of mortality and ASCVD.

Protection Against Oxidative Stress

Oxidative stress induced by the production of excess reactive oxygen species (ROS) plays a key role in all stages of the development of atherosclerosis. Essential for vascular homeostasis, ROS can lead to a host of problems, such as oxidative modification of lipoproteins, endothelial dysfunction and activation, leukocyte migration and differentiation, and DNA damage, when an imbalance in oxidant-to-anti-oxidant ratios occurs [29]. Oxidized LDL in the plasma is a prognostic marker for subclinical atherosclerosis and can predict acute CHD in healthy patients and patients with known CHD [40]. A dietary pattern that is low in antioxidants may increase the risk of vascular injury and subsequent development of atherosclerotic plaques. Foods abundant in the MedDiet, such as fruits, vegetable, legumes, whole grains, nuts, EVOO, and red wine, are rich in antioxidant vitamins (vitamins E and C, β-carotene), folate, minerals (selenium), and polyphenols, and adherence to this dietary pattern is associated with improvement in inflammatory and oxidant biomarkers [45, 48, 59]. For example, in vitro studies have demonstrated that polyphenols, compounds found is plant-based foods and considered to be antioxidants, scavenge and neutralize ROS, protecting against oxidation of LDL, platelet aggregation, and vascular inflammation [48].

The specific foods or nutrients that provide anti-inflammatory and antioxidant properties from the MedDiet are not known, but there is likely a synergistic effect of multiple nutrients from a wide variety of diverse foods [59]. Avoiding pro-inflammatory foods and nutrients, such as refined sugars and starches, trans-fatty acids, and following a MedDiet that is rich in anti-inflammatory nutrients and compounds, such as vitamins, minerals, antioxidants, fiber, and polyphenols, improves inflammation and reduces the inflammatory state. The current evidence suggests that the foods consumed by people adherent to the MedDiet not only reduce ASCVD risk factors but also are associated with improved endothelial function, decreased inflammatory biomarkers, and decreased oxidative stress. The MedDiet can be a dietary therapy prescribed to individuals for the primary prevention of inflammatory diseases and those at risk of and with low-grade chronic inflammatory diseases [3].

Protection Against Endothelial Dysfunction

Endothelial dysfunction is a key step in the pathogenesis of atherosclerosis and is an independent risk factor for the development of ASCVD [50, 59]. A RCT by Esposito et al. found that a MedDiet improved endothelial function in patients with MetS. As discussed

previously, 180 patients with MetS were randomized to either a MedDiet or a low-fat control diet. Endothelial function was assessed with the L-arginine test, because L-arginine is the natural precursor of nitric oxide. BP and platelet aggregation response to adenosine diphosphate were measured before and after L-arginine injection. At the end of 2 years, the participants in the MedDiet group had significantly improved endothelial function compared to the control group [13]. The ability of a MedDiet to impact endothelial function was also demonstrated in a meta-analysis by Schwingshackl et al. Participants that adhered to a MedDiet showed significant improvement in endothelial function, as measured by flow mediated dilatation and ICAM-1; however, the authors noted that the results should be interpreted conservatively given only two trials reported outcomes on these parameters [50]. The meta-analysis by Shannon et al. also found a beneficial effect of the MedDiet on endothelial function by measurement of flow-mediated dilatation in those adherent to a MedDiet [standardized mean difference (SMD): 0.35; 95% CI: 0.17, 0.53; $P < 0.001$; I2 = 73.68%] [53].

Lastly, through synergistic effects of the reduction in inflammation, oxidative stress, and endothelial dysfunction, the MedDiet is thought to have anti-platelet properties as well [39, 48]. This may be due to the increased consumption of foods high in fish oil and polyphenol-rich nutrients, such as EVOO, fruits, vegetables, and wine [61].

Pathways on the Horizon: Impact on Gut Microbiome, Nutrigenomics, and Genetic Stability

The gut microbiome is heavily influenced by alterations in diet, especially by protein and insoluble fiber [7]. The MedDiet, with a low consumption of red meat and a high consumption of legumes, nuts, fruits, and vegetables, has been shown to modulate gut microbiota and influence the production of metabolites [8]. People who follow a MedDiet pattern typically consume 50% less choline and L-carnitine, which are found in red meat, eggs, and cheese, compared to those following a typical Western diet, which leads to decreased gut microbial production of trimethylamine N-oxide (TMAO) and fecal short-chain fatty acids (SCFAs) [59]. TMAO influences macrophages and foam cells in plaque development and is thought to increase the risk of ASCVD independent of cardiometabolic risk factors although data to suggest definite causation are still lacking [55].

Intake of insoluble fiber is almost two times higher in the MedDiet compared to the Western diet due to the high consumption of legumes, fruits, and vegetables [59]. High fiber intake influences an alteration in specific gut microbiota that results in an increase in fecal (SCFAs), which are thought to be protective against inflammatory diseases [56, 59]. A study by De Fillipis et al. showed that higher adherence to a MedDiet increases the production of SCFAs in the gut and lower adherence to the MedDiet resulted in higher levels of urinary TMAO [8].

Another exciting area of research includes the field of nutrigenomics which examines how diet and genes interact. Nutrigenomic studies have shown that the MedDiet is able to impact gene expression, protecting against the proatherogenic gene expression involved in vascular inflammation, foam cell formation, and thrombosis [34, 38]. It is postulated that the high antioxidant content in the MedDiet is involved in the mechanism because antioxidants have been shown to modulate gene and protein expression, which then impacts metabolite production [19]. The benefits of the MedDiet on ASCVD have been evaluated; however, additional, larger studies are still needed to better understand the mechanisms of nutritional genomics before nutrigenomic-based recommendations may be given.

Section 5: Conclusion

There appear to be multiple benefits of the MedDiet, not only for CV health, but also other chronic diseases including cancer, diabetes, and neurodegenerative disorders [47].

However, determining whether the beneficial effects are due to single components of the dietary pattern, a combination of the dietary components in the MedDiet, or other factors remains challenging. In fact, some benefit is believed to be from the more balanced, active, community-oriented lifestyle that often is found in the European populations included in the studies examining the MedDiet. In addition, the types of animal products and fresh produce consumed in European countries may also differ from that of the USA and other countries. Aside from the potential benefit of lifestyle, the beneficial effects seen with higher adherence to the MedDiet is likely in part due to the multiple components of the dietary pattern that have an impact beyond improving CV risk factors. Indeed, the degree of ASCVD risk factor improvement appears to be modest for the benefits conferred on health outcomes. This suggests that other metabolic and molecular effects may be more influential, such as those on inflammation, endothelial function, TMAO production, and genomic stability [59]. Lastly, the degree to which individuals consume specific food components of the MedDiet (fruits, vegetables, fish, legumes, wine, and animal products) may make a substantial difference on the observed health benefits as some health benefits appear to be more closely linked to the provegetarian options. Although future studies may help to better understand the mechanisms of the MedDiet benefits, facilitating the implementation of this dietary pattern in patients with health conditions shown to be improved with adherence to the MedDiet is strongly encouraged at this time.

References

1. Alberti KGMM, Eckler RH, Grundy SM, Zimmet PZ, Cleeman JI, Donato KA, Fruchart JC, James WPT, Loria CM, Smith Jr SC. Harmonizing the Metabolic SyndromeA Joint Interim Statement of the International Diabetes Federation Task Force on Epidemiology and Prevention; National Heart, Lung, and Blood Institute; American Heart Association; World Heart Federation; International Atherosclerosis Society; and International Association for the Study of Obesity. Circulation. 2009;120:1640–45. https://doi.org/10.1161/CIRCULATIONAHA.109.192644

2. American Diabetes Association. 5. Lifestyle management: standards of medical care in diabetes—2019.
   Diabetes Care. 2019;42(Supplement 1):S46–60.
   https://doi.org/10.2337/dc19-S005.
3. Casas R, Sacanella E, Estruch R. The immune protective effect of the Mediterranean diet against
   chronic low-grade inflammatory diseases. Endocr
   Metab Immune Disord Drug Targets. 2016;14(4):
   245–54. https://doi.org/10.2174/18715303146661409
   22153350.
4. Chrysohoou C, Panagiotakos DB, Pitsavos C, Das
   UN, Stefanadis C. Adherence to the Mediterranean
   diet attenuates inflammation and coagulation process in healthy adults: the ATTICA study. J Am Coll
   Cardiol. 2004;44(1):152–8. https://doi.org/10.1016/j.
   jacc.2004.03.039.
5. Crous-Bou M, Fung TT, Prescott J, Julin B, Meng-
   meng D, Qi S, Rexrode KM, Frank BH, De Vivo
   I. Mediterranean diet and telomere length in
   nurses' health study: population based cohort study.
   BMJ (Clin Res Ed). 2014;349:g6674. https://doi.
   org/10.1136/bmj.g6674.
6. D'Alessandro A, De Pergola G. Mediterranean diet
   and cardiovascular disease: a critical evaluation of a
   priori dietary indexes. Nutrients. 2015;7(9):7863–88.
   https://doi.org/10.3390/nu7095367.
7. David LA, Maurice CF, Carmody RN, Gootenberg
   DB, Button JE, Wolfe BE, Ling AV, et al. Diet rapidly and reproducibly alters the human gut microbiome. Nature. 2014;505(7484):559–63. https://doi.
   org/10.1038/nature12820.
8. De Filippis F, Pellegrini N, Vannini L, Jeffery IB, La
   Storia A, Laghi L, Serrazanetti DI, et al. High-level
   adherence to a Mediterranean diet beneficially impacts
   the gut microbiota and associated metabolome. Gut.
   2016;65(11):1812–21. https://doi.org/10.1136/gutjnl-
   2015-309957.
9. de Lorgeril M, Salen P, Martin JL, Monjaud I, Delaye
   J, Mamelle N. Mediterranean diet, traditional risk factors, and the rate of cardiovascular complications after
   myocardial infarction: final report of the Lyon diet
   heart study. Circulation. 1999;99(6):779–85. https://
   doi.org/10.1161/01.cir.99.6.779.
10. De Pergola G, D'Alessandro A. Influence of Mediter-
    ranean diet on blood pressure. Nutrients. 2018;10(11)
    https://doi.org/10.3390/nu10111700.
11. Dinu M, Pagliai G, Casini A, Sofi F. Mediterranean
    diet and multiple health outcomes: an umbrella review
    of meta-analyses of observational studies and ran-
    domised trials. Eur J Clin Nutr. 2018;72(1):30–43.
    https://doi.org/10.1038/ejcn.2017.58.
12. Dinu M, Pagliai G, Angelino D, Rosi A, Dall'Asta M,
    Bresciani L, Ferraris C, et al. Effects of popular diets
    on anthropometric and cardiometabolic parameters:
    an umbrella review of meta-analyses of randomized
    controlled trials. Adv Nut (Bethesda, MD). 2020, Feb-
    ruary; https://doi.org/10.1093/advances/nmaa006.
13. Esposito K, Marfella R, Ciotola M, Di Palo C, Giug-
    liano F, Giugliano G, D'Armiento M, D'Andrea F,
    Giugliano D. Effect of a Mediterranean-style diet
    on endothelial dysfunction and markers of vascular

14. inflammation in the metabolic syndrome: a random-
    ized trial. JAMA. 2004;292(12):1440–6. https://doi.
    org/10.1001/jama.292.12.1440.
14. Esposito K, Kastorini C-M, Panagiotakos DB, Giug-
    liano D. Mediterranean diet and weight loss: meta-
    analysis of randomized controlled trials. Metab
    Syndr Relat Disord. 2011;9(1):1–12. https://doi.
    org/10.1089/met.2010.0031.
15. Esposito K, Maiorino MI, Bellastella G, Chiodini P,
    Panagiotakos D, Giugliano D. A journey into a Medi-
    terranean diet and type 2 diabetes: a systematic review
    with meta-analyses. BMJ Open. 2015;5(8) https://doi.
    org/10.1136/bmjopen-2015-008222.
16. Estruch R. Anti-inflammatory effects of the Medi-
    terranean diet: the experience of the PREDIMED
    study. Proc Nutr Soc. 2010;69(3):333–40. https://doi.
    org/10.1017/S0029665110001539
17. Estruch R, Ros E, Salas-Salvadó J, Covas M-I,
    Corella D, Arós F, Gómez-Gracia E, et al. Retraction
    and republication: primary prevention of cardiovascu-
    lar disease with a Mediterranean diet. N Engl J Med.
    2018;2013(368):1279–90." N Engl J Med 378 (25):
    2441–42. https://doi.org/10.1056/NEJMc1806491.
18. Evert AB, Dennison M, Gardner CD, Timothy Garvey
    W, Ka HKL, MacLeod J, Mitri J, et al. Nutrition ther-
    apy for adults with diabetes or prediabetes: a consen-
    sus report. Diabetes Care. 2019;42(5):731–54. https://
    doi.org/10.2337/dci19-0014.
19. Fitó M, Konstantinidou V. Nutritional genomics
    and the Mediterranean diet's effects on human car-
    diovascular health. Nutrients. 2016;8(4) https://doi.
    org/10.3390/nu8040218.
20. Flock MR, Fleming JA, Kris-Etherton PM. Mac-
    ronutrient replacement options for saturated fat:
    effects on cardiovascular health. Curr Opin Lipidol.
    2014;25(1):67–74.
21. Fontana L, Partridge L. Promoting health and longev-
    ity through diet: from model organisms to humans.
    Cell. 2015;161(1):106–18. https://doi.org/10.1016/j.
    cell.2015.02.020.
22. Franquesa M, Pujol-Busquets G, García-Fernández
    E, Rico L, Shamirian-Pulido L, Aguilar-Martínez A,
    Medina FX, Serra-Majem L, Bach-Faig A. Mediter-
    ranean diet and cardiodiabesity: a systematic review
    through evidence-based answers to key clinical ques-
    tions. Nutrients. 2019;11(3) https://doi.org/10.3390/
    nu11030655.
23. Fung TT, McCullough ML, Newby PK, Manson
    JE, Meigs JB, Rifai N, Willett WC, Frank BH. Diet-
    quality scores and plasma concentrations of markers of
    inflammation and endothelial dysfunction. Am J Clin
    Nutr. 2005;82(1):163–73. https://doi.org/10.1093/
    ajcn.82.1.163.
24. Garcia M, Bihuniak JD, Shook J, Kenny A, Kerstet-
    ter J, Huedo-Medina TB. The effect of the traditional
    Mediterranean-style diet on metabolic risk factors: a
    meta-analysis. Nutrients. 2016;8(3):168. https://doi.
    org/10.3390/nu8030168.
25. Godos J, Zappalà G, Bernardini S, Giambini I, Bes-
    Rastrollo M, Martinez-Gonzalez M. Adherence to
    the Mediterranean diet is inversely associated with

metabolic syndrome occurrence: a meta-analysis of observational studies. Int J Food Sci Nutr. 2017;68(2):138–48. https://doi.org/10.1080/0963748 6.2016.1221900.

26. Guasch-Ferré M, Liu G, Li Y, Sampson L, Manson JAE, Salas-Salvadó J, Martínez-González MA, et al. Olive oil consumption and cardiovascular risk in U.S. adults. J Am Coll Cardiol. 2020;75(15):1729–39. https://doi.org/10.1016/j.jacc.2020.02.036.

27. Huo R, Du T, Xu Y, Xu W, Chen X, Sun K, Yu X. Effects of Mediterranean-style diet on glycemic control, weight loss and cardiovascular risk factors among type 2 diabetes individuals: a meta-analysis. Eur J Clin Nutr. 2015;69(11):1200–8. https://doi.org/10.1038/ejcn.2014.243.

28. Kastorini C-M, Milionis HJ, Esposito K, Giugliano D, Goudevenos JA, Panagiotakos DB. The effect of Mediterranean diet on metabolic syndrome and its components: a meta-analysis of 50 studies and 534,906 individuals. J Am Coll Cardiol. 2011;57(11):1299–313. https://doi.org/10.1016/j.jacc.2010.09.073.

29. Kattoor AJ, Pothineni NVK, Palagiri D, Mehta JL. Oxidative stress in atherosclerosis. Curr Atheroscler Rep. 2017;19(11):42. https://doi.org/10.1007/s11883-017-0678-6.

30. Kesse-Guyot E, Ahluwalia N, Lassale C, Hercberg S, Fezeu L, Lairon D. Adherence to Mediterranean diet reduces the risk of metabolic syndrome: a 6-year prospective study. Nutr Metab Cardiovasc Dis. 2013;23(7):677–83. https://doi.org/10.1016/j.numecd.2012.02.005.

31. Keys A, Menotti A, Karvonen MJ, Aravanis C, Blackburn H, Buzina R, Djordjevic BS, Dontas AS, Fidanza F, Keys MH. The diet and 15-year death rate in the seven countries study. Am J Epidemiol. 1986;124(6):903–15. https://doi.org/10.1093/oxfordjournals.aje.a114480.

32. Kirkpatrick CF, Bolick JP, Kris-Etherton PM, Sikand G, Aspry KE, Soffer DE, Willard K-E, Maki KC. Review of current evidence and clinical recommendations on the effects of low-carbohydrate and very-low-carbohydrate (including ketogenic) diets for the management of body weight and other cardiometabolic risk factors: a scientific statement from the national lipid association nutrition and lifestyle task force. J Clin Lipidol. 2019;13(5):689–711.e1. https://doi.org/10.1016/j.jacl.2019.08.003.

33. Koloverou E, Esposito K, Giugliano D, Panagiotakos D. The effect of Mediterranean diet on the development of type 2 diabetes mellitus: a meta-analysis of 10 prospective studies and 136,846 participants. Metab Clin Exp. 2014;63(7):903–11. https://doi.org/10.1016/j.metabol.2014.04.010.

34. Konstantinidou V, Covas M-I, Muñoz-Aguayo D, Khymenets O, de la Torre R, Saez G, del Carmen Tormos M, et al. In vivo Nutrigenomic effects of virgin olive oil polyphenols within the frame of the Mediterranean diet: a randomized controlled trial. FASEB J Off Publ Fed Am Soc Exper Biol. 2010;24(7):2546–57. https://doi.org/10.1096/fj.09-148452.

35. Lăcătuşu CM, Grigorescu ED, Floria M, Onofriescu A, Mihai BM. The Mediterranean Diet: from an environment-driven food culture to an emerging medical prescription. Int J Environ Res Public Health. 2019;16(6):942. https://doi.org/10.3390/ijerph16060942. PMID: 30875998; PMCID: PMC6466433.

36. Liday C, Kirkpatrick C. Optimal dietary strategies for prevention of atherosclerotic cardiovascular disease in diabetes: evidence and recommendations. Curr Cardiol Rep. 2019;21(11):132. https://doi.org/10.1007/s11886-019-1232-7.

37. Liu G, Guasch-Ferré M, Hu Y, Li Y, Hu FB, Rimm EB, Manson JAE, Rexrode KM, Sun Q. Nut consumption in relation to cardiovascular disease incidence and mortality among patients with diabetes mellitus. Circ Res. 2019;124(6):920–9. https://doi.org/10.1161/CIRCRESAHA.118.314316.

38. Llorente-Cortés V, Estruch R, Mena MP, Ros E, González MAM, Fitó M, Lamuela-Raventós RM, Badimon L. Effect of Mediterranean diet on the expression of pro-atherogenic genes in a population at high cardiovascular risk. Atherosclerosis. 2010;208(2):442–50. https://doi.org/10.1016/j.atherosclerosis.2009.08.004.

39. Loffredo L, Perri L, Nocella C, Violi F. Antioxidant and antiplatelet activity by polyphenol-rich nutrients: focus on extra virgin olive oil and cocoa. Br J Clin Pharmacol. 2017;83(1):96–102. https://doi.org/10.1111/bcp.12923.

40. Meisinger C, Jens B, Natalie K, Hannelore L, Wolfgang K. Plasma oxidized low-density lipoprotein, a strong predictor for acute coronary heart disease events in apparently healthy, middle-aged men from the general population. Circulation. 2005;112(5):651–7. https://doi.org/10.1161/CIRCULATIONAHA.104.529297.

41. Neuenschwander M, Hoffmann G, Schwingshackl L, Schlesinger S. Impact of different dietary approaches on blood lipid control in patients with type 2 diabetes mellitus: a systematic review and network meta-analysis. Eur J Epidemiol. 2019;34(9):837–52. https://doi.org/10.1007/s10654-019-00534-1.

42. Nissensohn M, Román-Viñas B, Sánchez-Villegas A, Piscopo S, Serra-Majem L. The effect of the Mediterranean diet on hypertension: a systematic review and meta-analysis. J Nutr Educ Behav. 2016;48(1):42–53.e1. https://doi.org/10.1016/j.jneb.2015.08.023.

43. Ornish D, Scherwitz LW, Billings JH, Brown SE, Gould KL, Merritt TA, Sparler S, et al. Intensive lifestyle changes for reversal of coronary heart disease. JAMA. 1998;280(23):2001–7. https://doi.org/10.1001/jama.280.23.2001.

44. Pett KD, Willett WC, Vartiainen E, Katz DL. The seven countries study. Eur Heart J. 2017;38(42):3119–21. https://doi.org/10.1093/eurheartj/ehx603.

45. Razquin C, Martinez JA, Martinez-Gonzalez MA, Mitjavila MT, Estruch R, Marti A. A 3 years follow-up of a Mediterranean diet rich in virgin olive oil is associated with high plasma antioxidant capacity and reduced body weight gain. Eur J Clin Nutr.

2009;63(12):1387–93. https://doi.org/10.1038/ejcn.2009.106.

46. Rees K, Takeda A, Martin N, Ellis L, Wijesekara D, Vepa A, Das A, Hartley L, Stranges S. Mediterranean-style diet for the primary and secondary prevention of cardiovascular disease. Cochrane Database Syst Rev. 2019;3:CD009825. https://doi.org/10.1002/14651858.CD009825.pub3.

47. Romagnolo DF, Selmin OI. Mediterranean Diet and Prevention of Chronic Diseases. Nutr Today. 2017 Sep;52(5):208-222. https://doi.org/10.1097/NT.0000000000000228. Epub 2017 Aug 15. PMID: 29051674; PMCID: PMC5625964.

48. Salas-Salvadó J, Becerra-Tomás N, García-Gavilán JF, Bulló M, Barrubés L. Mediterranean diet and cardiovascular disease prevention: what do we know? Prog Cardiovasc Dis. 2018;61(1):62–7. https://doi.org/10.1016/j.pcad.2018.04.006.

49. Sala-Vila A, Romero-Mamani E-S, Gilabert R, Núñez I, de la Torre R, Corella D, Ruiz-Gutiérrez V, et al. Changes in ultrasound-assessed carotid intima-media thickness and plaque with a Mediterranean diet: a substudy of the PREDIMED trial. Arterioscler Thromb Vasc Biol. 2014;34(2):439–45. https://doi.org/10.1161/ATVBAHA.113.302327.

50. Schwingshackl L, Hoffmann G. Mediterranean dietary pattern, inflammation and endothelial function: a systematic review and meta-analysis of intervention trials. Nutr Metab Cardiovasc Dis. 2014;24(9):929–39. https://doi.org/10.1016/j.numecd.2014.03.003.

51. Schwingshackl L, Missbach B, König J, Hoffmann G. Adherence to a Mediterranean diet and risk of diabetes: a systematic review and meta-analysis. Public Health Nutr. 2015;18(7):1292–9. https://doi.org/10.1017/S1368980014001542.

52. Schwingshackl L, Chaimani A, Hoffmann G, Schwedhelm C, Boeing H. A network meta-analysis on the comparative efficacy of different dietary approaches on glycaemic control in patients with type 2 diabetes mellitus. Eur J Epidemiol. 2018;33(2):157–70. https://doi.org/10.1007/s10654-017-0352-x.

53. Shannon OM, Mendes I, Köchl C, Mazidi M, Ashor AW, Rubele S, Minihane A-M, Mathers JC, Siervo M. Mediterranean diet increases endothelial function in adults: a systematic review and meta-analysis of randomized controlled trials. J Nutr. 2020;150(5):1151–9. https://doi.org/10.1093/jn/nxaa002.

54. Sofi F, Dinu M, Pagliai G, Cesari F, Gori AM, Sereni A, Becatti M, Fiorillo C, Marcucci R, Casini A. Low-calorie vegetarian versus Mediterranean diets for reducing body weight and improving cardiovascular risk profile: CARDIVEG study (cardiovascular prevention with vegetarian diet). Circulation. 2018;137(11):1103–13. https://doi.org/10.1161/CIRCULATIONAHA.117.030088.

55. Tang W, Wilson H, Wang Z, Levison BS, Koeth RA, Britt EB, Xiaoming F, Wu Y, Hazen SL. Intestinal microbial metabolism of phosphatidylcholine and cardiovascular risk. N Engl J Med. 2013;368(17):1575–84. https://doi.org/10.1056/NEJMoa1109400.

56. Thorburn AN, Macia L, Mackay CR. Diet, metabolites, and 'Western-Lifestyle' inflammatory diseases. Immunity. 2014;40(6):833–42. https://doi.org/10.1016/j.immuni.2014.05.014.

57. Toledo E, Hu FB, Estruch R, Buil-Cosiales P, Corella D, Jordi S-S, Isabel Covas M, et al. Effect of the Mediterranean diet on blood pressure in the PREDIMED trial: results from a randomized controlled trial. BMC Med. 2013;11(September):207. https://doi.org/10.1186/1741-7015-11-207.

58. Tong TYN, Wareham NJ, Khaw K-T, Imamura F, Forouhi NG. Prospective association of the Mediterranean diet with cardiovascular disease incidence and mortality and its population impact in a non-Mediterranean population: the epic-Norfolk study. BMC Med. 2016;14(1):135. https://doi.org/10.1186/s12916-016-0677-4.

59. Tosti V, Bertozzi B, Fontana L. Health benefits of the Mediterranean diet: metabolic and molecular mechanisms. J Gerontol A Biol Sci Med Sci. 2018;73(3):318–26. https://doi.org/10.1093/gerona/glx227.

60. Trichopoulou A, Kouris-Blazos A, Wahlqvist ML, Gnardellis C, Lagiou P, Polychronopoulos E, Vassilakou T, Lipworth L, Trichopoulos D. Diet and overall survival in elderly people. Br Med J. 1995;311(7018):1457–60.

61. Violi F, Pignatelli P, Basili S. Nutrition, supplements, and vitamins in platelet function and bleeding. Circulation. 2010;121(8):1033–44. https://doi.org/10.1161/CIRCULATIONAHA.109.880211.

62. Willett WC, Sacks F, Trichopoulou A, Drescher G, Ferro-Luzzi A, Helsing E, Trichopoulos D. Mediterranean diet pyramid: a cultural model for healthy eating. Am J Clin Nutr. 1995;61(6 Suppl):1402S–6S. https://doi.org/10.1093/ajcn/61.6.1402S.

63. Wu L, Sun D. Adherence to Mediterranean diet and risk of developing cognitive disorders: an updated systematic review and meta-analysis of prospective cohort studies. Sci Rep. 2017;7(January) https://doi.org/10.1038/srep41317.

Dietary Approaches to Hypertension: Dietary Sodium and the DASH Diet for Cardiovascular Health

4

Keith C. Ferdinand, Samar A. Nasser, Daphne P. Ferdinand, and Rachel M. Bond

Introduction: Design and Results of the DASH Diet

The Dietary Approaches to Stop Hypertension (DASH) trial was a multicenter, randomized feeding study that tested the effects of dietary patterns on blood pressure (BP) [1]. At the time of the DASH trial inception, there was inconsistent evidence reflecting the BP effects by modifying single nutrients; however, there was generally positive evidence in the vegetarian diets with observational studies on diet and BP. Given that the DASH trial assessed dietary patterns rather than individual nutrients, overall, it tested the combined effects of nutrients that occur concurrently in food. The DASH trial encompassed a 7-day menu cycle with 21 meals at four-calorie levels (1600, 2100, 2600, and 3100 kcal) developed for each diet and identical at all centers. The study cohort consisted of nearly 50% female, over 50% black participants who, on average, were in their mid-40s with BPs roughly 130/80 mm Hg. The hypothesis was that the change in BP would differ between the fruits and vegetables and the combination compared to control diets.

The DASH diet, sponsored by the National Heart, Lung, and Blood Institute (NHLBI), incorporated randomized, controlled participants who were selected for a feeding intervention with DASH foods and closely monitored. For 3 weeks, participants were fed a control diet that was low in fruits, vegetables, and dairy products, with a fat content typical of the average diet in the USA. Next, they were randomly assigned to receive 8 weeks on the control diet, a diet rich in fruits and vegetables, or a combination diet rich in fruits, vegetables, and low-fat dairy products and with reduced saturated and total fat. Throughout the trial, sodium intake and body weight were maintained at constant levels.

The NHLBI promotes the DASH eating pattern to prevent and control BP without the use of pharmacotherapy and is promoted as a healthy option for the general population [2–4]. The NHLBI's DASH eating plan encourages foods that are low in saturated fat, total fat, cholesterol,

K. C. Ferdinand (✉)
Gerald S. Berenson Endowed Chair in Preventive Cardiology, Tulane University School of Medicine, New Orleans, LA, USA
e-mail: kferdina@tulane.edu

S. A. Nasser
Department of Clinical Research & Leadership, School of Medicine and Health Sciences, The George Washington University, Washington, DC, USA
e-mail: snasser@gwu.edu

D. P. Ferdinand
Healthy Heart Community Prevention Project, Inc, New Orleans, LA, USA
e-mail: daphnep@healthyheartcpp.org

R. M. Bond
Dignity Health, Chandler Regional Medical Center, Chandler, AZ, USA

Creighton University School of Medicine, Omaha, NE, USA

© Springer Nature Switzerland AG 2021
M. J. Wilkinson et al. (eds.), *Prevention and Treatment of Cardiovascular Disease*, Contemporary Cardiology, https://doi.org/10.1007/978-3-030-78177-4_4

and sodium and high in potassium, calcium, magnesium, fiber, and protein. This plan was originally developed from studies demonstrating that the DASH diet lowers BP and low-density lipoprotein cholesterol (LDL-C) [5]. The number of servings recommended is based upon one's caloric need, and the nutrient goals of the DASH eating pattern are as follows:

- Total fat: 27% of calories
- Saturated fat: 6% of calories
- Protein: 18% of calories
- Carbohydrates: 55% of calories
- Cholesterol: 150 mg
- Sodium: 2300 mg
- Potassium: 4700 mg
- Calcium: 1250 mg
- Magnesium: 500 mg
- Fiber: 30 g

Current Evidence-Based Guideline Recommendations: DASH and DASH Sodium Eating Patterns

With a focus on the primary prevention of cardiovascular disease (CVD), lifestyle modifications are the bedrock of appropriate cardiovascular therapy. According to the 2019 American College of Cardiology (ACC)/American Heart Association (AHA) Multisociety Guidelines on the Primary Prevention of Cardiovascular Disease, a healthy diet emphasizes the intake of vegetables, fruits, legumes, nuts, whole grains, lean vegetable or animal protein, and fish and minimizes the intake of trans fats, processed meats, refined carbohydrates, and sweetened beverages [6]. Adherence to these recommendations can be enhanced by shared decision-making among the healthcare team and patients, with patient engagement in selecting interventions based on individual values, preferences, and associated conditions and co-morbidities.

Accordingly, the DASH diet is one of the best proven nonpharmacological interventions for the prevention and treatment of hypertension (HTN) with an overall 11 mm Hg reduction in systolic BP (SBP) in hypertensives and a 3 mm Hg reduction in SBP in normotensives following the DASH dietary intervention [6]. Furthermore, with the 2017 ACC/AHA Multisociety Guideline for the Prevention, Detection, Evaluation, and Management of High Blood Pressure [7], the DASH eating plan demonstrated effectiveness in BP lowering. Additionally, interventions to reduce sodium also demonstrate lower BP in those with hypertension, specifically those with elevated levels of BP, African Americans, older persons, and those who are salt sensitive [7] (Table 4.1), and thus may have a synergistic impact with DASH eating plans.

Recommendations from the 2017 ACC/AHA Multisociety High BP Guideline described the DASH diet as an exemplary diet that facilitates achieving a desirable weight as well as sodium reduction, which is recommended for adults with hypertension. Moreover, dietary modification to incorporate an increase in potassium is recommended as well. Nevertheless, potassium supplementation is contraindicated if in the presence of chronic kidney disease (CKD) or the use of medications that limit potassium excretion [7]. Studies demonstrate that dietary behavior is an important lifestyle factor impacting the risk of HTN development [8]. Individuals living in acculturated societies, given free access to salt, invariably consume between 100 and 200 mmol of sodium daily [9]. Several meta-analyses indi-

Table 4.1 Summary of benefits of using the DASH diet

Diet	Includes	Restricts	Health benefits	Special considerations
Dietary approaches to stop hypertension	52–55% carbohydrates, 16–18% proteins, and 30% total fats; rich in fruits, vegetables, whole grains, and low-fat dairy products	Limits saturated fats, cholesterol, refined grains, and sugars; suggested sodium intake is less than 2400 mg per day	Decreased CVD risk factors, blood pressure, obesity, and type 2 diabetes	African Americans CKD Diabetes Children

cate that among hypertensive and older subjects, a 3–5 mm Hg systolic and approximately 1 mm Hg diastolic change in pressure is associated with a 75–100 mmol/24 h difference in sodium intake. The effect on younger and normotensive subjects is less with approximately 2–3 mm Hg for systolic and <1 mm Hg for diastolic [9].

Recently, Welsh and colleagues conducted a 7-year prospective cohort study on 457,484 United Kingdom Biobank participants (mean age, 56.3 years; 44.7% men) without CVD to determine if urinary sodium excretion affects mortality or CVD development [10]. Participants were assessed in quintiles of mean arterial BP and urinary sodium excretion; however, no association was found between urinary sodium (high or low) and risk of developing CVD, including heart failure. Thus, although urinary sodium excretion correlated with elevated BP in participants at low cardiovascular risk, there was no pattern of increased CVD, heart failure, or mortality risk demonstrated.

Data have suggested, a long period of exposure to increased sodium intake may be required for BP manifestations to be apparent, with the age of the population studied influencing these observations as well [11, 12]. Over a period of time, both sodium and chloride in salt lead to extracellular volume expansion, which eventually causes BP to rise. Thus, information from more dramatic manipulations of sodium balance in an older cohort may provide greater insight into the relationship between BP and salt.

Effectiveness of the DASH Sodium Approach: Low Sodium, High Potassium

Although the original DASH diet was not low in sodium at 2400 mg of sodium per day, BP was effectively lowered. Therefore, the DASH-Sodium trial, supported by the NHLBI, was conducted to understand the effect of BP on sodium restriction and included 412 subjects who were randomized to a control diet (typical American diet) or the DASH diet [13]. Within each group, subjects were then assigned to three diets: a high-

sodium diet (3.5 g/day), a moderate-sodium diet (2.3 g/day), or a low-sodium diet (1.2 g/day), each for 30 days.

The results of the DASH-Sodium study [13] demonstrated that reducing daily sodium lowered BP for participants on either diet. However, the DASH diet lowered BP more than the typical American diet at all three daily sodium levels. Finally, by reducing sodium intake and following the DASH diet, a greater BP-lowering effect was observed than following the DASH diet alone or sodium reduction alone. Finally, a follow-up study demonstrated that combining the DASH diet with sodium reduction benefited those with a higher than normal BP and those who started out with the highest BP readings experienced the greatest benefits [14].

In additional to sodium intake, dietary potassium is also important and inversely related to BP. Diets rich in fruits and vegetables are associated with lower BP, 2–5 mm Hg, especially in those patients consuming an excess of sodium and in African Americans [15]. Increased intake of potassium is associated with decreased BP independent of sodium intake [16]. Moreover, increased consumption of potassium can mitigate the negative effects of high sodium consumption on BP and is more effective in the setting of higher salt intake. Thus, the dietary sodium–potassium ratio is a major determinant of BP. There are several methods to replace sodium, and potassium chloride is often used as the key ingredient in salt substitutes as it is similar to sodium chloride in terms of its physical and functional properties [17]. According to a meta-analysis by the Evidence-based Practice Centers, data demonstrate that potassium-enriched salt substitutes lower systolic and diastolic BP (DBP) (average net Δ [95% CI] in mm Hg: −5.58 [−7.08 to −4.09] and −2.88 [−3.93 to −1.83], respectively) [18]. On the other hand, more data are needed to assess the effects of potassium-enriched salt on serum potassium levels and the occurrence of hyperkalemia, especially in those with CDK. Accordingly, Greer and colleagues reviewed the use of potassium-enriched salt substitutes and evidence on their potential benefits and risks. Although replacing potassium-enriched salt substitutes lowers BP, the safety and acceptance were with ≤30% of potassium chloride [19]. To reduce salt intake, empirical data support salt substitutes, such as potassium-enriched, as a potential alternative to managing HTN while maintaining taste [19]; however, empirical research is necessary to evaluate the effect on serum potassium levels and to estimate the population-wide impact of potassium-enriched salt substitutes.

DASH Diet Impact in Special Populations: Blacks/African Americans, Persons with Diabetes and CKD, Youth

Despite a clear epidemiological and clinical relationship between salt intake and HTN, the BP response to changes in dietary salt is heterogeneous among individuals. For example, baseline BP levels in the DASH sodium diet were similar for blacks and whites, and average SBP/DBP was 135.3/86.1 and 134.1/85.1 mm Hg, respectively; however, those participants on the lower (vs. higher) sodium intake decreased SBP by 8.0 mm Hg (95% CI 6.5–9.4 mm Hg) in blacks and by 5.1 mm Hg (3.4–6.7) in whites (P < 0.01). Moreover, for those on the DASH-sodium diet, lower (vs. higher) sodium intake decreased SBP by 3.6 mm Hg (95% CI 2.2–5.1) in blacks and by 2.2 mm Hg (0.5–3.8) in whites [20, 21].

In 2003, it was projected that if the US population successfully adopted the DASH diet and experienced the DASH trial effect of lower SBP by 5.5 mm Hg, then 668,000 coronary heart disease events could be prevented over a decade [22]. Accordingly, Thomas and colleagues recently utilized the CARDIA (Coronary Artery Risk Development in Young Adults) data to determine the cumulative incidence of HTN and to identify risk factors associated with a greater HTN risk in blacks and whites aged 18–30 years who were followed until 55 years of age [23]. To investigate lifestyle and other factors that influence, favorably or unfavorably, the evolution of coronary heart disease risk factors during young adulthood, the CARDIA study comprised 5115 African American and Caucasian men and women 18–30 years of age across urban areas in the USA in 1985 [24]. Thomas and colleagues determined that a higher DASH diet adherence score was associated with a lower risk for HTN in both African Americans and Caucasians, and within each SBP/DBP category. The results support the importance of focusing on modifiable risk factors, including adherence to a DASH diet at an early age, for the prevention of hypertension, regardless of race.

The American Diabetes Association (ADA) Standards of Medical Care in Diabetes—2020 highlights the need for lifestyle Intervention recommendations. Recommendations for patients with BP more than 120/80 mm Hg include lifestyle intervention consisting of weight loss if overweight or obese, a DASH-style eating pattern including reduced sodium and increased potassium intake, moderation of alcohol intake, and increased physical activity [25]. Thus, the ADA also promotes the use of a variety of eating patterns to help with the management of diabetes, given that the DASH trials support a nutritious, balanced, and sustainable eating plan that can improve HTN which is often prevalent in diabetes.

Given that the protective role of DASH dietary patterns in the development of CKD, as measured by estimated glomerular filtration rate, is not consistent in the literature, Mozaffari and colleagues completed a systematic review and meta-analysis of observational studies [26]. In their review, a significant inverse association was observed between DASH dietary pattern and CKD risk. The combined risk estimates for two cross-sectional and four prospective cohort studies demonstrated an inverse association between DASH dietary patterns and risk of CKD (pooled risk estimate: 0.77, 95% CI 0.63–0.94; P = 0.01) [26]. Thus, adherence to DASH dietary patterns may have beneficial effects against CKD development and progression.

There are complex interactions among lifestyle factors and genetic markers which play important roles in determining an individual's risk of HTN. Zafarmand evaluated the interaction between dietary patterns and genetic markers in relation to children's BP. Based upon a population-based cohort study of 1068 Dutch children, aged 5–7, they analyzed the association between a DASH-type diet, genetic variants, and their interaction on BP [27]. They showed that adherence to the DASH-type diet, as well as a low genetic risk profile for BP, is associated with lower BP in children, thus portraying evidence of a gene–diet interaction on BP in children.

Beneficial Cardiometabolic Effects of DASH Eating Plans: Glucose, Lipids, Obesity

Evidence from randomized controlled trials (RCTs) and prospective cohort studies in the US populations established DASH diet's benefits on BP, plasma glucose, lipid profiles as well as the risk of and CVD mortality [28–31]. According to a recent analysis of systematic reviews and meta-analyses, Chiavaroli and colleagues confirmed that the DASH dietary pattern had CVD benefit which was reflected by reductions in BP, HbA1c, and LDL-C in those with and without diabetes [32].

The overall prevalence of CVD (comprising coronary heart disease [CHD], congestive heart failure [CHF], cerebrovascular accident [CVA], and HTN) in adults ≥20 years of age is 48.0% overall and increases with advancing age [33]. Importantly, CHD (42.6%) is the leading cause of deaths attributable to CVD in the USA, followed by CVA (17%), HTN (10.5%), CHF (9.4%), diseases of the arteries (2.9%), and other CVDs (17.6%), all of which boast high cholesterol as a significant risk factor [34]. Given that 28.5 million adults ≥20 years of age have serum total cholesterol levels ≥240 mg/dL, with a prevalence of 11.9% [33], the impact of sustained and population-level reduction in cholesterol levels on cardiovascular co-morbidities and mortality could be profound.

According to the 2018 ACC/AHA Multisociety Guideline on the Management of Blood Cholesterol, lifestyle counseling is recommended as part of the treatment utilizing principles of plant-based diets such as DASH and Mediterranean diets. Moreover, a personalized approach with more detailed risk assessments and new cholesterol-lowering medication options are presented for people at the highest CVD risk [35]. In addition to traditional risk factors such as smoking, HTN, and diabetes, the guideline now includes additional CVD risk enhancers such as family history and race/ethnicity, as well as specific co-morbidities such as metabolic syndrome, CKD, chronic inflammatory conditions, female-specific conditions including premature menopause, premature labor, gestational hypertension, diabetes or pre-eclampsia, and high lipid biomarkers, to help clinicians better determine individualized risk and treatment options. Recognizing the cumulative effect of LDL-C over the full lifespan, the guideline also suggests elective cholesterol screening for children along with the aggressive diagnosis and management of familial hypercholesterolemia in children, adolescents, and young adults. Accordingly, 21% of youths 6–19 years of age have at least one abnormal cholesterol measure [33].

Obesity is a potent risk factor for multiple co-morbidities including diabetes, CVD, and hyperlipidemia and the rates among adults have been steadily rising since the 1980s. Among adults aged 20 years and older, obesity is defined as a body mass index (BMI) of 30 or more and severe obesity is defined as a BMI of 40 or more. Obesity rates in the USA have been consistently rising, age-standardized prevalence of obesity among adults increased from 33.7% (95% CI 31.5–36.1%) in 2007–2008 to 39.6% (95% CI 36.1–43.1%) in 2015–2016 ($P = 0.001$) [36]. Additionally, severe obesity in adults has increased with age-standardized prevalence increasing from 5.7% (95% CI 4.9–6.7%) in 2007–2008 to 7.7% (95% CI 6.6–8.9%) in 2015–2016 ($P = 0.001$). According to the Centers for Disease Control [37], every state in the USA had more than 20% of adults with obesity.

Although overweight status and obesity contribute significantly to HTN risk in all racial/ethnic populations, many racial and ethnic minorities manifest obesity disproportionately with marked ethnic and age-based differences in the rates of weight accumulation. Relative to white women, the onset of obesity occurred sooner for black and Hispanic women. After 28 years of age, black men develop obesity more rapidly than white men [38]. Anthropometric measures, such as obesity, especially in women, can also influence biologic systems involved in BP regulation and the expression of pressure-related target-organ damage (i.e., chronic renal injury).

Practical and Novel Approaches to Implementation of the DASH Diet: Current Perspectives and Future Directions

Comparing BP Reduction Over Time: Sodium Reduction and DASH Diet

In an RCT of 412 pre- or stage 1 hypertensive participants (not currently on any antihypertensive medications and without any prior CVD), a combination of a low sodium diet with the DASH diet significantly lowered SBP, especially in those with higher baseline systolic readings [14]. In this study, the mean age was 48 years with 57% women and 57% African American, and the mean SBP/DBP was 135/86 mm Hg. With either the DASH or a control diet, participants were exposed to three sodium levels (50, 100, and 150 mmol/day at 2100 kcal) in random order over 4 weeks separated by 5-day breaks. While the effects of the DASH diet occurred within 1 week, sodium reduction continued to lower BP up through 4 weeks of initiation. The combination of the low sodium-DASH diet versus the high sodium-control diet on SBP were −5.3, −7.5, −9.7, and −20.8 mm Hg ($P < 0.001$), respectively.

Impressively, a participant with a baseline SBP of 150 mm Hg or greater who consumed a low-sodium plus DASH diet had an average reduction of 21 mm Hg in SBP compared to the high-sodium control diet. The novel approach here to examining the combination of two diets in adults with early or modest forms of hypertension provides evidence that dietary interventions are as, or even more effective, than antihypertensive agents in those at greatest risk

for hypertension, and should be incorporated as a routine first-line treatment option. In Journal of the American College of Cardiology health promotion series, Carey and colleagues state that the combination of low-sodium intake and the DASH diet provides substantially greater BP reduction than sodium restriction or the DASH diet alone [39]. Thus, in adults with elevated BP, the DASH diet and sodium reduction are concomitantly recommended, especially to those at the greatest risk.

One potential reason the DASH diet has not been adopted generally is due to the financial constraint of maintaining a high-quality diet. There is evidence reflecting the DASH-accordant diets were generally more costly; however, ethnic eating patterns may be the key to making healthy diets economically feasible for all [40]. Recently, longitudinal data from 1466 adult urban participants from Healthy Aging in Neighborhoods of Diversity Across the Life Span (HANDLS) study were analyzed for the association between the monetary value of the diet (MVD) and the overall dietary quality across sex, race, and income groups [41]. Beydoun and colleagues demonstrated a positive overall association between the rate of change in MVD and indices of dietary quality, and whites had a better diet quality compared with African Americans [41]. In a follow-up study, Beydoun and colleagues examined the overall association between cumulative exposure to MVD and DASH diet scores over 5 years and rates of change and follow-up allostatic load (AL) using the HANDLS study [42]. The AL is considered a more precise alternative to the term stress. Overall by using the structural equation modeling, the study demonstrated an independent pathway linking MVD to AL through DASH. Therefore, the energy-adjusted increase in MVD may have a significant impact on the DASH diet score, which could reduce the AL.

Given how scalable the DASH diet is and the considerable impact that it could make on the general population, research must integrate how best to deliver the DASH diet while incorporating diverse dietary regimens and digital health tools for the full dissemination and implementation.

Novel Use of App-Based Approaches: WHEELS for DASH

Health apps are widely used on smart phone devices by the US adult populations (58%) with 66% using these apps at least once a day to track their diet and physical activity [43]. Although health apps have been helpful to engage the public with monitoring health activities, most of these health apps do not focus on managing chronic conditions such as hypertension. Novel approaches to health interventions can offer alternative methods to garner patient adherence to treatment regimens. The WHEELS for DASH mobile app research study was conducted to examine adherence to the DASH diet program and to also determine patient user satisfaction or enjoyment with the app [44]. There were 72 participants recruited from an outpatient registry (19–73 years, 78% female, 18% African American, 33% diagnosis of hypertension). Although 66 participants completed the study, all users who tracked their dietary adherence demonstrated improvement in their adherence to the DASH diet during 1–6 weeks and 1–8 weeks ($P \leq 0.001$ and $P \leq 0.05$). The app had excellent reliability estimates (Intraclass correlation coefficient (ICC) [2.66] = 0.85; 95% CI 0.66–0.97, $P < 0.001$) and good user satisfaction (75%) with a very useful or useful rating.

The app's core feature is the cognitive behavioral intervention (CBI) program which captures assessment data based on the "DASH Eating Plan" as users respond to morning and evening tailored text messages. Conceptual components of self-regulation theory provided the framework for this behavioral intervention, which was tested in a previous study testing tailored messages to increase the adherence to the DASH diet [45]. In the WHEELS app study, patient users were allowed to manage and regulate their own behavior, which guided their decision making to achieve the goal of adhering to the DASH dietary plan. User responses were threefold in accordance with goal attainment, (1) adhering to one DASH food group; (2) current attitude, behavior, and skill associated with the DASH diet; and (3) reading DASH messages to increase knowledge, attitude,

and reinforcement. Although there are a number of DASH mobile apps available to patients, the WHEELS for DASH mobile app is the only app derived from a behavioral theoretical framework researched on outpatients with HTN allowing users to evaluate their eating behavior, app utility, and BP improvement in less than 8 min per day. This app provided an alternative approach to improve the adherence to the DASH diet.

According to study researchers, the WHEELS app is a potential value-added resource that can be integrated into existing treatment regimens for patients with hypertension.

There are concerns to be considered with how these health apps are evaluated and chosen for intervention use [46], with third-party development companies focused on commercial benefits and lacking expert content [45]. Due to this, there is a need to develop criteria for evaluating health apps such as involving health professional input, assessing educational content and quality, ease of use, and behavior change [47]. The standards for evaluation of the WHEELS DASH app were evidence-based, and evaluated by content experts such as the University of Michigan registered dietitians, the ADA, the ADA Evidence Analysis Library, the Cochrane Systematic Review of Best Dietary Intervention, and Science Direct [48]. The benefit in such performance measures has a potential expectancy in hypertension management and control.

Relationship of Diet, Social Determinants of Health, and Genetics (Fig. 4.1)

Although hypertension is a consequence of a combination of environmental and genetic risk factors, social determinants of health (SDOH) are also common risk factors which require acknowledgment [49]. Specifically, SDOH is broadly defined as the circumstances in which people are born, grow up, live, work, and age that may affect health [33]. The social factors that affect different behaviors, risk factors, and conditions are so important that information on SDOH was included and highlighted in all chapters with a

Fig. 4.1 Genetic/
epigenetic,
environmental, and
social determinants
interact to increase BP
in virtually all
hypertensive individuals
and populations. *BP*
blood pressure, *SD*
social determinants.
(Reprinted from Carey
et al. [60], with
permission from
Elsevier)

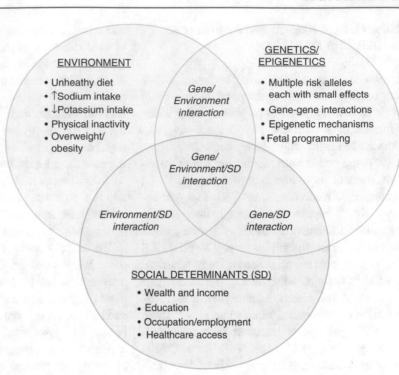

ENVIRONMENT
• Unhealthy diet
• ↑Sodium intake
• ↓Potassium intake
• Physical inactivity
• Overweight/obesity

GENETICS/EPIGENETICS
• Multiple risk alleles each with small effects
• Gene-gene interactions
• Epigenetic mechanisms
• Fetal programming

Gene/Environment interaction

Gene/Environment/SD interaction

Environment/SD interaction

Gene/SD interaction

SOCIAL DETERMINANTS (SD)
• Wealth and income
• Education
• Occupation/employment
• Healthcare access

subsection in the Heart Disease and Stroke 2020 Statistical Update [33]. Examples include low income, unemployment, discrimination, unsafe neighborhoods, substandard education, among others.

In the USA, a strong association exists between SDOH and hypertension, especially in under-represented minority populations such as blacks and Hispanics [50]. A common example has to do less with where we are born, but more so with where we are raised. Research has shown that neighborhood characteristics may affect hypertension prevalence. Individuals residing in the most economically deprived neighborhoods have greater odds of having hypertension [51]. An association also exists between residences in certain geographic areas, such as the Southeastern USA. This may be due to the higher abundance of the classic Southern diet in these locations.

Adverse Effects of the Southern Dietary Eating Pattern

The classic Southern diet, composed of high amounts of saturated fat, cholesterol, sugar,

fried foods, is considered a major contributor to the high prevalence of hypertension in the African American population. The Reasons for Geographic and Racial Differences in Stroke (REGARDS) trial researched this phenomenon attempting to explain the association between the traditional Southern diet and influence on BP and HTN [52]. Researchers conducted a prospective study examining a cohort of black and white adults selected from the original REGARDS longitudinal study. Approximately 6897 men and women with a mean age of 62 years participated in the research study (26% black; 55% women). Forty-six percent of black participants and 33% of white participants developed HTN. The black male participants had a high Southern diet score of 0.81 adjusted mean (95% CI 0.72–0.90) versus white males, −0.26 (95% CI −0.31 to −0.21), black women 0.27 (95% CI 0.20–0.33), and white women −0.57 (95% CI −0.61 to −0.54). There was a statistically significant association with the incidence of HTN and the Southern diet in black men (odds ratio 1.16 per 1 SD [95% CI 1.06–1.27]). Among all of the 12 mediating factors analyzed in this study, the Southern diet was the most significant factor for incident HTN attributing to excess risk in black men versus black women, and white men and women. Also, black men demonstrated a higher dietary ratio of sodium to potassium accounting for 12.3% of the excess hypertension incidence. Black women although expressed a much lower Southern diet score (0.27 [95% CI 0.20–0.33]) than black men, they had a high dietary sodium to potassium ratio of 6.8%, higher BMI mediated an 18.3% excess risk of incident hypertension, larger waist circumference, 15.2%; with poor adherence to the DASH diet 11.2%.

The Southern diet in the REGARDS study included high consumption of processed meats which are already high in sodium, fried foods, organ meats, high fat dairy, sugary drinks, and refined bread products. Although Southern diet is rooted in the culture and tradition of African American history, it predisposes this population to not only HTN but also to CVD [53] as compared to whites. The DASH eating plan which is high in potassium, fresh fruits and vegetables, whole grains, low fat dairy, and low in sodium becomes the likely choice for blacks.

The Oldways African Heritage Diet

Oldways is a nonprofit organization in 1990 Massachusetts invested in improving the public health of individuals and organizations promoting the "old way," or diets historically eaten in various ethnic groups or the healthy aspects of these diets (https://oldwayspt.org/programs). The focus is more on bringing back the joy of eating healthy versus adopting a so-called diet to support health to reduce the development of chronic disease associated with the typical American diet. The dietary program includes the Mediterranean, Latin American, African Heritage, Vegetarian/ Vegan and Asian styles of ethnic food consumption which use the concept of traditional foods as means of a healthier approach to eating. The Oldways site is based on the concept that foods eaten by ancestral relatives were abundant in fruits, vegetables, whole grains, nuts, seeds, with a healthy balance of seafood, yogurt, and cheese and meat with the addition of healthy oils and spices; devoid of highly processed meats, salt, and fat. Grounded in African, African American, Caribbean, and South American recipes, the diet incorporates traditional spices, ingredients and cooking techniques where they can eat healthy without giving up their traditional foods familiar to family history. The Oldways African Heritage Diet provides another alternative approach to nutritional interventions used by clinicians as a primary prevention effort to reduce chronic diseases in African American communities [54]. The benefit of traditional diets in some ethnic populations demonstrated positive effects on risk factors associated with diabetes. A randomized crossover feeding trial with first and second generation healthy Mexican women ($n = 53$) descent was conducted looking at metabolic responses when comparing a traditional Mexican diet to the US diet [55]. It was found the Mexican diet improved insulin sensitivity, reduced insulin by 14% ($P = 0.02$) and IGFBP-3 by 6% ($P = 0.006$). These studies demonstrate that clinicians, dieticians, and healthcare professionals need to consider patient traditional values, culture, and social norms when planning dietary interventions for the treatment of hypertension.

Translating DASH Eating Patterns Research into Real-World Settings

In summary, to translate the DASH trial results and develop effective strategies for increasing uptake of and adherence to the DASH diet among individuals in community-based settings, more research is needed. Although the NHLBI has developed simplified websites and pamphlets of the DASH diet for the public, application and uptake must be addressed. One method is on the feasibility of applying the DASH diet by comparing the process of preparing at-home meals as opposed to proceeding to a clinic daily to obtain prepared meals in a randomized-controlled fashion. Notably, food-related knowledge and skills differ among populations which may affect their ability to adopt healthy diets. However, evidence has demonstrated that preparing foods from scratch is associated with more adequate dietary intakes and greater food security especially among low-income populations [56].

Moreover, increased food preparation instruction, including cooking and meal-planning skills are positively associated with fruit and vegetable intake and negatively with BMI [57]. On the other hand, there is also substantial evidence that lower-income and/or minority areas have less access to healthier foods close-by, with a lower likelihood of supermarkets and more likelihood for fast food restaurants [58]. One example of an effective approach is the Association of Black Cardiologists, Inc., an organization that offers simple and tasty, heart-healthy plant-based recipes in their "Cooking for Your Heart and Soul Cookbook" [59] providing patients with additional sources to create plant-based meals as components of the DASH diet. Additionally, the NHLBI has educational resources to inform patients on the DASH eating plan to not only help control BP but also learn more about other aspects to a heart-healthy lifestyle. Educational interventions, culturally tailored and literacy appropriate, are instrumental to effecting positive change in health behavior and to hypertension treatment, control, and management. Without these readily available resources, compliance on the DASH diet will be difficult, however, with the proper meal-planning skills and food truck interventions, there is the potential of obtaining the necessary food resources in a coordinated effort to maximize DASH interventions on a community level.

References

1. Appel LJ, Moore TJ, Obarzanek E, et al. A clinical trial of the effects of dietary patterns on blood pressure. DASH collaborative research group. N Engl J Med. 1997;336(16):1117–24.
2. Sacks FM, Svetkey LP, Vollmer WM, et al. Effects on blood pressure of reduced dietary sodium and the dietary approaches to stop hypertension (DASH) diet. N Engl J Med. 2001;3–10(5):344.
3. U.S. Department of Health and Human Services and U.S. Department of Agriculture. 2015–2020 dietary guidelines for Americans. 8 December 2015. Available at: https://health.gov/dietaryguidelines/2015/guidelines/. Accessed 2 Jan 2019.
4. Appel LJ, Sacks FM, Carey VJ, et al. Effects of protein, monounsaturated fat, and carbohydrate intake on blood pressure and serum lipids: results of the Omni-Heart randomized trial. JAMA. 2005;294:2455–64.
5. NHLBI. DASH eating plan: also known as dash diet. https://www.nhlbi.nih.gov/health-topics/dash-eating-plan. Accessed 10 Mar 2020.
6. Arnett DK, Blumenthal RS, Albert MA, Michos ED, Buroker AB, Miedema MD, Goldberger ZD, Muñoz D, Hahn EJ, Smith SC, Himmelfarb CD. 2019 ACC/AHA guideline on the primary prevention of cardiovascular disease. J Am Coll Cardiol. 2019 Mar;17:26029.
7. Whelton PK, Carey RM, Aronow WS, et al. 2017 ACC/AHA/AAPA/ABC/ACPM/AGS/APhA/ASH/ASPC/NMA/PCNA guideline for the prevention, detection, evaluation, and management of high blood pressure in adults: a report of the American College of Cardiology/American Heart Association task force on clinical practice guidelines. Circulation. 2018;138(17):e426–81.
8. Appel LJ, Brands MW, Daniels SR, Karanja N, Elmer PJ, Sacks FM, et al. Dietary approaches to prevent and treat hypertension: a scientific statement from the American Heart Association. Hypertension. 2006;47:296–308.
9. Whelton PK, Appel LJ, Sacco RL, et al. Sodium, blood pressure, and cardiovascular disease: further evidence supporting the American Heart Association sodium reduction recommendations. Circulation. 2012 Dec 11;126(24):2880–9. https://doi.org/10.1161/CIR.0b013e318279acbf.
10. Welsh CE, Welsh P, Jhund P, Delles C, Celis-Morales C, Lewsey JD, et al. Urinary sodium excretion, blood pressure, and risk of future cardiovascular disease and mortality in subjects without prior cardiovascular disease. Hypertension. 2019;73:1202–9.
11. Choi HY, Park HC, Ha SK. Salt sensitivity and hypertension: a paradigm shift from kidney malfunction to vascular endothelial dysfunction. Electrolyte Blood Press. 2015 Jun 1;13(1):7–16.
12. Pimenta E, Gaddam KK, Oparil S, Aban I, Husain S, Dell'Italia LJ, Calhoun DA. Effects of dietary sodium reduction on blood pressure in subjects with resistant hypertension: results from a randomized trial. Hypertension. 2009 Sep 1;54(3):475–81.
13. Frank MS, Svetkey LP, Vollmer WM, et al. Effects on blood pressure of reduced dietary sodium and the dietary approaches to stop hypertension (DASH) diet. N Engl J Med. 2001;344:3–10. https://doi.org/10.1056/NEJM200101043440101.
14. Juraschek SP, Miller ER, Weaver CM, Appel LJ. Effects of sodium reduction and the DASH diet in relation to baseline blood pressure. J Am Coll Cardiol. 2017 Dec 4;70(23):2841–8.
15. Whelton PK, He J, Cutler JA, et al. Effects of oral potassium on blood pressure. Meta-analysis of randomized controlled clinical trials. JAMA. 1997;277:1624–32.

16. Aburto NJ, Hanson S, Gutierrez H, Hooper L, Elliott P, Cappuccio FP. Effect of increased potassium intake on cardiovascular risk factors and disease: systematic review and meta-analyses. BMJ. 2013;346:f1378.

17. Cepanec K, Vugrinec S, Cvetković T, Ranilović J. Potassium chloride-based salt substitutes: a critical review with a focus on the patent literature. Comp Rev Food Sci Food Safe. 2017;16(5):881–94.

18. Newberry SJ, Chung M, Anderson CAM, et al. Sodium and potassium intake: effects on chronic disease outcomes and risks. Comparative effectiveness review no. 206. (prepared by the RAND Southern California evidence-based practice Center under contract no. 290–2015-00010-I.) AHRQ publication no. 18-EHC009-EF. Rockville: Agency for Healthcare Research and Quality; June 2018. Posted final reports are located on the Effective Health Care Program search page. DOI: https://doi.org/10.23970/AHRQEPCCER206.

19. Greer RC, Marklund M, Anderson CAM, Cobb LK, Dalcin AT, Henry M, Appel LJ. Potassium-enriched salt substitutes as a means to lower blood pressure: benefits and risks. Hypertension. 2019 Dec 16; https://doi.org/10.1161/HYPERTENSIONAHA.119.13241. [Epub ahead of print]

20. Vollmer WM, Sacks FM, Ard J, Appel LJ, Bray GA, SimonsMorton DG, et al. Effects of diet and sodium intake on blood pressure: subgroup analysis of the DASH-sodium trial. Ann Intern Med. 2001;135(37):1019–28.

21. Bray GA, Vollmer WM, Sacks FM, Obarzanek E, Svetkcy LP, Appel LJ, et al. A further subgroup analysis of the effects of the DASH diet and three dietary sodium levels on blood pressure: results of the DASH-sodium trial. Am J Cardiol. 2004;94:222–7.

22. Erlinger TP, Vollmer WM, Svetkey LP, Appel LJ. The potential impact of nonpharmacologic population-wide blood pressure reduction on coronary heart disease events: pronounced benefits in African-Americans and hypertensives. Prev Med. 2003;37(4):327–33.

23. Thomas SJ, Booth IIIJN, Dai C, Li X, Allen N, Calhoun D, Carson AP, Gidding S, Lewis CE, Shikany JM, Shimbo D. Cumulative incidence of hypertension by 55 years of age in blacks and whites: the CARDIA study. J Am Heart Assoc. 2018 Jul 17;7(14):e007988.

24. Friedman GD, Cutter GR, Donahue RP, Hughes GH, Hulley SB, Jacobs DR, Liu K, Savage PJ. CARDIA: study design, recruitment, and some characteristics of the examined subjects. J Clin Epidemiol. 1988;41:1105–16.

25. Standards of Medical Care in Diabetes—2020. Diabetes Care. 2020 Jan;43(Supplement 1):S1–S122. https://doi.org/10.2337/dc20-Sint.

26. Mozaffari H, Ajabshir S, Alizadeh S. Dietary approaches to stop hypertension and risk of chronic kidney disease: a systematic review and meta-analysis of observational studies. Clin Nutr. 2019;39(7):2035–44. pii: S0261-5614(19)33076-6.

27. Zafarmand MH, Spanier M, Nicolaou M, Winhoven HAH, van Schaik BDC, Uitterlinden AG, et al. Influence of dietary approaches to stop hypertension-type diet, known genetic variants and their interplay on blood pressure in early childhood: ABCD study. Hypertension. 2020 Jan;75(1):59–70. https://doi.org/10.1161/HYPERTENSIONAHA.118.12292.

28. Asemi Z, Samimi M, Tabassi Z, Sabihi S, Esmaillzadeh A. A randomized controlled clinical trial investigating the effect of DASH diet on insulin resistance, inflammation, and oxidative stress in gestational diabetes. Nutrition. 2013;29:619–24.

29. Struijk EA, May AM, Wezenbeek NLW, Fransen HP, Soedamah-Muthu SS, Geelen A, et al. Adherence to dietary guidelines and cardiovascular disease risk in the EPIC-NL cohort. Int J Cardiol. 2014;176:354–9.

30. George SM, Ballard-Barbash R, Manson JE, Reedy J, Shikany JM, Subar AF, et al. Comparing indices of diet quality with chronic disease mortality risk in postmenopausal women in the women's health initiative observational study: evidence to inform national dietary guidance. Am J Epidemiol. 2014;180:616–25.

31. Blumenthal JA, Babyak MA, Hinderliter A, Watkins LL, Craighead L, Lin PH, et al. Effects of the DASH diet alone and in combination with exercise and weight loss on blood pressure and cardiovascular biomarkers in men and women with high blood pressure: the ENCORE study. Arch Intern Med. 2010;170:126–35.

32. Chiavaroli L, Viguiliouk E, Nishi SK, Mejia SB, Rahelić D, Kahleová H, Salas-Salvadó J, Kendall CW, Sievenpiper JL. DASH dietary pattern and cardiometabolic outcomes: an umbrella review of systematic reviews and meta-analyses. Nutrients. 2019 Feb;11(2):338.

33. Virani SS, Alonso A, Benjamin EJ, Bittencourt MS, Callaway CW, et al. Heart disease and stroke statistics- 2020 update: a report from the American Heart Association. Circulation. 2020;141:e1–e458.

34. Benjamin EJ, Virani SS, Callaway CW, Chamberlain AM, Chang AR, Cheng S, et al. Heart disease and stroke statistics—2018 update: a report from the American Heart Association. Circulation. 2018 Mar 20;137(12):e67–492.

35. Grundy SM, Stone NJ, Bailey AL, Beam C, Birtcher KK, Blumenthal RS, Braun LT, de Ferranti S, Faiella-Tommasino J, Forman DE, Goldberg R. 2018 AHA/ACC/AACVPR/AAPA/ABC/ACPM/ADA/AGS/APhA/ASPC/NLA/PCNA guideline on the management of blood cholesterol: a report of the American College of Cardiology/American Heart Association task force on clinical practice guidelines. J Am Coll Cardiol. 2018 Nov;10:25709.

36. Hales CM, Fryar CD, Carroll MD, Freedman DS, Ogden CL. Trends in obesity and severe obesity prevalence in US youth and adults by sex and age, 2007-2008 to 2015-2016. JAMA. 2018;319(16):1723–5.

37. Centers for Disease Control website.: division of nutrition, physical activity, and obesity, national cen-

ter for chronic disease prevention and health promotion, Accessed 19 Nov 2019.

38. McTigue KM, Garrett JM, Popkin BM. The natural history of the development of obesity in a cohort of young U.S. adults between 1981 and 1998. Ann Intern Med. 2002;136:857–64.

39. Carey RM, Muntner P, Bosworth HB, Whelton PK. Prevention and control of hypertension: JACC health promotion series. J Am Coll Cardiol. 2018 Sep 11;72(11):1278–93.

40. Monsivais P, Rehm CD, Drewnowski A. The DASH diet and diet costs among ethnic and racial groups in the United States. JAMA Intern Med. 2013 Nov 11;173(20):1922–4.

41. Beydoun MA, Fanelli-Kuczmarski MT, Poti J, Allen A, Beydoun HA, Evans MK, Zonderman AB. Longitudinal change in the diet's monetary value is associated with its change in quality and micronutrient adequacy among urban adults. PLoS One. 2018 Oct 12;13(10):e0204141.

42. Beydoun HA, Huang S, Beydoun MA, Hossain S, Zonderman AB. Mediating-moderating effect of allostatic load on the association between dietary approaches to stop hypertension diet and all-cause and cause-specific mortality: 2001–2010 national health and nutrition examination surveys. Nutrients. 2019 Oct;11(10):2311.

43. Krebs P, Duncan DT. Health app use among US mobile phone owners: a national survey. JMIR Mhealth Uhealth. 2015;3(4):e101. https://doi.org/10.2196/mhealth.4924. PMID: 26537656. PMCID: 4704953

44. Steigerwalt A, Hummel S, DiFillipo K, Scisney-Matlock M. A novel mobile app's reliability, end user satisfaction, and changes in DASH diet eating patterns over 8 weeks. Paper presented at: American Heart Association Hypertension 2019 Scientific Sessions; September 5–8, 2019: New Orleans, LA. https://www.abstractsonline.com/pp8/#!/7943/presentation/639

45. Scisney-Matlock M, Glazewhi L, McClerking C, Kachorek L. Development and evaluation of DASH diet tailored messages for hypertension treatment. Appl Nurs Res. 2006;19:78–87.

46. Parati, G., Torlasco, C. Omboni S, Pellegrini, D. Smartphone applications for hypertension management: a potential game-changer that needs more control. Curr Hypertens Rep. 2017;19(48). DOI https://doi.org/10.1007/s11906-017-0743-0.

47. McKay FH, Cheng C, Wright A, Shill J, Stephens H, Uccellini M. Evaluating mobile phone applications for health behaviour change: a systematic review. J Telemed Telecare. 2018;24(1):22–30. https://doi.org/10.1177/1357633X16673538.

48. Cardiology consultants 360. 4 Questions about the WHEELS for DASH App. https://www.consultant360.com/print-version/253310

49. Havranek EP, Mujahid MS, Barr DA, et al. American Heart Association Council on quality of care and outcomes research, council on epidemiology and prevention, council on cardiovascular and stroke nursing, council on lifestyle and cardiometabolic health, and stroke council. Social determinants of risk and outcomes for cardiovascular disease: a scientific statement from the American Heart Association. Circulation. 2015;132:873–98.

50. Rodriguez F, Ferdinand KC. Hypertension in minority populations: new guidelines and emerging concepts. Adv Chronic Kidney Dis. 2015;22:145–53.

51. Keita AD, Judd SE, Howard VJ, Carson AP, Ard JD, Fernandez JR. Associations of neighborhood area level deprivation with the metabolic syndrome and inflammation among middle- and older-age adults. BMC Public Health. 2014;14:1319.

52. Howard G, Cushman M, Moy CS, Oparil S, Muntner P, Lackland DT, Manly JJ, Flaherty ML, Judd SE, Wadley VG, Long DL, Howard VJ. Association of clinical and social factors with excess hypertension risk in black compared with white US adults. JAMA. 2018;320(13):1338–48.   https://doi.org/10.1001/jama.2018.13467. Corrected on 8 Oct 2018.

53. Shikany JM, Safford MM, Newby PK, Durant RW, Brown TM, Judd SE. Southern dietary pattern is associated with hazard of acute coronary heart disease in the reasons for geographic and racial differences in stroke (REGARDS) study. Circulation. 2015;132:804–14.   https://doi.org/10.1161/CIRCULATIONAHA.114.014421.

54. Kuehn BM. Heritage diets and culturally appropriate dietary advice May help combat chronic diseases. JAMA. 2019;322(23):2271–3.

55. Santiago-Torres M, Kratz M, Lampe JW, et al. Metabolic responses to a traditional Mexican diet compared with a commonly consumed US diet in women of Mexican descent: a randomized crossover feeding trial. Am J Clin Nutr. 2016;103(2):366–74. https://doi.org/10.3945/ajcn.115.119016.

56. McLaughlin C, Tarasuk V, Kreiger N. An examination of at-home food preparation activity among low-income, food-insecure women. J Am Diet Assoc. 2003;103(11):1506–12.

57. Hanson AJ, Kattelmann KK, McCormack LA, et al. Cooking and meal planning as predictors of fruit and vegetable intake and BMI in first-year college students. Int J Environ Res Public Health. 2019;16(14):2462.

58. Gailey S, Bruckner TA. Obesity among black women in food deserts: an "omnibus" test of differential risk. SSM Popul Health. 2019;7:100363.

59. Cooking for Your Heart and Soul. Association of Black Cardiologists. Krames Publishing. http://www.abc-patient.com/

60. Carey RM, Muntner P, Bosworth HB, Whelton PK. Prevention and control of hypertension: JACC health promotion series. J Am Coll Cardiol. 2018;72(11):1278–93. https://doi.org/10.1016/j.jacc.2018.07.008.

The Impact of Carbohydrate Restriction and Nutritional Ketosis on Cardiovascular Health

5

Dylan Lowe, Kevin C. Corbit, and Ethan J. Weiss

Introduction

Defining Cardiovascular Risk and Nutritional Ketosis

For the purposes of this chapter, we will highlight the effects of low-carbohydrate, high-fat (LCHF) diets on the following cardiovascular (CV) disease risk factors: obesity [1], hypertension [2], glycemia [3], cholesterol [4], insulin resistance [5], and non-alcoholic fatty liver disease [6]. We will focus specifically on cardiometabolic risks given the findings of the Global Burden of Diseases, Injuries, and Risk Factors Study 2016 [7].

The most recent USDA nutritional guidelines recommend that 45–65% of caloric intake derive from carbohydrates, which translates to ~225–325 g per day (standardized to a 2000 calories per diem diet). Thus, we define low-carbohydrate (LC) diets as those <200 g per day. We will distinguish LC diets from overtly ketogenic diets (KD), where possible, by studies reporting ketonemia (here, defined at total ketones or beta-hydroxybutyrate levels in serum, plasma, or whole blood) instead of dietary composition per se. While there is no clinical definition of what constitutes nutritional ketosis, a sustained level of venous blood total ketones of more than 0.5 mM in the prandial state is a common standard [8]. However, we feel a more precise definition should be arrived at through appropriate clinical trials, possibly applying different levels of ketosis to varying outcomes (e.g., weight loss, insulin, and glucose homeostasis, low-density lipoprotein cholesterol [LDL-C]). Further, defining the composition of the high-fat component of low-carbohydrate diets is of importance given the potential association of saturated fat intake with adverse CV outcomes [9].

Ketogenesis and Ketolysis

The ketone bodies (KB) acetoacetate, beta-hydroxybutyrate (BOHB), and acetone are generated predominently in the liver from acetyl-CoA, utilizing ketogenic amino acids or fatty acids (FA) as substrates. Catabolism of ketogenic amino acids accounts for only ~4% of KB formation, meaning FA are the dominant ketogenic substrate [10]. FA acyl chains are transported across mitochondrial membranes by carnitine palmitoyltransferase 1 and 2 (CPT1 and CPT2) to undergo beta-oxidation, resulting in acetyl-CoA formation and condensation by thiolase to acetoacetyl-CoA (AcAc-CoA). Mitochondrial 3-hydroxymethylglutaryl-CoA synthase (HMGCS2) subsequently drives the condensation of AcAc-CoA with acetyl-CoA to

D. Lowe · K. C. Corbit · E. J. Weiss (✉)
The Cardiovascular Research Institute, University of California, San Francisco, CA, USA
e-mail: Dylan.lowe@ucsf.edu; Kevin.corbit@ucsf.edu; Ethan.weiss@ucsf.edu

© Springer Nature Switzerland AG 2021
M. J. Wilkinson et al. (eds.), *Prevention and Treatment of Cardiovascular Disease*, Contemporary Cardiology, https://doi.org/10.1007/978-3-030-78177-4_5

generate HMG-CoA, the fate-committing step of ketogenesis. HMG-CoA is cleaved by HMG-CoA lysase (HMGCL) to generate acetyl-CoA and the KB acetoacetate, which can be further reversibly reduced to BOHB by BOHB dehydrogenase (BDH1). Acetoacetate can further spontaneously decarboxylate to acetone, which can be detected in breath in extreme cases such as ketoacidosis (i.e., serum ketones >5 mM with hyperglycemia >250 mg/dL and arterial blood pH <7.3). KBs are finally exported from hepatocytes into the circulation via the MCT1 and MCT2 transporters.

KB are avidly taken up from blood into peripheral tissues by monocarboxylate transporter-mediated activity and mitochondrially oxidized. Acetoacetate is converted to AcAc-CoA by succinyl-CoA-dependent transferase (succinyl-CoA:3-ketoacid-CoA transferase, SCOT), the key reaction permitting utilization of KB as fuel. AcAc-CoA is cleaved by ACAT1 to produce two molecules of acetyl-CoA, which are then oxidized in the TCA cycle and respiratory chain for ATP synthesis.

The Physiological Uses of Ketones

KB are produced during times of fasting and starvation, when relative hypoglycemia persists. Further, lack of nutrient intake suppresses insulin secretion, promoting adipocyte lipolysis and consequently FA (i.e., ketogenic substrate) liberation and release. KB are also used as alternative fuel sources during the neo-natal period, post-exercise, pregnancy, and during LCHF diets (nutritional ketosis). In addition to energy substrates, KB act as signaling molecules, inhibiting histone deacetylases, suppressing sympathetic tone, and reducing metabolic rate [11]. Interestingly, KB inhibit adipocyte lipolysis, and hence their own ketogenic substrates, possibly as a negative feedback loop to prevent ketoacidosis [12].

The Rationale for and Against Low Carbohydrate-Based Nutrition

High intake of carbohydrates has been associated with CV risk factors including hyperinsulinemia, hyperglycemia, and hypertriglyceridemia. Diets high in fat, especially saturated fats, have also been associated with increased mortality and CV events [13]. Many rationales have been proposed to support both LC and low-fat (especially saturated fat)-based diets and here we highlight two.

Carbohydrate-Insulin Model (CIM) This model posits that high carbohydrate intake induces postprandial hyperinsulinemia and a sequalae of events leading to adiposity and obesity. Further, the carbohydrate-insulin model (CIM) suggests that carbohydrate restriction (and replacement with fat) leads to decreased insulin levels in the fasting and fed state and thus a decrease in lipogenesis leading to weight loss and primarily fat loss. Comprehensive clinical reviews supporting [14] and falsifying [15] the CIM have been published, leading to equivocal conclusions. In contrast, the uniformly positive association of hyperinsulinemia—dietary [16], pharmacological [17], and genetic [18]—with CV disease risk is less confounding (discussed below). However, it is challenging to dissociate the effects of insulin from glycemia on ultimate CV outcomes.

Diet-Heart Hypothesis Proposed by Dr. Ancel Keys in the 1950s, this hypothesis links dietary saturated fat with hypercholesterolemia and incidence of CV disease. It follows from this, then, that reducing saturated fat intake attenuates blood cholesterol levels and, thereby, the risk of CV disease. Many randomized controlled trial (RCT) support the hypothesis and the American Heart Association (AHA) recommends lowering dietary saturated fat [13]. However, as with the CIM, the validity of the diet-heart hypothesis has been called into question [19, 20]. Much of the debate centers on the effect of replacing dietary saturated with polyunsaturated fats in regards to CV outcomes and mortality. Meta-analyses have supported both sides of the debate, highlighting the challenges around proper design, and interpretation of human interventional dietary studies (discussed in detail below).

Collectively, it is currently not possible to definitely associate high fat-based KD regimens with CV disease risk. There is consensus, however, that calorie-for-calorie replacement of saturated fat with unspecified carbohydrate does not result in reduced CV disease events, for example, [13]. Thus, a potential unifying approach would be a low carbohydrate (LC), moderate protein diet enriched in unsaturated fats, and following current AHA guidelines to not exceed 5–6% of daily calories derived from saturated fats.

Ketonemia: Nutritional Ketosis Versus Diabetic Ketoacidosis (DKA)

Hyperketonemia is associated with pathological diabetic ketoacidosis (DKA), a life-threatening complication of diabetes manifesting with blood ketone levels of >10 mM. Nutritional ketosis occurs in the context of very LC intake, generally less than 50 g/day, and achieves blood levels of 0.5–3 mM [8]. The main clinical difference between the two is the co-presentation of hyperglycemia with DKA while dietary ketosis is coincident with eu- or hypoglycemia. This suggests functional insulin signaling in the latter but not the former. Ketogenesis self-regulates via a negative feedback mechanism of ketones on adipocyte lipolysis [12], and it has been suggested that insulin attenuates ketogenesis (though the precise mechanism remains unknown), in addition to inhibiting adipocyte lipolysis-mediated substrate liberation, in a liver-autonomous manner [21]. Thus, DKA may result from loss of insulin-mediated inhibition of adipocyte lipolysis and anti-ketogenic mechanisms within the hepatocyte itself. In contrast, reduced-insulin levels in the setting of preserved or enhanced adipose insulin sensitivity may promote benign nutritional ketosis when dietary carbohydrate is limited.

Where Do the Potential Benefits of KD Come from?

There are two macronutrient variables in a KD: low carbohydrate (LC) and high fat (HF). However, it is not known if one or both variables drive potential metabolic benefits and, how much, if any, the benefit derives from ketones themselves. Further, it remains to be clarified if any weight loss realized following a KD intervention is solely responsible for improvements in metabolic markers. LCHF diets often result in reduced total caloric intake and, hence, weight loss. Thus, the most parsimonious explanation for reduced CV disease risk markers with LCHF diets is weight reduction. Indeed, several studies have demonstrated statistical weight loss following KD feeding in obese individuals with or without type 2 diabetes (Table 5.1).

Only one study, to our knowledge, attempted to dissociate weight loss from the metabolic benefit of KD. In this study, daily caloric intake was fixed at ~2950 kcal for obese patients with metabolic syndrome, while the subjects (N = 16 for each diet) were randomized to high (~420 g/day), medium (~234 g/day), or low (~45 g/day) carbohydrate diets at a fixed protein intake of ~146 g/day for 4 weeks [37]. Interestingly, saturated fat accounted for ~50% of total fat intake in all three diets. While weight remained constant, 9/16 patients on the LC diet no longer met the requirements of a metabolic syndrome diagnosis. Of the 16 patients, 3 and 1 patients in the mid and high carbohydrate cohorts, respectively, also were no longer classified as having metabolic syndrome

Table 5.1 Clinical trials of low-carbohydrate or ketogenic diet in overweight/obese or diabetes with >25 subjects for controlled trials or >15 subjects for crossover studies

Author year	Population (n)	Design	Duration	Dietary intervention	Calorie matched?	Weight loss	Body composition	CVD markers	Glucose homeostasis	Comments
Samaha et al. [22]	132 obese subjects	RCT	6 months	<30 g carb intake vs 30% TE from fat	Not matched	−5.8 ± 8.6 kg vs −1.9 ± 4.2 kg		TG (mg/dL) −38 ± 80 vs −7 ± 54; TC NS; HDL NS; LDL NS	Glu (mg/dL) −11 ± 24 vs −2 ± 21; ins (mM/L) −6 ± 16 vs 1 ± 10	
Yancy et al. [23]	120 overweight, hyperlipidemic subjects	RCT	24 weeks	<20 g carb intake vs 30% TE from fat	Not matched	−12.0 kg vs −6.5 kg		TG (mg/dL) −74.2 vs −27.9 TC NS; HDL (mg/dL) 5.5 vs −1.6; LDL NS		Subjects in KD group with urinary ketones of trace or greater was 86% (47 of 55) at 2 weeks and 42% (19 of 45) at 24 weeks. Subjects in this group with moderate or greater urinary ketones 64% (35 of 55) at 2 weeks and 18% (8 of 45) at 24 weeks.
Johnstone et al. [24]	17 obese men	Crossover	4 weeks/arm	30% P, 4% C, 66% F vs 30% P, 35% C, 35% F	Not matched	−5.8% vs −4.0%	FM NS; FFM NS	TG NS; TC (mmol/L) −3.9 vs −0.92; HDL NS; LDL (mmol/L) −0.18 vs −0.67	Glu (mmol/L) −0.62 vs −0.35; ins (IU/L) −3.98 vs −1.41; HOMA-IR −1.22 vs −0.52	*ad libitum* eating, KD subjects ate less but reported higher satiation
Saslow et al. [25]	34 overweight/obese and Prediabetes/T2DM	RCT	3 months	20–50 g net carbs vs 45–50% TE from carbs	Not matched (−696.9 kcal/day vs −792.1 kcal/day difference from baseline)	Not significant (−5.5 kg vs −2.6 kg)		TG NS; HDL NS; LDL NS; sBP NS; dBP NS	Glu NS; ins NS; HOMA2-IR NS; HbA1C −0.6 vs 0.0	

Study	Subjects	Design	Duration	Intervention	Matched	Weight change	WC/FM	Lipids/BP	Glucose	Notes
Moreno et al. [26]	79 obese subjects	RCT	12 months	<50 g carbs vs 45–55% carbs	Not matched	−19.9 ± 12.3 kg vs −7.0 ± 56 kg	WC (cm) −18.4 ± 10.4 vs −7.0 ± 6.3; FM (kg) −16 vs −5.6	TG NS; TC (mg/dL) −14 vs −1.9; HDL NS; LDL NS.	Glu NS; HbA1C NS	KD group went through severe calorie restriction with gradual increase in calorie intake. Control arm aimed for a 10% calorie deficit. TC was significantly different at baseline (207.2 vs 185.9)
Yancy et al. [27]	146 overweight/obese subjects	RCT	48 weeks	<20 g carb intake vs <30% TE from fat + Orlistat	Not matched	Not significant (−9.5 kg vs −11.4 kg)	WC NS	TG NS; TC NS; HDL NS; LDL NS sBP (mmHg) −5.94 vs 1.50; dBP (mmHg) −4.53 vs 0.43	Glu NS; ins NS; HbA1C NS	Only 13% of KD subjects had urinary ketones >0.9 mmol/L at 48 weeks
Moreno et al. [28]	45 obese subjects	RCT	24 months	<50 g carbs vs 45–55% carbs	Not matched	−12.5 kg vs −5.2 kg	WC (cm) −11.6 vs −4.1; FM (kg) −8.8 vs −3.8; VAT (g) −666 vs −200			Follow up to Moreno et al. [28] KD group went through severe calorie restriction with gradual increase in calorie intake. Control arm aimed for a 10% calorie deficit.
Goday et al. [29]	89 obese with T2DM	RCT	4 months	<50 g carbs vs 45–60% carbs	Not matched	−14.7 kg vs −5.05 kg	WC (cm) −12 vs −5.4	TG NS; TC NS; HDL NS; LDL NS	Glu NS, ins NS, HOMA-IR −3.4 vs −1.2; HbA1C NS	KD group went through severe calorie restriction with gradual increase in calorie intake. Control arm aimed for a 500-1000 kcal/day deficit.

(continued)

Table 5.1 (continued)

Author year	Population (n)	Design	Duration	Dietary intervention	Calorie matched?	Weight loss	Body composition	CVD markers	Glucose homeostasis	Comments
Hall et al. [30]	17 overweight/obese men	Crossover	4 weeks/arm	15% P, 5% C, 80% F vs 15% P, 50% C, 35% F	Calorie matched			TG decreased from 104 ± 6.4 to 85.4 ± 6	Glu NS; ins (mU/L) decreased from 7.92 to 6.27	Energy expenditure increased by ~100 kcal/day on KD
Saslow et al. [31]	25 overweight subjects with T2DM	RCT	32 weeks	20–50 g net carbs vs ADA "create your plate" diet	Not matched	−12.7 kg vs −3.0 kg		TG (mg/dL) −60.1 vs −6.2; HDL NS; LDL NS		
Saslow et al. [31]	34 overweight/obese and Prediabetes/T2DM	RCT	12 months	20–50 g net carbs vs 45–50% TE from carbs	Not matched	−7.0 kg vs −1.7 kg		TG NS; HDL NS; LDL NS; sBP NS; dBP NS	Ins NS; HOMA2-IR NS; HbA1c −0.5 vs −0.2	
Cohen et al. [32]	45 women with ovarian/endometrial cancer (average BMI >30)	RCT	12 weeks	<20 g carbs vs American Cancer Society dietary guidelines	Not matched		FM (kg) −5.2 vs −2.9, VAT (g) −177 vs −126		Glu NS, Ins (mU/L) −3.8 vs −2.1	
Genco et al. [33]	80 obese subjects	RCT	2 months	<800 kcal/day, <100 g carbs vs 1000 kcal/day, ~160 g carbs	Not matched	−8.1 ± 1.1 vs −3.0 ± 1.2		Improved TG levels	Greater diabetes remission	Diet intervention began 4 months after intragastric balloon surgery (Orbera)
Bhanpuri et al. [34]	349 T2DM patients	NRCT	12 months	Virta continuous care intervention vs usual care (ADA guidelines)	Not matched	−13.8 kg vs −1.1 kg		Change from baseline: TG −24.4%; HDL-C +18.1%; LDL-C +9.9%; LDL particle size +1.1%; decreased 10-year ASCVD risk		

Phillips et al. [35]	RCT	8 weeks	1750 kcal/day. 16 g net carbs vs 246 g net carbs	Calorie matched	Not significant (−4.37 kg vs −4.87 kg)		TG NS; TC (mmol/L) +0.94 vs −0.63; HDL (mmol/L) +0.40 vs −0.11; LDL (mmol/L) +0.70 vs −0.40	Bedtime glucose (mmol/L) 5.70 ± 1.20 vs 6.28 ± 0.73; HbA1C NS
Di Lorenzo et al. [36]	Crossover	1 month	30–50 g carbs vs >70 g carbs	Not matched	Not significant			Glu NS; ins NS
Hyde et al. [37]	Crossover	4 weeks/arm	Eucaloric, protein constant between groups. Low carb (6% TE), medium carb (32% TE), high carb (57% TE)	Calorie matched	No change between groups	No change in FM or WC	TG (mg/dL) −57 vs +12 vs +22; HDL (mg/dL) +3 vs −2 vs −3. Low-carb diet increases LDL size and decreased small, dense LDL particles	

RCT Randomized controlled trial, *NRCT* Non-random controlled trial, *%TE* Percentage of total energy intake from macronutrient, *P* Protein, *C* Carbohydrate, *F* Fat, *NS* Not significantly different between groups, *FM* Fat Mass, *FFM* Fat-free mass, *WC* Waist circumference, *VAT* Visceral adipose tissue, *TG* Triglyceride, *TC* Total cholesterol, *HDL* High-density lipoprotein, *LDL* Low-density lipoprotein, *sBP* Systolic blood pressure, *dBP* Diastolic blood pressure, *Glu* Fasting glucose, *Ins* Fasting insulin

after the 4-week study. LDL-C was in the clinically normal range for all participants, with the LC cohort having a preponderance of less atherogenic large, buoyant LDL particles (phenotype A). The authors concluded that adherence to an LC diet improved metabolic syndrome independent of weight loss. While promising, we encourage more similar trials with longer adherence to validate and extend the findings of this study.

To our knowledge, no trials using a diet fixed on total calories and LC (e.g., <50 g/day) with variable fat have been reported. Such a study would be important in unraveling the relative contributions of LC and HF. Further, the relative benefit of ketones themselves needs resolution, as a cause-and-effect conundrum exists for LC and ketonemia. Given the reported benefits of exogenous ketones on HF [38] coupled with studies demonstrating glycemic and lipemic effects of LC diets without ketogenesis (see below), it is tempting to speculate that ketones will influence some but not all of the potential benefits of LC diets.

The Historical Clinical Uses of Low Carbohydrate Diets

Modern clinical employment of starvation to treat epilepsy goes back at least a century [39] and has, in general, been successful. Given the difficulties of adhering to prolonged fasting, attempts to mimic physiological starvation by dietary intervention were made. Woodyatt, in 1921, noted that both fasting and high-fat low-carbohydrate diets increased ketonemia and proposed that excessive carbohydrate exacerbated diabetes [40]. Concurrently, Wilder proposed the use of ketonemia-inducing diets to treat epilepsy [41]. Fifty years later, a longitudinal survey of over 1000 epilepsy patients treated by ketogenic diet found 52% and 27% of patients exhibited complete and partial control, respectively [39].

The most prevalent clinical use of ketogenic diets, arguably, is for GLUT1 deficiency syndrome. GLUT1 is encoded by *SLC2A1* and is responsible for glucose uptake into neurons;

hence loss of GLUT1 function results in neuroglycopenia and seizures [42]. Induction of dietary ketosis has been successfully employed to provide an alternative neuronal energy source and reduce symptoms [42]. However, growth suppression during adolescence has been observed, presumably due to the low amount of protein in ketogenic diets [43]. Regardless, chronic use of KD regimens in GLUT1 deficient syndrome demonstrates long-term safety and efficacy.

Low-Carbohydrate "Fad" Diets

A number of nutritional trends centered on carbohydrate restriction have attracted attention in popular culture. Three in particular—Atkins, Paleo, and KD—have gained commercial and some scientific consideration.

Atkins Developed in the 1960s by cardiologist Robert Atkins and first popularly published in 1972, the Atkins diet is an LC diet based on unrestricted protein and caloric intake. The diet centers on a restrictive induction phase of <20 g of carbohydrate per day to achieve target weight loss, and gradually increasing by ~5 g per week, reaching a value of 40–90 g per day to maintain weight loss [44]. It is unclear if Atkins diet adherents achieve nutritional ketosis, and a "modified" Atkins diet has been used that promotes fat over protein intake to, specifically, induce nutritional ketosis [45].

The first RCT specifically evaluating the Atkins diet was published in 2003 [46]. This 1-year study examined weight loss and cardiovascular risk markers in 63 obese men and women who were randomized to an Atkins-style diet or a high-carb, low-fat "conventional" diet. While weight loss was greater in the Atkins group at 3 and 6 months, there was no significant difference in weight at 1 year between the two diets. Serum triglycerides were lower in the Atkins group at 3 and 12 months. However, total cholesterol and LDL-C were significantly higher in the Atkins group at 3 months, but there was no significant difference at 6 and 12 months. HDL was significantly higher in the Atkins group at 6 and 12 months. It is important to note that protein and fiber intake between groups was not controlled in this study, so while carbohydrate and fat intake was the focus of this study, protein and fiber content was not held constant and likely varied between study groups. Additionally, type of fat (animal vs plant, saturated vs unsaturated, etc.) was not included in the diet prescriptions. Attrition for this study was high; of the 63 subjects that started the study, 14 dropped out prior to the 3-month mark, another 7 before the 6-month mark, and 5 more before the end of the 1-year study (only 59% of participants completed the full year). The caveats listed here are not unique to this study. Rather, these caveats are systemic to dietary clinical trials and should be considered when interpreting results.

Other studies examining the Atkins diet found similar results. In one, the high-fat (HF) Atkins diet, high-protein (HP) Zone diet, and a high-carbohydrate (HC) diet found HF and HP diets lead to greater weight loss than the HC diet and was accompanied by lowered serum triglycerides [47]. However, LDL-C levels in the HF Atkins group were significantly higher than in the HP group. Likewise, a study of 262 overweight premenopausal women found that changes in LDL-C levels were less favorable in the Atkins group compared to other diets at 2 months but normalized by 6 and 12 months [44]. In obese patients with type 2 diabetes, the Atkins diet improved glucose homeostasis but resulted in increased HDL, LDL-C, and total cholesterol and decreased triglycerides after 24 weeks [48]. In normal-weight subjects, an LCHF Atkins diet also raised LDL-C as well as apolipoprotein B, total cholesterol, and HDL [49]. In this study, there was no difference in triglycerides between groups.

Taken together, the majority of studies examining the Atkins diet demonstrate a decrease in serum triglycerides and an increase in serum LDL-C that is typically transient and normalizes after a few months. However, not all studies reached the same conclusions. One study found that LDL-C levels are unaffected by the Atkins

diet, but LDL particle size increased following an Atkins-style diet [50]. Another study found that while the Atkins diet had no effect on cholesterol levels, triglycerides decreased in subjects in the LC Atkins group [51]. This study also reported that the LC Atkins diet leads to reduced flow-mediated dilation relative to low-fat diets indicating that LC Atkins-style diets may have negative effects on cardiovascular risk.

Paleo Credited to gastroenterologist Walter Voegtlin, this diet mimics a supposed "paleolithic" way of eating, emphasizing increased consumption of lean meat, fruits, vegetables, nuts, and seeds, while excluding grains, legumes, refined sugars, added salt, and dairy [52]. Although no specific macronutrient guidance has been uniformly agreed upon, attempts to estimate Paleo diet macronutrient composition has been given as 38% protein, 23% carbohydrate, and 39% fat (https://nutrition.ucdavis.edu/sites/g/files/dgvnsk426/files/inline-files/fact-pro-paleo-diet.pdf). If followed, the Paleo diet will not result in nutritional ketosis.

The first clinical trial examining the effects of the Paleo diet was published in 2009 [53]. The study was small; only nine non-obese healthy adults were recruited for this short-term (10-day) study. By design, subjects did not lose any weight throughout the study yet experienced significant reductions in blood pressure, improved arterial distensibility, reduced total cholesterol, LDL-C and triglycerides, and improved insulin sensitivity [53]. Other short-term studies also found promising improvements in blood lipid profiles following a Paleo diet relative to control diets. When compared to control diets, the Paleo diet leads to reductions in weight and triglyceride levels in five out of eight studies examined [54–58], decreased total cholesterol in five out of eight studies [54–57, 59], and improved HDL in 4 out of 8 studies examined [54–57]. Two of these studies also reported decreased LDL-C in Paleo subjects [56, 57]. Other studies revealed that while the Paleo diet did improve blood lipid profiles, the changes were not significantly different than control diets [60, 61]. Out of the seven studies that examined markers of insulin sensitivity, one found significant changes in HbA1C [54] and one found changes in fasting insulin and HOMA-IR [55]. One study found that HOMA-IR was significantly improved in the Paleo group relative to baseline, but significance was lost when compared to the control group [58]. It is difficult to determine if these changes are unique to Paleo or just a result of calorie deficit-induced weight loss.

While these results seemed promising, long-term RCT studies revealed that the Paleo diet did not fare much better than control diets. One study found that while the Paleo diet provided a modest improvement in weight loss in the short-term (6 months) in overweight and obese subjects, there was no difference in weight loss between diets at 24 months (a familiar trend in weight loss trials) [59]. Likewise, systolic and diastolic blood pressure and total cholesterol decreased at 6 months but returned to baseline by 24 months. Triglycerides and LDL-C decreased throughout the 24-month study, but this was not significantly different in the Paleo group than the reference diet [59]. A second long-term study revealed that although the Paleo diet improved weight, body fat, liver fat, total cholesterol, triglycerides, and LDL-C at 6 months, only triglycerides were significantly improved at 24 months [57]. Although both of these studies showed some improvement in fasting insulin and/or glucose at 6 months, no significant differences were observed at the end of the 24-month studies [57, 59]. Thus, it is unclear at this time if the Paleo diet offers any cardiometabolic effects independent of calorie restriction and weight loss.

Ketogenic Diet This term was coined and the diet developed in the 1920s to mimic fasting, which had been shown to be beneficial in reducing epileptic seizures [39]. The KD has been used extensively in the setting of epilepsy, while it began to be adopted clinically for diabetes treatment by Woodyatt and others in the early- to mid-twentieth century. The goal of the KD is to induce a level of ketonemia well below pathological ketoacidosis by dietary instead of starvation-based means, leading to "nutritional ketosis". The KD requires sustained intake of very LC (20–50 g per day) and is considered moderate protein (~1.5 g/day per kg of reference weight) [8]. The remainder of the diet is composed of fat, and no guidance on the type of dietary fat has been provided. Given the long history of use in epilepsy, a more comprehensive clinical picture has developed for the KD compared to other LC diets; hence, this chapter will concentrate primarily on the effects of KD on CV health and disease risk. Although KD regimens have been around for many years, its popularity has exploded recently. A PubMed search of human clinical trials with "Ketogenic Diet" in the title or abstract yields 164 results, 67 of which were published in just the past 5 years (2015–2019). We find the most pressing question to be whether a KD is superior to other weight loss methods when calories are controlled. In other words, does a KD confer additional benefits independently of weight loss?

Effects of KD in the Overweight/Obese and T2D Population

To comprehensively address the efficacy of KD regimens in this population, we examined only clinical trials that had a control arm and >25 subjects for controlled trials or >15 subjects for crossover studies (Table 5.1). Of the 16 studies that reported weight loss, 10 studies reported significant reductions in weight conferred by KD compared to a control diet [22–24, 26–29, 31, 33, 34, 62]. Additionally, out of the six long-term trials (>6 months), five demonstrated significant weight loss at the end of the study [26, 28, 31, 34, 62]. Of the six studies that also measured body composition, three studies demonstrated a greater loss in fat mass [26, 28, 32]. Both studies that measured visceral adipose tissue found significant decreases [28, 32]. It is important to note that calorie intake between diets was not matched in any of these studies. Only three studies were calorie-matched between diet arms, and all three studies found no difference in weight loss or fat loss between

KD and control diets [30, 37, 63]. One study aimed to determine how energy expenditure is affected by KD and reported a significant albeit minor increase in energy expenditure [30]. Whether this minor change in energy expenditure has any effect on weight loss in patients is unclear. Together, these data confirm that KD is effective for weight loss but is not superior to other diets in terms of weight loss and fat loss when matched for calories.

Thirteen out of sixteen studies reported improvements in one or more markers of insulin sensitivity after KD (fasting insulin, glucose, HOMA-IR, HbA1C, or diabetes remittance) [22, 24, 25, 29–37, 62–64]. HbA1C was the most commonly improved marker in 50% of studies [25, 31, 34, 62] and was improved in three out of five long-term studies [31, 34, 62]. Importantly, insulin sensitivity improved in four out of the six studies where no weight change was observed [25, 30, 37, 63], suggesting that improvements in insulin sensitivity may occur independently of weight loss in KD subjects.

The effects of KD on markers of CVD risk are less clear. Total cholesterol decreased in one study [26], increased in one study [63], and did not change in the other six studies [22–24, 29, 33, 65]. HDL increased in 4 out of 12. LDL-C was unchanged in most studies but did increase in two studies (which were associated with increased HDL as well) [34, 63]. Triglycerides decreased in half of the studies that measured it [22, 23, 30, 33–37, 62] and blood pressure decreased in a third of the studies that reported it [34, 65]. C-reactive protein significantly decreased in only one study [34]. The only study that examined a calorie-matched KD and reported in-depth CV markers demonstrated that KD increased LDL size and decreased small, dense LDL particles even though total LDL-C was unchanged [37]. Together, these data do not suggest that a KD is inherently harmful to CV health in the context of weight loss in overweight and obese subjects. However, the effects of a KD on CV health in the context of weight maintenance in normal-weight subjects remain to be explored. Importantly, no study of the KD has yet evaluated effects on hard CV outcomes.

Are there Weight-Loss-Independent Effects with KD Feeding?

As mentioned previously, when matched for calories, most studies report that a KD does not lead to greater weight loss than other diets [30, 37, 63]. Yet, even without weight loss, KD improved markers of insulin sensitivity in all three studies [30, 37, 63] and triglycerides decreased in two [30, 37]. One study reported an increase in total cholesterol, HDL and LDL-C [63] while another only saw a significant increase in HDL as well as a significant improvement in LDL particle size [37]. The discrepancy in CVD outcomes between these studies is likely due to differences in fat intake composition which will be described in more detail later.

While it is generally agreed that calorie consumption is key for weight and fat loss, a few studies have found conflicting results. One study examining a KD versus a low-fat diet found a significant decrease in weight and fat loss in men on KD even though their daily energy intake was higher [66]. Men on a KD lost approximately 5 kg of fat while the low-fat group lost ~3 kg fat over the ~50-day study. The discrepancy between this study and other studies is unclear. One possibility is the room for error in self-reported energy-intake. Another possibility is that a KD leads to increased resting energy expenditure/total energy expenditure, although this study reported no change in resting energy expenditure; however, other studies have found a small but significant increase in total energy expenditure after KD [30]. It is possible that, over time, this small increase in energy expenditure may provide a slight advantage for weight loss.

Should Healthy Individuals Follow a KD?

Although much is known about how a KD affects overweight and T2D subjects, how a KD affects healthy, normal weight subjects with normal insulin sensitivity—arguably the largest adherents to commercialized KD regimens—remains unknown. Additionally, the majority of KD studies are performed with the intention of weight loss; little is known how a KD affects health after long-term weight maintenance.

There are a few studies examining KD in metabolically healthy individuals. One study found that just 3 days of a eucaloric KD increases the metabolic clearance rate of insulin by 10%, which corresponded to a 10% decrease in steady-state insulin levels [67]. Another single-arm KD study reported a significant decrease in fasting glucose, insulin, and IGF-1 [68]. This study also reported decreased alkaline phosphatase and alanine transaminase, suggesting that liver health may be improved. However, there was no control arm and the study participants lost 2 kg body weight, so it is difficult to determine if these changes are unique to KD or simply the result of weight loss. A potentially worrisome trend in the few studies of KD in healthy individuals is a significant increase in LDL-C and total cholesterol [68–70]. However, one study suggests that lipid composition of a KD determines the CV risk outcomes [71]. This study compared two KD that were matched for all macronutrients except polyunsaturated and saturated fats (POLY = 60%, 15% and SAT = 15%, 60%, respectively). This study demonstrated that the SAT diet did not improve glucose, insulin, or triglyceride levels, and it did raise LDL-C and total cholesterol. On the other hand, the POLY diet decreased glucose and triglyceride levels and improved insulin sensitivity and had no effect on cholesterol levels. It is also interesting to note that the POLY diet increased circulating ketones significantly more than SAT, even though total fat, carbohydrate, and protein intake were the same [71]. More studies would need to confirm these findings, and long-term studies investigating if KD has a negative impact on CVD risk are warranted.

KD: Potential Mechanisms and Emerging Questions

Obesity: Is Satiety the Key to Weight Loss?

Obesity has one of the strongest associations with negative CV outcomes, and is an indepen-dent risk factor for dyslipidemia, insulin resistance, hypertension, and atherosclerosis [1]. As little as 5% weight loss improves CV disease risk markers in obese patients [72]. Acute weight loss is a common event observed following KD feeding, and hypophagia has been reported by several trials interrogating the efficacy of KD in obesity, which suggests that KD may increase satiation [73]. However, the mechanism driving satiety is unknown. Given the difficulties of attaining and maintaining weight loss due to hunger drive, the ultimate benefit of a KD may be caloric restriction through increased satiation and decreased food intake [24, 74].

Type 2 Diabetes: Weight Loss Versus Insulinopenia?

KD feeding has shown remarkable efficacy in the setting of type 2 diabetes [75–77]. The simplest explanation for reductions and even cessation of diabetic medication following long-term KD feeding is weight loss [78]. However, glycemic benefit independent of weight loss has been reported for an LC diet [37], although if these patients achieved nutritional ketosis was not reported. Another common finding with KD feeding in both healthy and type 2 diabetics is insulinopenia [77]. Reductions in circulating insulin levels, especially in the setting of hyperinsulinemia, promote both weight loss [79] and insulin sensitivity [80]. Thus, a KD may improve type 2 diabetic traits by weight loss-dependent (e.g., satiety and subsequent caloric restriction) as well as independent (e.g., reduced insulin levels due to reduced carbohydrate intake) mechanisms.

Non-alcoholic Fatty Liver Disease (NAFLD): The Heart of the Matter?

An emerging condition is non-alcoholic fatty liver disease (NAFLD), affecting 25–30% of adults in Western countries where it often co-exists with obesity and type 2 diabetes [6]. Weight loss was reported to improve not only liver disease but also cardio-metabolic risk factors in NAFLD patients

[81]. However, meta-analyses of 34,000 patients linked NAFLD as an independent predictor of long-term CV outcomes, suggesting that fatty liver in itself is tightly correlated with CV disease risk [82]. The process of *de novo lipogenesis* (DNL), the production of triglycerides from non-fat sources (e.g., glucose, fructose) has been implicated in the etiology of NAFLD, and clinical trials with small molecule inhibitors of DNL have demonstrated efficacy in both NAFLD and its manifestation non-alcoholic steatohepatitis [83]. Interestingly, ketogenesis is inhibited with the increasing hepatic fat burden [84] and the DNL product, malonyl-CoA, directly inhibits ketogenesis by blocking the mitochondrial entry of fatty acids [85]. Thus, carbohydrate restriction will simultaneously decrease or even inhibit DNL via loss of substrate (e.g., glucose, fructose) while increasing ketogenesis by reducing malonyl-CoA (a product of DNL)-mediated inhibition of CPT1. KD regimens, in particular, have been employed successfully to reduce the hepatic fat burden and disease severity in NASH [86, 87].

Hyperinsulinemia: Cause or Consequence?

A major goal of LC diets is to lower circulating insulin levels. Hyperinsulinemia and insulin therapy promote adiposity [88], while insulin insufficiency, in the setting of type 1 diabetes, is associated with reduced fat mass [89]. In addition to adiposity, potential links between hyperinsulinemia and other CV disease risk factors have been documented for at least 40 years, but is not without controversy [90, 91]. Several confounding factors may be at the root of the disparate interpretations, including the definition of hyperinsulinemia (fasting vs oral glucose load-stimulated), sex, diabetic status, and co-segregating factors such as hyperglycemia, hypertriglyceridemia, hypercholesterolemia, and insulin resistance [92]. This classic "chicken or egg" conundrum derives from the complicated and inter-connected nature of regulatory and counter-regulatory metabolism. In addition, endogenous

and pharmacological hyperinsulinemia have mitogenic effects in both the vascular and cardiomyocyte compartments [93], further challenging the prospects of isolating the independent effects of hyperinsulinemia, which has been reported to increase CV disease risk [94]. To our knowledge, no adverse CV outcomes have been reported for either hypoinsulinemia or insulin sensitivity. Thus, reducing insulin levels should, at worse, be benign.

Beyond Diets: Are Exogenous Ketones a Therapy for Heart Failure?

Myocardial tissue from patients with severe heart failure utilizes the ketone body BOHB [95]. This observation may be phenomenological or a metabolic adaptation, either beneficial or maladaptive. To determine this, 16 patients with chronic heart failure and reduced ejection fraction (HFrEF) were randomized in a crossover design to placebo or experimental BOHB infusions [38]. The 3-hour experimental infusion during the study reached steady-state levels of plasma BOHB between ~0.4 and 3.0 mM, the same levels achieved via dietary ketosis. BOHB significantly increased cardiac output, stroke volume, heart rate, oxygen consumption, and left ventricular ejection fraction. Myocardial external energy efficiency was unaffected. It was concluded that BOHB has beneficial hemodynamic effects in the setting of HFrEF at a physiologically relevant concentration. This suggests that LC, KD regimens may be protective or even therapeutic for heart failure.

Beyond Diets: Sodium-Glucose Co-Transporter 2 Inhibitors (SGLT2i)

Sodium-glucose co-transporter 2 inhibitors (SGLT2i) have entered the clinical toolbox for type 2 diabetes treatment. This class of drugs lowers glycemia by preventing glucose reabsorption from renal tubules [96]. An interesting manifestation of SGLT2i treatment is euglycemic ketoacidosis [97], which has been attributed to dehydration and insulinopenia [98]. Outcome trials with SGLT2i have demonstrated lower rates of primary composite CV outcomes and all-cause mortality, accompanied by reductions in HF hospitalizations [99]. It has been hypothesized that the reductions in CV disease are due, in part, to ketosis [100]. Given the similarities between SGLT2i and KD—reductions in glycemia and insulinemia coupled with increased ketonemia—the CV outcomes, including HF, upon long-term KD feeding should be determined. Importantly, there is a significant risk of euglycemic ketoacidosis in patients taking SGLT2 inhibitors and also following a ketogenic diet [101, 102]. For this reason, ketogenic diets should be avoided in patients taking these drugs.

Beyond Diets: Lessons from Human Genetics

Medium-Chain Acyl-CoA Dehydrogenase Deficiency (MCADD)

Homozygous and compound heterozygous loss-of-function mutations in *ACADM,* encoding mitochondrial medium-chain acyl-CoA dehydrogenase, are characterized by fasting intolerance, episodes of hypoglycemia coma, and impaired ketogenesis [103]. Medium-chain acyl-CoA dehydrogenase deficiency (MCADD) is the most common disorder of fatty acid oxidation and is associated with hepatomegaly and fatty liver [104]. Thus, it is tempting to speculate that reduced ketogenesis is more cause than consequence of fatty liver (see section on NAFLD). Interestingly, MCADD has been found to be associated with prolonged QTc interval [105]. In summary, genetic attenuation of ketogenesis correlates with hepatic and electrocardiographic abnormalities.

Long-Chain 3-Hydroxyacyl-CoA Dehydrogenase Deficiency (LCHADD)

Homozygous and compound heterozygous loss-of-function mutations in *HADHA,* encoding a

component of the mitochondrial trifunctional protein complex controlling fatty acid oxidation, is characterized by early-onset cardiomyopathy, hypoglycemia, neuropathy, hepatomegaly, and sudden death [106]. As with MCADD, long-chain 3-hydroxyacyl-CoA dehydrogenase deficiency (LCHADD) is associated with fatty liver [107], further supporting the notion that impaired ketogenesis leads to hepatosteatosis. The physiological basis of cardiomyopathy is unknown, but may involve the build-up of toxic partially oxidized fatty acid esters [108]. Given the high energy needs of cardiac muscle it will be interesting to determine the role of ketogenic insufficiency in manifestation of cardiomyopathy, especially in light of the effects of ketones on cardiac energetics [38].

Future Directions and Challenges

LDL Risk: Saturated Versus Unsaturated Fats

A major concern of the ketogenic diet is the potential for elevated LDL-C levels and CV risk due to the relatively high consumption of dietary fats. Some studies have demonstrated positive effects on LDL-C from a KD while others have shown negative effects. The discrepancy between these results is not immediately clear; however, it is likely that the composition of dietary fats consumed plays a role. In fact, a trial comparing two KD regimens differing only in saturated and polyunsaturated fat content (total fat, carbohydrate, protein, and calories were matched) showed that the KD high in saturated fats raised LDL-C, while the KD high in polyunsaturated fats did not affect LDL-C [71]. It is unclear from this study alone if saturated fats have negative effects or polyunsaturated fats have protective effects (or both), but other studies have explored this topic extensively.

A meta-analysis examining the associations of fat intake and mortality in over 500,000 people concluded that intake of saturated fats, trans-fatty acids, animal MUFAs, α-linolenic acid, and arachidonic acid was associated with higher mortality [109]. Consumption of fish-based omega-3 PUFA was inversely associated with CVD mortality, and replacing saturated fats with plant MUFAs or linoleic acid was associated with lower total, CVD, and certain cause-specific mortality [109]. While this was designed to only detect associations, other RCTs have found similar results. The OmniHeart study examined how replacing 10% of the carbohydrates from the DASH diet with unsaturated fat affected CV disease risk outcomes [110]. This study found that replacing a small amount of carbohydrates with unsaturated fats decreased LDL-C and reduced estimated 10-year coronary artery disease risk greater than the already heart-healthy DASH diet. The MUFFIN study examined two calorically restricted diets, one enriched for MUFA and one enriched for PUFA [111]. Both diets led to weight loss, but only the PUFA-enriched diets reduced triglyceride and blood pressure and improved flow-mediated dilation. However, this study demonstrated that there were no changes between diets in total cholesterol, LDL-C, or HDL and levels did not change from baseline. The DIVAS study substituted a portion of saturated fats (10% of total energy intake) with either MUFA or omega-6 PUFA and demonstrated a reduction in total cholesterol, LDL-C, and total cholesterol: HDL ratio reported a 17–20% reduction in CVD mortality risk [112]. A follow-up report showed that replacing saturated fats with MUFA or omega-6 PUFA reduced endothelial microparticles and platelet microparticles [113]. The RESET trial replaced some saturated fat in dairy with MUFA, which lead to improvements in LDL-C and endothelial function in patients with moderate CV disease risk [114]. There are many more studies exploring how replacing saturated fats with unsaturated fats affects CVD risk, and the general consensus is that unsaturated fats reduced LDL-C and cardiovascular risk with PUFAs being even more beneficial over MUFAs. Additionally, there is evidence that omega-3 PUFAs are beneficial to omega-6 PUFAs.

Dietary Interventions: Study Design and Considerations

What Is a Proper Control in Dietary Trials?

Nutrition and dietary clinical trials are notoriously difficult to perform, and researchers face many obstacles to perform well-controlled clinical trials. The need for proper control groups in a dietary intervention is vital. The only exception is pilot studies studying the safety of a dietary intervention in a certain population. Many single-arm dietary interventions ultimately conclude efficacy findings in their study; however, it is unclear if the benefits reported are unique to the dietary intervention of interest or general benefits related to caloric restriction and weight loss. Additionally, it had been postulated that the act of participating in a weight loss trial could change behaviors that inadvertently lead to weight loss independently of the dietary intervention in question. This is due to the so-called Hawthorne effect [115]. Many trials examining the effects of the ketogenic diet have been single arm or uncontrolled and thus warrant caution in interpretation.

RCT or Cross-Over?

Many dietary intervention trials use randomized cross-over study designs where half of the participants will undergo treatment A, undergo a washout period, then treatment B (or visa-versa for the other half of participants). This design has a few strengths over RCTs. First, crossover trials allow the response of treatment A to be contrasted with the response of treatment B *within the same subject*. This reduces inter-subject variability, and, in theory, treatment effects can be estimated with greater precision than an RCT with the same number of subjects [116]. Second, fewer participants are required for adequate power. There are also negative aspects including that one treatment may carry over and alter the response of another treatment. Therefore, a sufficient washout period must be pre-calculated and employed to ensure that effects from treatment A do not interfere with the effectiveness of treatment B. By design, crossover studies take much longer to complete than RCTs with the same treatment duration. Therefore, crossover studies are typically reserved for studying short-term outcomes of chronic diseases.

RCTs are considered the "gold-standard" in biomedical research. When factors that may bias outcomes are randomly distributed across intervention groups, the results of the study will not be confounded by inherent biases. Some dietary studies run "non-randomized" controlled trials that allow subjects to self-select into intervention groups, often to improve compliance. This is especially common in KD clinical trials where compliance can be especially low in certain patient populations. However, this introduces great bias to the study and should generally be avoided except for exploratory studies.

Lack of Placebo

One important obstacle is the lack of placebo or control groups. In a blinded pharmaceutical clinical trial, the treatment group will receive the medication and the control group will receive a placebo and the participants of the study are not aware which group they are in. Even surgical studies will have a "sham surgery" placebo group. There is no such placebo group for a dietary intervention study and we, therefore, have no good way of "blinding" a subject in a dietary clinical trial; the subject will always know what intervention they are receiving. However, it can be possible to randomize to a treatment and an alternate active comparator and it is critical that investigators interpreting data are blinded to the treatment allocation.

Controlling Macronutrient and Calorie Intake

Along the same lines, specific aspects of a diet cannot be studied in isolation. For instance, to understand the effects of saturated fats on blood LDL cholesterol, would a daily bolus of saturated fats be given? In this example, would any observed effect be due to increased saturated fats or simply augmented caloric intake or replacement of another nutrient? To study more broadly the effects of a high-fat diet, varying levels of fat should be administered, akin to a dose-escalation study. In this context, the amount of protein and/ or carbohydrate must vary in proportion to the degree of dietary fat and, further, the total caloric composition will deviate. Therefore, it is impossible to unequivocally conclude that any outcome observed is not due to the capricious intake of one variable over another. Ultimately, there is no proper placebo-control for calorie-containing substances. It is impossible to perform a perfectly controlled dietary study.

Concluding Remarks

Clinically speaking, weight loss improves most, if not all, CV disease risk markers. Beyond the "walk more, eat less" paradigm, a universal weight loss regimen is unlikely. Thus, the desire to achieve weight reduction promotes a revolving door of fad diets. Coupled with evolving recommendations from authoritative agencies, the average consumer is often left confused. This is probably driven in part by the inherent pitfalls of dietary intervention trials. Our analysis of available clinical trial data leads us to the conclusion that the biggest potential danger of LCHF diets is increased LDL-C. However, if the fat component of LC diets is primarily devoid of saturated fat and, therefore, enriched in plant and fish-based unsaturated fatty acids, it might be possible to mitigate this risk. Otherwise, there appears to be no significant down-side to LC diets and, at worst, they appear to be benign. Indeed, the majority of studies find improved glycemic control with LCHF diets, and the few studies examining the efficacy of exogenous ketones are promising enough to warrant follow-up. At this point, there appears to be enough traction that LC diets will be around for the foreseeable future, and, with appropriately designed trials, more evidence will become available to inform clinician-based guidance. We are most excited by the potential to use LCHF diets to treat metabolic diseases beyond obesity and diabetes—most notably non-alcoholic fatty liver disease and heart failure with preserved ejection fraction.

References

1. Cercato C, Fonseca FA. Cardiovascular risk and obesity. Diabetol Metab Syndr. 2019;11:74.

2. Lamprea-Montealegre JA, Zelnick LR, Hall YN, Bansal N, de Boer IH. Prevalence of hypertension and cardiovascular risk according to blood pressure thresholds used for diagnosis. Hypertension. 2018;72(3):602–9.

3. Giugliano D, Maiorino MI, Bellastella G, Chiodini P, Esposito K. Glycemic control, preexisting cardiovascular disease, and risk of major cardiovascular events in patients with type 2 diabetes mellitus: systematic review with meta-analysis of cardiovascular outcome trials and intensive glucose control trials. J Am Heart Assoc. 2019;8(12):e012356.

4. Brunner FJ, Waldeyer C, Ojeda F, Salomaa V, Kee F, Sans S, et al. Application of non-HDL cholesterol for population-based cardiovascular risk stratification: results from the multinational cardiovascular risk consortium. Lancet. 2019;394(10215):2173–83.

5. Adeva-Andany MM, Martinez-Rodriguez J, Gonzalez-Lucan M, Fernandez-Fernandez C, Castro-Quintela E. Insulin resistance is a cardiovascular risk factor in humans. Diabetes Metab Syndr. 2019;13(2):1449–55.

6. Tana C, Ballestri S, Ricci F, Di Vincenzo A, Ticinesi A, Gallina S, et al. Cardiovascular risk in non-alcoholic fatty liver disease: mechanisms and therapeutic implications. Int J Environ Res Public Health. 2019;16(17):3104.

7. Collaborators GBDRF. Global, regional, and national comparative risk assessment of 84 behavioural, environmental and occupational, and metabolic risks or clusters of risks, 1990-2016: a systematic analysis for the global burden of disease study 2016. Lancet. 2017;390(10100):1345–422.

8. Miller VJ, Villamena FA, Volek JS. Nutritional ketosis and mitohormesis: potential implications for mitochondrial function and human health. J Nutr Metab. 2018;2018:5157645.

9. Forouhi NG, Krauss RM, Taubes G, Willett W. Dietary fat and cardiometabolic health: evidence, controversies, and consensus for guidance. BMJ. 2018;361:k2139.

10. Puchalska P, Crawford PA. Multi-dimensional roles of ketone bodies in fuel metabolism, Signaling, and therapeutics. Cell Metab. 2017;25(2):262–84.

11. Newman JC, Verdin E. Ketone bodies as signaling metabolites. Trends Endocrinol Metab. 2014;25(1):42–52.

12. Senior B, Loridan L. Direct regulatory effect of ketones on lipolysis and on glucose concentrations in man. Nature. 1968;219(5149):83–4.

13. Sacks FM, Lichtenstein AH, Wu JHY, Appel LJ, Creager MA, Kris-Etherton PM, et al. Dietary fats and cardiovascular disease: a presidential advisory from the American Heart Association. Circulation. 2017;136(3):e1–e23.

14. Ludwig DS, Ebbeling CB. The carbohydrate-insulin model of obesity: beyond "calories in, calories out". JAMA Intern Med. 2018;178(8):1098–103.

15. Hall KD. A review of the carbohydrate-insulin model of obesity. Eur J Clin Nutr. 2017;71(5):679.

16. DiNicolantonio JJ, JH OK. Added sugars drive coronary heart disease via insulin resistance and hyperinsulinaemia: a new paradigm. Open Heart. 2017;4(2):e000729.

17. Braffett BH, Dagogo-Jack S, Bebu I, Sivitz WI, Larkin M, Kolterman O, et al. Association of insulin dose, cardiometabolic risk factors, and cardiovascular disease in type 1 diabetes during 30 years of follow-up in the DCCT/EDIC study. Diabetes Care. 2019;42(4):657–64.

18. Tikkanen E, Pirinen M, Sarin AP, Havulinna AS, Mannisto S, Saltevo J, et al. Genetic support for the causal role of insulin in coronary heart disease. Diabetologia. 2016;59(11):2369–77.

19. DuBroff R, de Lorgeril M. Fat or fiction: the diet-heart hypothesis. BMJ Evid Based Med. 2019;26:3–7.

20. Calder PC. Lipids: a hole in the diet-heart hypothesis? Nat Rev Cardiol. 2016;13(7):385–6.

21. McGarry JD, Foster DW. The regulation of ketogenesis from octanoic acid. The role of the tricarboxylic acid cycle and fatty acid synthesis. J Biol Chem. 1971;246(4):1149–59.

22. Samaha FF, Iqbal N, Seshadri P, Chicano KL, Daily DA, McGrory J, et al. A low-carbohydrate as compared with a low-fat diet in severe obesity. N Engl J Med. 2003;348(21):2074–81.

23. Yancy WS Jr, Olsen MK, Guyton JR, Bakst RP, Westman EC. A low-carbohydrate, ketogenic diet versus a low-fat diet to treat obesity and hyperlipidemia: a randomized, controlled trial. Ann Intern Med. 2004;140(10):769–77.

24. Johnstone AM, Horgan GW, Murison SD, Bremner DM, Lobley GE. Effects of a high-protein ketogenic diet on hunger, appetite, and weight loss in obese men feeding ad libitum. Am J Clin Nutr. 2008;87(1):44–55.

25. Saslow LR, Kim S, Daubenmier JJ, Moskowitz JT, Phinney SD, Goldman V, et al. A randomized pilot trial of a moderate carbohydrate diet compared to a very low carbohydrate diet in overweight or obese individuals with type 2 diabetes mellitus or prediabetes. PLoS One. 2014;9(4):e91027.

26. Moreno B, Bellido D, Sajoux I, Goday A, Saavedra D, Crujeiras AB, et al. Comparison of a very low-calorie-ketogenic diet with a standard low-calorie diet in the treatment of obesity. Endocrine. 2014;47(3):793–805.

27. Yancy et al. 2015: PMCID: PMC4470323. https://www.ncbi.nlm.nih.gov/pmc/articles/PMC4470323/.

28. Moreno B, Crujeiras AB, Bellido D, Sajoux I, Casanueva FF. Obesity treatment by very low-calorie-ketogenic diet at two years: reduction in visceral fat and on the burden of disease. Endocrine. 2016;54(3):681–90.

29. Goday A, Bellido D, Sajoux I, Crujeiras AB, Burguera B, Garcia-Luna PP, et al. Short-term safety, tolerability and efficacy of a very low-calorie-ketogenic diet interventional weight loss program versus hypocaloric diet in patients with type 2 diabetes mellitus. Nutr Diabetes. 2016;6(9):e230.

30. Hall KD, Chen KY, Guo J, Lam YY, Leibel RL, Mayer LE, et al. Energy expenditure and body composition changes after an isocaloric ketogenic diet in overweight and obese men. Am J Clin Nutr. 2016;104(2):324–33.

31. Saslow LR, Daubenmier JJ, Moskowitz JT, Kim S, Murphy EJ, Phinney SD, et al. Twelve-month outcomes of a randomized trial of a moderate-carbohydrate versus very low-carbohydrate diet in overweight adults with type 2 diabetes mellitus or prediabetes. Nutr Diabetes. 2017;7(12):304.

32. Cohen CW, Fontaine KR, Arend RC, Alvarez RD, Leath CA III, Huh WK, et al. A ketogenic diet reduces central obesity and serum insulin in women with ovarian or endometrial cancer. J Nutr. 2018;148(8):1253–60.

33. Genco A, Ienca R, Ernesti I, Maselli R, Casella G, Bresciani S, et al. Improving weight loss by combination of two temporary antiobesity treatments. Obes Surg. 2018;28(12):3733–7.

34. Bhanpuri NH, Hallberg SJ, Williams PT, McKenzie AL, Ballard KD, Campbell WW, et al. Cardiovascular disease risk factor responses to a type 2 diabetes care model including nutritional ketosis induced by sustained carbohydrate restriction at 1 year: an open label, non-randomized, controlled study. Cardiovasc Diabetol. 2018;17(1):56.

35. Phillips et al. 2018. PMCID: PMC6175383. https://www.ncbi.nlm.nih.gov/pmc/articles/PMC6175383/.

36. Di Lorenzo et al. 2019. PMCID: PMC6722531. https://www.ncbi.nlm.nih.gov/pmc/articles/PMC6722531/.

37. Hyde PN, Sapper TN, Crabtree CD, LaFountain RA, Bowling ML, Buga A, et al. Dietary carbohydrate restriction improves metabolic syndrome independent of weight loss. JCI Insight. 2019;4(12):e128308.

38. Nielsen R, Moller N, Gormsen LC, Tolbod LP, Hansson NH, Sorensen J, et al. Cardiovascular effects of treatment with the ketone body 3-Hydroxybutyrate in chronic heart failure patients. Circulation. 2019;139(18):2129–41.

39. Wheless JW. History of the ketogenic diet. Epilepsia. 2008;49(Suppl 8):3–5.

40. Woodyatt RT. Objects and method of diet adjustment in diabetics. Arch Intern Med. 1921;28:125–41.

41. Wilder RM. The effect on ketonemia on the course of epilepsy. Mayo Clin Bull. 1921;2:307.

42. Gras D, Roze E, Caillet S, Meneret A, Doummar D, Billette de Villemeur T, et al. GLUT1 deficiency syndrome: an update. Rev Neurol (Paris). 2014;170(2):91–9.

43. Ferraris C, Guglielmetti M, Pasca L, De Giorgis V, Ferraro OE, Brambilla I, et al. Impact of the ketogenic diet on linear growth in children: a single-Center retrospective analysis of 34 cases. Nutrients. 2019;11(7):1442.

44. Gardner CD, Kiazand A, Alhassan S, Kim S, Stafford RS, Balise RR, et al. Comparison of the atkins, zone, ornish, and LEARN diets for change in weight and related risk factors among overweight premenopausal women: the a TO Z weight loss study: a randomized trial. JAMA. 2007;297(9):969–77.

45. Kossoff EH, McGrogan JR, Bluml RM, Pillas DJ, Rubenstein JE, Vining EP. A modified Atkins diet is effective for the treatment of intractable pediatric epilepsy. Epilepsia. 2006;47(2):421–4.

46. Foster GD, Wyatt HR, Hill JO, McGuckin BG, Brill C, Mohammed BS, et al. A randomized trial of a low-carbohydrate diet for obesity. N Engl J Med. 2003;348(21):2082–90.

47. McAuley KA, Hopkins CM, Smith KJ, McLay RT, Williams SM, Taylor RW, et al. Comparison of high-fat and high-protein diets with a high-carbohydrate diet in insulin-resistant obese women. Diabetologia. 2005;48(1):8–16.

48. Krebs JD, Bell D, Hall R, Parry-Strong A, Docherty PD, Clarke K, et al. Improvements in glucose metabolism and insulin sensitivity with a low-carbohydrate diet in obese patients with type 2 diabetes. J Am Coll Nutr. 2013;32(1):11–7.

49. Retterstol K, Svendsen M, Narverud I, Holven KB. Effect of low carbohydrate high fat diet on LDL cholesterol and gene expression in normal-weight, young adults: a randomized controlled study. Atherosclerosis. 2018;279:52–61.

50. Morgan LM, Griffin BA, Millward DJ, DeLooy A, Fox KR, Baic S, et al. Comparison of the effects of four commercially available weight-loss programmes on lipid-based cardiovascular risk factors. Public Health Nutr. 2009;12(6):799–807.

51. Phillips SA, Jurva JW, Syed AQ, Syed AQ, Kulinski JP, Pleuss J, et al. Benefit of low-fat over low-carbohydrate diet on endothelial health in obesity. Hypertension. 2008;51(2):376–82.

52. Hoffman R. Can the paleolithic diet meet the nutritional needs of older people? Maturitas. 2017;95:63–4.

53. Frassetto LA, Schloetter M, Mietus-Synder M, Morris RC Jr, Sebastian A. Metabolic and physiologic improvements from consuming a paleolithic, hunter-gatherer type diet. Eur J Clin Nutr. 2009;63(8):947–55.

54. Jonsson T, Granfeldt Y, Ahren B, Branell UC, Palsson G, Hansson A, et al. Beneficial effects of

a Paleolithic diet on cardiovascular risk factors in type 2 diabetes: a randomized cross-over pilot study. Cardiovasc Diabetol. 2009;8:35.

55. Boers I, Muskiet FA, Berkelaar E, Schut E, Penders R, Hoenderdos K, et al. Favourable effects of consuming a Palaeolithic-type diet on characteristics of the metabolic syndrome: a randomized controlled pilot-study. Lipids Health Dis. 2014;13:160.

56. Pastore RL, Brooks JT, Carbone JW. Paleolithic nutrition improves plasma lipid concentrations of hypercholesterolemic adults to a greater extent than traditional heart-healthy dietary recommendations. Nutr Res. 2015;35(6):474–9.

57. Otten J, Mellberg C, Ryberg M, Sandberg S, Kullberg J, Lindahl B, et al. Strong and persistent effect on liver fat with a Paleolithic diet during a two-year intervention. Int J Obes. 2016;40(5):747–53.

58. Blomquist C, Chorell E, Ryberg M, Mellberg C, Worrsjo E, Makoveichuk E, et al. Decreased lipogenesis-promoting factors in adipose tissue in postmenopausal women with overweight on a Paleolithic-type diet. Eur J Nutr. 2018;57(8):2877–86.

59. Stomby A, Simonyte K, Mellberg C, Ryberg M, Stimson RH, Larsson C, et al. Diet-induced weight loss has chronic tissue-specific effects on glucocorticoid metabolism in overweight postmenopausal women. Int J Obes. 2015;39(5):814–9.

60. Genoni A, Lyons-Wall P, Lo J, Devine A. Cardiovascular, metabolic effects and dietary composition of ad-libitum Paleolithic vs. Australian guide to healthy eating diets: a 4-week randomised trial. Nutrients. 2016;8(5):314.

61. Masharani U, Sherchan P, Schloetter M, Stratford S, Xiao A, Sebastian A, et al. Metabolic and physiologic effects from consuming a hunter-gatherer (Paleolithic)-type diet in type 2 diabetes. Eur J Clin Nutr. 2015;69(8):944–8.

62. Saslow LR, Mason AE, Kim S, Goldman V, Ploutz-Snyder R, Bayandorian H, et al. An online intervention comparing a very low-carbohydrate ketogenic diet and lifestyle recommendations versus a plate method diet in overweight individuals with type 2 diabetes: a randomized controlled trial. J Med Internet Res. 2017;19(2):e36.

63. Phillips MCL, Murtagh DKJ, Gilbertson LJ, Asztely FJS, Lynch CDP. Low-fat versus ketogenic diet in Parkinson's disease: a pilot randomized controlled trial. Mov Disord. 2018;33(8):1306–14.

64. Crujeiras AB, Gomez-Arbelaez D, Zulet MA, Carreira MC, Sajoux I, de Luis D, et al. Plasma FGF21 levels in obese patients undergoing energy-restricted diets or bariatric surgery: a marker of metabolic stress? Int J Obes. 2017;41(10):1570–8.

65. Yancy WS Jr, Westman EC, McDuffie JR, Grambow SC, Jeffreys AS, Bolton J, et al. A randomized trial of a low-carbohydrate diet vs orlistat plus a low-fat diet for weight loss. Arch Intern Med. 2010;170(2):136–45.

66. Volek J, Sharman M, Gomez A, Judelson D, Rubin M, Watson G, et al. Comparison of energy-restricted very low-carbohydrate and low-fat diets on weight loss and body composition in overweight men and women. Nutr Metab (Lond). 2004;1(1):13.

67. Suzuki R, Tamura Y, Takeno K, Kakehi S, Funayama T, Furukawa Y, et al. Three days of a eucaloric, low-carbohydrate/high-fat diet increases insulin clearance in healthy non-obese Japanese men. Sci Rep. 2019;9(1):3857.

68. Urbain P, Strom L, Morawski L, Wehrle A, Deibert P, Bertz H. Impact of a 6-week non-energy-restricted ketogenic diet on physical fitness, body composition and biochemical parameters in healthy adults. Nutr Metab (Lond). 2017;14:17.

69. Kephart WC, Pledge CD, Roberson PA, Mumford PW, Romero MA, Mobley CB, et al. The three-month effects of a ketogenic diet on body composition, blood parameters, and performance metrics in crossFit trainees: a pilot study. Sports (Basel). 2018;6(1):1.

70. O'Neal EK, Smith AF, Heatherly AJ, Killen LG, Waldman HS, Hollingsworth A, et al. Effects of a 3-week high-fat-low-carbohydrate diet on lipid and glucose profiles in experienced, middle-age male runners. Int J Exerc Sci. 2019;12(2):786–99.

71. Fuehrlein BS, Rutenberg MS, Silver JN, Warren MW, Theriaque DW, Duncan GE, et al. Differential metabolic effects of saturated versus polyunsaturated fats in ketogenic diets. J Clin Endocrinol Metab. 2004;89(4):1641–5.

72. Magkos F, Fraterrigo G, Yoshino J, Luecking C, Kirbach K, Kelly SC, et al. Effects of moderate and subsequent progressive weight loss on metabolic function and adipose tissue biology in humans with obesity. Cell Metab. 2016;23(4):591–601.

73. Paoli A, Bosco G, Camporesi EM, Mangar D. Ketosis, ketogenic diet and food intake control: a complex relationship. Front Psychol. 2015;6:27.

74. Boden G, Sargrad K, Homko C, Mozzoli M, Stein TP. Effect of a low-carbohydrate diet on appetite, blood glucose levels, and insulin resistance in obese patients with type 2 diabetes. Ann Intern Med. 2005;142(6):403–11.

75. Hussain TA, Mathew TC, Dashti AA, Asfar S, Al-Zaid N, Dashti HM. Effect of low-calorie versus low-carbohydrate ketogenic diet in type 2 diabetes. Nutrition. 2012;28(10):1016–21.

76. Yancy WS Jr, Foy M, Chalecki AM, Vernon MC, Westman EC. A low-carbohydrate, ketogenic diet to treat type 2 diabetes. Nutr Metab (Lond). 2005;2:34.

77. Athinarayanan SJ, Adams RN, Hallberg SJ, McKenzie AL, Bhanpuri NH, Campbell WW, et al. Long-term effects of a novel continuous remote care intervention including nutritional ketosis for the Management of Type 2 diabetes: a 2-year non-randomized clinical trial. Front Endocrinol (Lausanne). 2019;10:348.

78. Dambha-Miller H, Day AJ, Strelitz J, Irving G, Griffin SJ. Behaviour change, weight loss and remission of type 2 diabetes: a community-based prospective cohort study. Diabet Med. 2019;37:681–88.

79. Lustig RH, Greenway F, Velasquez-Mieyer P, Heimburger D, Schumacher D, Smith D, et al. A multicenter, randomized, double-blind, placebo-controlled, dose-finding trial of a long-acting formulation of octreotide in promoting weight loss in obese adults with insulin hypersecretion. Int J Obes. 2006;30(2):331–41.
80. Orskov L, Moller N, Bak JF, Porksen N, Schmitz O. Effects of the somatostatin analog, octreotide, on glucose metabolism and insulin sensitivity in insulin-dependent diabetes mellitus. Metabolism. 1996;45(2):211–7.
81. Musso G, Cassader M, Rosina F, Gambino R. Impact of current treatments on liver disease, glucose metabolism and cardiovascular risk in non-alcoholic fatty liver disease (NAFLD): a systematic review and meta-analysis of randomised trials. Diabetologia. 2012;55(4):885–904.
82. Targher G, Byrne CD, Lonardo A, Zoppini G, Barbui C. Non-alcoholic fatty liver disease and risk of incident cardiovascular disease: a meta-analysis. J Hepatol. 2016;65(3):589–600.
83. Alkhouri N, Lawitz E, Noureddin M, DeFronzo R, Shulman GI. GS-0976 (Firsocostat): an investigational liver-directed acetyl-CoA carboxylase (ACC) inhibitor for the treatment of non-alcoholic steatohepatitis (NASH). Expert Opin Investig Drugs. 2020;29(2):135–41.
84. Fletcher JA, Deja S, Satapati S, Fu X, Burgess SC, Browning JD. Impaired ketogenesis and increased acetyl-CoA oxidation promote hyperglycemia in human fatty liver. JCI Insight. 2019;5:e127737.
85. Foster DW. Malonyl-CoA: the regulator of fatty acid synthesis and oxidation. J Clin Invest. 2012;122(6):1958–9.
86. Vilar-Gomez E, Athinarayanan SJ, Adams RN, Hallberg SJ, Bhanpuri NH, McKenzie AL, et al. Post hoc analyses of surrogate markers of non-alcoholic fatty liver disease (NAFLD) and liver fibrosis in patients with type 2 diabetes in a digitally supported continuous care intervention: an open-label, non-randomised controlled study. BMJ Open. 2019;9(2):e023597.
87. Luukkonen PK, Dufour S, Lyu K, Zhang XM, Hakkarainen A, Lehtimaki TE, et al. Effect of a ketogenic diet on hepatic steatosis and hepatic mitochondrial metabolism in nonalcoholic fatty liver disease. Proc Natl Acad Sci U S A. 2020;117(13):7347–54.
88. Carlson MG, Campbell PJ. Intensive insulin therapy and weight gain in IDDM. Diabetes. 1993;42(12):1700–7.
89. Rosenfalck AM, Almdal T, Hilsted J, Madsbad S. Body composition in adults with type 1 diabetes at onset and during the first year of insulin therapy. Diabet Med. 2002;19(5):417–23.
90. Pyorala M, Miettinen H, Laakso M, Pyorala K. Hyperinsulinemia predicts coronary heart disease risk in healthy middle-aged men: the 22-year follow-up results of the Helsinki policemen study. Circulation. 1998;98(5):398–404.
91. Lakka HM, Lakka TA, Tuomilehto J, Sivenius J, Salonen JT. Hyperinsulinemia and the risk of cardiovascular death and acute coronary and cerebrovascular events in men: the Kuopio ischaemic heart disease risk factor study. Arch Intern Med. 2000;160(8):1160–8.
92. Despres JP, Lamarche B, Mauriege P, Cantin B, Dagenais GR, Moorjani S, et al. Hyperinsulinemia as an independent risk factor for ischemic heart disease. N Engl J Med. 1996;334(15):952–7.
93. Muntoni S, Muntoni S, Draznin B. Effects of chronic hyperinsulinemia in insulin-resistant patients. Curr Diab Rep. 2008;8(3):233–8.
94. Herman ME, O'Keefe JH, Bell DSH, Schwartz SS. Insulin therapy increases cardiovascular risk in type 2 diabetes. Prog Cardiovasc Dis. 2017;60(3):422–34.
95. Bedi KC, Jr., Snyder NW, Brandimarto J, Aziz M, Mesaros C, Worth AJ, et al. Evidence for intramyocardial disruption of lipid metabolism and increased myocardial ketone utilization in advanced human heart failure. Circulation 2016;133(8):706–716.
96. Hsia DS, Grove O, Cefalu WT. An update on sodium-glucose co-transporter-2 inhibitors for the treatment of diabetes mellitus. Curr Opin Endocrinol Diabetes Obes. 2017;24(1):73–9.
97. Tentolouris A, Vlachakis P, Tzeravini E, Eleftheriadou I, Tentolouris N. SGLT2 inhibitors: a review of their antidiabetic and cardioprotective effects. Int J Environ Res Public Health. 2019;16(16):2965.
98. Perry RJ, Rabin-Court A, Song JD, Cardone RL, Wang Y, Kibbey RG, et al. Dehydration and insulin-openia are necessary and sufficient for euglycemic ketoacidosis in SGLT2 inhibitor-treated rats. Nat Commun. 2019;10(1):548.
99. Zinman B, Wanner C, Lachin JM, Fitchett D, Bluhmki E, Hantel S, et al. Empagliflozin, cardiovascular outcomes, and mortality in type 2 diabetes. N Engl J Med. 2015;373(22):2117–28.
100. Ferrannini E, Mark M, Mayoux E. CV protection in the EMPA-REG OUTCOME trial: a "thrifty substrate" hypothesis. Diabetes Care. 2016;39(7):1108–14.
101. Garay PS, Zuniga G, Lichtenberg R. A case of euglycemic diabetic ketoacidosis triggered by a ketogenic diet in a patient with type 2 diabetes using a sodium–glucose cotransporter 2 inhibitor. Clin Diabetes. 2020;38(2):204.
102. Rosenstock J, Ferrannini E. Euglycemic diabetic ketoacidosis: a predictable, detectable, and preventable safety concern with SGLT2 inhibitors. Diabetes Care. 2015;38(9):1638.
103. Bentler K, Zhai S, Elsbecker SA, Arnold GL, Burton BK, Vockley J, et al. 221 newborn-screened neonates with medium-chain acyl-coenzyme a dehydrogenase deficiency: findings from the inborn errors of metabolism collaborative. Mol Genet Metab. 2016;119(1–2):75–82.

104. Fishbein M, Smith M, Li BU. A rapid MRI technique for the assessment of hepatic steatosis in a subject with medium-chain acyl-coenzyme a dehydrogenase (MCAD) deficiency. J Pediatr Gastroenterol Nutr. 1998;27(2):224–7.
105. Wiles JR, Leslie N, Knilans TK, Akinbi H. Prolonged QTc interval in association with medium-chain acyl-coenzyme a dehydrogenase deficiency. Pediatrics. 2014;133(6):e1781–6.
106. L IJ, Ruiter JP, Hoovers JM, Jakobs ME, Wanders RJ. Common missense mutation G1528C in long-chain 3-hydroxyacyl-CoA dehydrogenase deficiency. Characterization and expression of the mutant protein, mutation analysis on genomic DNA and chromosomal localization of the mitochondrial trifunctional protein alpha subunit gene. J Clin Invest. 1996;98(4):1028–33.
107. Ibdah JA, Bennett MJ, Rinaldo P, Zhao Y, Gibson B, Sims HF, et al. A fetal fatty-acid oxidation disorder as a cause of liver disease in pregnant women. N Engl J Med. 1999;340(22):1723–31.
108. Dyke PC 2nd, Konczal L, Bartholomew D, McBride KL, Hoffman TM. Acute dilated cardiomyopathy in a patient with deficiency of long-chain 3-hydroxyacyl-CoA dehydrogenase. Pediatr Cardiol. 2009;30(4):523–6.
109. Zhuang P, Zhang Y, He W, Chen X, Chen J, He L, et al. Dietary fats in relation to Total and cause-specific mortality in a prospective cohort of 521 120 individuals with 16 years of follow-up. Circ Res. 2019;124(5):757–68.
110. Swain JF, McCarron PB, Hamilton EF, Sacks FM, Appel LJ. Characteristics of the diet patterns tested in the optimal macronutrient intake trial to prevent heart disease (OmniHeart): options for a heart-healthy diet. J Am Diet Assoc. 2008;108(2):257–65.
111. Miller M, Sorkin JD, Mastella L, Sutherland A, Rhyne J, Donnelly P, et al. Poly is more effective than monounsaturated fat for dietary management in the metabolic syndrome: the muffin study. J Clin Lipidol. 2016;10(4):996–1003.
112. Vafeiadou K, Weech M, Altowaijri H, Todd S, Yaqoob P, Jackson KG, et al. Replacement of saturated with unsaturated fats had no impact on vascular function but beneficial effects on lipid bio-markers, E-selectin, and blood pressure: results from the randomized, controlled dietary intervention and VAScular function (DIVAS) study. Am J Clin Nutr. 2015;102(1):40–8.
113. Weech M, Altowaijri H, Mayneris-Perxachs J, Vafeiadou K, Madden J, Todd S, et al. Replacement of dietary saturated fat with unsaturated fats increases numbers of circulating endothelial progen-itor cells and decreases numbers of microparticles: findings from the randomized, controlled dietary intervention and VAScular function (DIVAS) study. Am J Clin Nutr. 2018;107(6):876–82.
114. Vasilopoulou D, Markey O, Kliem KE, Fagan CC, Grandison AS, Humphries DJ, et al. Reformulation initiative for partial replacement of saturated with unsaturated fats in dairy foods attenuates the increase in LDL cholesterol and improves flow-mediated dil-atation compared with conventional dairy: the ran-domized, controlled REplacement of SaturatEd fat in dairy on Total cholesterol (RESET) study. Am J Clin Nutr. 2020;
115. McCambridge J, Witton J, Elbourne DR. Systematic review of the Hawthorne effect: new concepts are needed to study research participation effects. J Clin Epidemiol. 2014;67(3):267–77.
116. Sibbald B, Roberts C. Understanding controlled tri-als. Crossover trials BMJ. 1998;316(7146):1719.

Plant-Based Diets in the Prevention and Treatment of Cardiovascular Disease

6

Rajiv S. Vasudevan, Ashley Rosander, Aryana Pazargadi, and Michael J. Wilkinson

Introduction

A plant-based diet (PBD), or plant-based nutrition, is generally defined as a diet consisting mostly of plant derivatives and is low in animal-based products (e.g., meat, fish, dairy, eggs) in comparison to a Western-style diet, which consists of predominantly animal products, refined carbohydrates, and added fats [1]. While this definition encompasses a broad spectrum of possible diets, there is an emphasis on diets that are low in saturated fat, processed carbohydrates, and added sugars. Such diets emphasize plant-based food categories such as whole grains, fruits, vegetables, nuts, legumes, soy products, and seeds [1]. These foods are rich in macronutrients (carbohydrates, protein, healthy fats, fiber), micronutrients (vitamins and minerals), and bioactive compounds (e.g., flavonoids, plant sterols, and polyphenols) [2]. In particular, PBDs are rich in fiber, vitamin C and E, magnesium, folic acid, iron, and phytochemicals [2]. Nutrients like B12 and the more bioavailable vitamin D3 are found predominantly in animal products [3, 4] but can be sufficiently derived through supplementation and fortification of plant-based foods. Most importantly, a PBD typically involves limited intake of certain compounds found in animal products that can potentially exacerbate cardiometabolic disease. This includes saturated fats [5], heme-iron [6], chemical contaminants (hydrocarbons and heterocyclic amines) [7], advanced glycation end-products [8], and proinflammatory metabolites found in meat (e.g., L-carnitine [9] and N-glycolylneuraminic acid [10]).

A PBD encompasses many definitions, ranging from conventionally utilized terms (e.g., vegan, vegetarian, and pescatarian) to specific diet and lifestyle programs (e.g., Ornish, Pritikin, Esselstyn, Barnard) which encompass specific plant-based dietary approaches. Additionally, some diets including Mediterranean [11] and DASH (Dietary Approaches to Stop Hypertension) [12] emphasize plant-based nutrition to improve cardiovascular health. However, these diets include animal products, particularly low-fat dairy and lean animal proteins (e.g., fish, poultry, and eggs) in their recommendations.

Ashley Rosander and Aryana Pazargadi contributed equally.

R. S. Vasudevan
University of California, San Diego School of Medicine, La Jolla, CA, USA
e-mail: rvasudev@health.ucsd.edu

A. Rosander · A. Pazargadi · M. J. Wilkinson (✉)
Division of Cardiovascular Medicine, Department of Medicine, University of California San Diego, San Diego, CA, USA
e-mail: arosande@health.ucsd.edu;
apazarga@health.ucsd.edu; mjwilkinson@health.ucsd.edu

© Springer Nature Switzerland AG 2021
M. J. Wilkinson et al. (eds.), *Prevention and Treatment of Cardiovascular Disease*, Contemporary Cardiology, https://doi.org/10.1007/978-3-030-78177-4_6

Beyond specific PBDs, there are several terms one can encounter colloquially and in the scientific literature. Vegan (or veganism) is a diet that completely excludes animal products and relies exclusively on plant-derived foods. A lacto-vegetarian consumes dairy products (milk, cheese, yogurt, etc.) in addition to plant-based foods while a lacto-ovo-vegetarian involves the addition of eggs. A semivegetarian consumes dairy, eggs, and red meat/poultry ≥1 time/month and <1 time/week according to the Adventist Health Study-2 definition [13].

Often, emphasis is placed on the type of animal products present within a PBD, as indicated by the definitions above. However, the constitution of a PBD is important to consider in order to ensure a heart healthy PBD. A diet that is high in refined grains, saturated fat (e.g., coconut oil, palm oil, and palm kernel oil), potatoes, and added-sugar beverages still ascribes to the literal definition of a PBD. However, such a diet contributes to exacerbating cardiovascular and metabolic disease risk [14]. To address this, studies have proposed PBD scores/indices which can be used to assess both the animal-product constitution of the diet and its "healthiness." These scores rate healthier plant-based foods (fruits, vegetables, whole grains) positively and unhealthy plant-based foods (refined sugars, added fats) negatively [14, 15, 16].

Overall, scientific evidence supports that adhering to a healthy, low-saturated fat PBD is associated with beneficial cardiovascular outcomes. This includes mitigating coronary artery disease (CAD), hypertension (HTN), cerebrovascular accident (CVA) risk, type 2 diabetes mellitus (DM2), heart failure (HF), and death [1, 17, 18]. Reductions in serum atherogenic lipids play a significant role in these risk reductions. Low-fat PBDs have been associated with reductions in total cholesterol (TC), low-density lipoprotein (LDL-C), and non-high-density lipoprotein cholesterol (non-HDL-C) [19, 20]. Reductions in the "good" cholesterol high-density lipoprotein cholesterol (HDL-C) have also been observed in patients adhering to a PBD compared to an omnivorous diet [19, 20]. Beneficial effects on

hemoglobin A_{1c} [21], insulin resistance [22], and systemic inflammation [23] have also been reported.

The extensive evidence in support of a PBD has led to recommendations from the Academy of Nutrition and Dietetics [24], American Heart Association (AHA) [25], and 2015–2020 Dietary Guidelines for Americans [26] on adopting PBDs for weight loss and improvement of cardiometabolic health. The AHA advocates for a reduction in the consumption of animal products for protein, replacing it with protein-rich plant-based foods like tofu, quinoa, mushrooms, lentils, chickpeas, beans, and legumes [24]. They also recommend that only 5–6% of daily calories should come from saturated fat and warn against replacing an animal-based diet with unhealthy processed plant-based foods, such as fruit juices, potatoes (e.g., French fries), and sweets with high added sugar. The American Academy for Nutrition and Dietetics recommends a PBD that is low in saturated fat, given the association between saturated fat and cardiovascular disease (CVD) [24], which can come from plant-based oils such as palm oil, palm kernel oil, and coconut oil. The 2015–2020 Dietary Guidelines for Americans makes similar recommendations and provides serving-size recommendations for the consumption of plant and animal products, with an emphasis on limiting meat consumption [26].

There is overwhelming evidence in support of a PBD to reduce the risk of CVD. Despite recent advances in treatment and prevention, heart disease continues to be the leading cause of death worldwide [27]. Implementing a PBD has proven to be an effective measure, including in combination with other interventions, to reduce the risk of CVD and promote the overall health and well-being of patients.

Evidence Behind Plant-Based Diets

PBDs have been proven to have a beneficial effect on many types of CVD: CAD, HTN, CVA, and HF [1, 17, 18, 28, 29]. For example, some of the most potent contributors to CVD are serum atherogenic lipids, particularly LDL-C [19]. PBDs have been shown to significantly reduce LDL-C levels [19]. Thus, it is important to consider a PBD as an adjunct for the management of several CVDs.

Coronary Artery Disease

PBDs have been shown to both reduce the risk and improve the treatment of CAD by lowering atherogenic serum lipid levels [19] and reducing systemic inflammation [23]. Based on findings from the Lifestyle Heart Trial, which implemented a 10% fat vegetarian diet ($n = 28$) versus usual care ($n = 20$), it was also suggested that a PBD might reduce average percent diameter stenosis in CAD (measured by quantitative coronary angiography (QCA)) (-3.1% vs. 11.8%, $p = 0.001$ at 5 years) [32]. However, it is important to note that coronary plaque regression in the setting of PBDs remains controversial and substantial evidence of this effect is lacking. Also, the assessment of coronary artery plaque by QCA has been largely replaced by more advanced imaging modalities in contemporary studies, including coronary computed tomographic angiography and intravascular ultrasound [30, 31]. Nevertheless, the Lifestyle Heart Trial demonstrated a cardiac event rate of 0.86 per patient (25 events among 28 patients) in the experimental arm versus 2.25 (45 events among 20 patients) in the usual care arm [32]. An analysis of participants from the Nurses' Health Study (NHS1) ($n = 73,710$ women), NHS2 ($n = 92,329$ women), and the Health Professionals Follow-Up Study ($n = 43,259$ men) found that plant-based diet index scores (PDI) had an inverse relationship with CHD risk, with the highest PDI scores (10th decile) being associated with significantly reduced risk of CHD in a multivariate adjusted model (HR: 0.93; 95% CI = [0.90, 0.97]; p trend = 0.003). Scores on a healthy plant-based diet (healthy plant-based diet index [hPDI]) had a significant association with lowering CHD risk with increasing scores (HR: 0.75; 95% CI = [0.68, 0.83]; p trend <0.001).

Conversely, increasing unhealthy plant-based index scores (uPDI) had a significant association with increasing CHD risk (HR: 1.32; 95% CI = [1.20, 1.46]; p trend <0.001) [14]. Kwok et al. performed a systematic review and meta-analysis of eight studies where cardiovascular outcomes were assessed when comparing vegetarian versus nonvegetarian diets. When analyzing a subgroup of the Adventist Health studies [13, 33, 34], there was a reduced risk of ischemic heart disease (RR: 0.60; 95% CI = [0.43, 0.80]) [35]. Thus, a PBD may be one important tool for helping patients to reduce their risk of CAD and related events.

Hypertension

Consumption of just one serving of meat per day, including seafood, has been shown to have an association with increased HTN risk [36]. Conversely, PBDs are associated with significant reductions in blood pressure [37]. A study by Steffen et al. found that a PBD (whole grains, refined grains, fruit, vegetables, nuts, or legumes) reduces the risk of HTN, with higher levels of plant consumption being associated with further reductions in risk for HTN incidence (5th quintile plant consumption: HR: 0.64; 95% CI = [0.53, 0.90]) [38]. Consumption of ≥4 servings of vegetables and fruits was associated with HTN hazard ratios of 0.95 (95% CI = [0.86, 1.04]) and 0.92 (95% CI = [0.87, 0.97]), respectively [39]. A meta-analysis of 7 clinical trials and 32 observational studies found that vegetarian diets are associated with reductions in both systolic blood pressure (SBP) and diastolic blood pressure (DBP). From the seven clinical trials, there was a mean SBP reduction of -4.8 mmHg (95% CI = [-6.6, -3.1]; p <0.001) and DBP by -2.2 mmHg (95% CI = [-3.5, -1.0]; p <0.001). From the 32 observational studies, there was a mean SBP reduction of -6.9 mmHg (95% CI = [-9.1, -4.7]; p < 0.001) and DBP of -4.7 mmHg (95% CI = [-6.3, -3.1]; p < 0.001) [37]. Overall consumption of a healthful PBD is associated with a reduction in blood pressure and risk for HTN.

Cerebrovascular Accident (Stroke)

Stroke is one of the leading causes of death and disability in the world [27]. Among the many risk factors associated with stroke, HTN is the strongest risk factor (OR: 2.98; 99% CI = [2.72, 3.28]) [40]. Given the association between PBDs and reduction of several aspects of CVD, including HTN [37], a PBD is also implicated in the reduction of stroke risk. A meta-analysis from Hu et al. found that higher consumption of fruits and vegetables was associated with reduced stroke risk (RR: 0.79; 95% CI = [0.75, 0.84]) [41]. Studies have found that dietary intake of fish might be protective against stroke [42, 43]. These findings corroborate studies on stroke prevention using the Mediterranean Diet, which includes fish along with a high fruit/vegetable diet. The Mediterranean Diet has been strongly associated with stroke risk reduction [11]. Analysis of the Adventist Health-2 study found a pescovegetarian diet to be superior to a nonvegetarian diet in reducing all-cause mortality [13], but not superior in reducing DM2 risk [44]. Further studies comparing a "plant-strict" diet to a "plant-with-fish" diet are warranted to assess stroke and CVD risk overall.

Heart Failure

Evidence for the use of a PBD in HF prevention and treatment is somewhat limited. An analysis of the REGARDS (REasons for Geographic and Racial Differences in Stroke) study cohort assessed cardiovascular outcomes from 16,068 participants with no baseline CAD or HF who were categorized based on their general dietary pattern. The highest quartile of individuals adhering to a "plant-based" diet category (vegetables, fruits, beans, fish) had a 41% lower risk of HF (both reduced (HFrEF) and preserved (HFpEF) ejection fraction) (HR: 0.59; 95% CI = [0.41, 0.86]; $p = 0.004$) compared to the lowest quartile. This was in contrast to those adhering to the highest quartile of a "southern-diet" (fried food, organ meats, processed meats, added fats, sugar sweetened beverages), which had 72% higher

risk of HF (HR: 1.72; 95% CI = [1.20, 2.46]; $p = 0.005$) [45]. Although the "plant-based" category in this study included fish, the study supports the protective effect of fruits and vegetables in preventing HF. While other studies have also implicated the beneficial effects of fruits and vegetables in preventing HF [46], further evidence is needed to support a PBD specifically in the prevention and treatment of HF.

Cardiovascular and All-Cause Mortality

Despite evidence supporting PBDs for reduction of certain cardiovascular outcomes (CAD, stroke, HTN, HF), evidence for the reduction of cardiovascular death (myocardial infarction, HF, stroke, hemorrhage, CV procedures) [47] and all-cause death is not definitive. An analysis from the Adventist Health Study-2 (AHS-2; $n = 73,308$) found that a vegetarian diet reduced the risk of all-cause death when compared to a nonvegetarian diet (HR: 0.88; 95% CI = [0.80, 0.97]). However, a significant reduction in cardiovascular mortality was only observed for men (HR: 0.71; 95% CI = [0.57, 0.90]) and not women (HR: 0.99; 95% CI = [0.83, 1.18]) [13]. In an analysis of the NHANES III (National Health and Nutrition Examination Survey III) dataset, mortality risk was stratified based on scores on a general PDI, hPDI and uPDI. Neither PDI nor uPDI was associated with all-cause mortality; however, there was a reduction in all-cause mortality for every 10-point increase in the hPDI for individuals above the median score (HR per 10-unit increase in hPDI: 0.95; 95% CI = [0.91, 0.98]). There was no association between PDI, uPDI, or hPDI and cardiovascular mortality [15].

A meta-analysis of five studies by Huang et al. found that a vegetarian diet was associated with a lower risk for ischemic heart disease mortality (RR: 0.71; 95% CI = [0.56, 0.87]) when compared to nonvegetarian diets. However, reduction in CVA (RR: 0.88; 95% CI = [0.70, 1.06]) and all-cause mortality (RR: 0.91; 95% CI = [0.66, 1.16]) was not significant [48]. Furthermore, another meta-analysis of seven studies by Kwok et al. found similar results: a significant reduction in ischemic heart disease risk (RR: 0.71; 95% CI = [0.57, 0.87]), but not cerebrovascular (RR: 0.93; 95% CI = [0.70, 1.23]) or all-cause death (RR: 0.87; 95% CI = [0.68, 1.11]) [35]. While there appears to be evidence in support of PBDs lowering ischemic heart disease mortality, further studies are needed to elucidate more conclusive evidence in favor of a PBD for both overall cardiovascular and all-cause mortality reduction.

Type 2 Diabetes Mellitus

PBDs have been shown to lower the risk of developing DM2. The Adventists Health Study-2 documented the incidence of diabetes in 15,200 men and 26,187 women over 2 years. Participants did not have diabetes at the time of enrollment and were grouped based on their self-reported dietary practices. The following diets had a lower risk of incident diabetes compared to nonvegetarians in the following order: vegans (OR: 0.381; 95% CI = [0.236, 0.617]), lacto-ovo-vegetarians (OR: 0.618; 95% CI = [0.503, 0.760]), and semivegetarians (OR: 0.486; 95% CI = [0.312, 0.755]). A pesco-vegetarian diet (OR: 0.790; 95% CI = [0.575, 1.086]) was not statistically superior to a nonvegetarian diet in preventing diabetes [44]. An analysis of participants from the Nurses' Health Study 2 ($n = 90,239$ women) and the Health Professionals Follow-Up Study ($n = 40,539$ men) assessed risk of DM2 based on stratification of diet using plant-based diet indices (PDI = plant-based diet index; hPDI = healthful plant-based diet index; uPDI = unhealthful plant-based diet index). These indices value healthy plant-based foods positively and unhealthy plant-based or animal products unfavorably. They found that PDI and hPDI scores were inversely associated with DM2 (HR: 0.51; 95% CI = [0.47, 0.55], $p < 0.001$), and uPDI scores were directly associated with DM2 risk (HR: 1.16; 95% CI = [1.08, 1.25], $p < 0.001$). The same associations were found between these dietary indices and the risk of CHD [49]. Thus, a diet that is more limited in animal products confers the lowest risk of developing diabetes, a vegan diet conferring the low-

est risk and a nonvegetarian diet conferring the highest risk.

Other studies have demonstrated the benefit of a PBD in lowering HbA_{1C} [50, 51, 52]. Yokoyama et al. performed meta-analysis of six controlled trials/randomized control trials (RCTs) studying the use of vegetarian diets in glycemic control in DM2. Consumption of a vegetarian diet was associated with a significant reduction in HbA_{1C} (−0.39%; 95% CI = [−0.62, −0.15]; $p = 0.001$) [21]. Reductions in insulin resistance have also been reported in association with PBDs [22].

Atherogenic Lipids (LDL-C and non-HDL-C)

Elevated atherogenic lipid levels, particularly LDL-C, are strongly associated with vascular endothelial cell dysfunction, progression of atherosclerotic disease, and poor cardiovascular outcomes [1]. Foods that are high in saturated fat and cholesterol, such as meat and dairy products [5], can promote both the elevation of LDL-C and its oxidation [53]. Thus, the benefits of a PBD in lowering LDL-C are partly related to consuming a diet that is low in saturated fat and cholesterol, which is found in much smaller quantities in plant foods.

The association between plant-based nutrition and lowering of LDL-C, TC, and non-HDL-C has been thoroughly reported in the literature over the past few decades [19, 32, 54, 55]. The Lifestyle Heart Trial (1998) conducted by Ornish et al. was among the first RCTs to test a PBD intervention in lieu of lipid-lowering (statin) therapy. The intervention consisted of a 10% fat vegetarian diet in addition to moderate aerobic exercise, stress management, and smoking cessation. Whereas there were no significant differences at baseline, at 1 year there were significant differences in atherogenic lipid levels between the experimental and control groups; LDL-C (143.8 mg/dL vs. 86.56 mg/dL, $p = 0.003$) and TC (225.1 mg/dL vs. 162.9 mg/dL, $p = 0.004$) were reported in the experimental group ($n = 20$) compared to control ($n = 15$), respectively [32]. The GEICO study was a more recent multicenter

RCT (2013) conducted with employees from a large insurance company, implementing a low fat (<3 g fat per serving), PBD free from animal products, and encouraging foods of low glycemic index [56]. After the 18-week study period, there was a significant difference between the intervention (n = 142) and control group (n = 149) in the reduction of LDL-C (-8.1 mg/dL vs. -0.9 mg/dL, $p < 0.0001$) and TC (-8.0 vs. -0.1 mg/dL, $p < 0.0001$) [50].

A meta-analysis performed by Yokohama et al. assessed 19 clinical trials and 30 observational studies in which a plant-based/vegetarian diet was implemented, and serum lipid levels were assessed. Amongst the observational studies (n = 30), a vegetarian diet was associated with significant reductions in mean TC (-29.2 mg/dL; 95% CI = [-34.6, -23.8]; $p < 0.001$); LDL-C (-22.9 mg/dL; 95% CI = [-27.9, -17.9]; $p < 0.001$); HDL-C (-3.6 mg/dL; 95% CI = [-4.7, -2.5]; $p < 0.001$); and a nonsignificant reduction in triglycerides (-6.5 mg/dL; 95% CI = [-14.0, 1.1]; $p = 0.092$) compared with consumption of omnivorous diets. Among the clinical trials (n = 19), vegetarian diets were associated with reduction in mean TC (-12.5 mg/dL; 95% CI = [-17.8, -7.2]; $p < 0.001$); LDL-C (-12.2 mg/dL; 95% CI = [-17.7, -6.7]; $p < 0.001$); and HDL-C (-3.4 mg/dL; 95% CI = [-4.3, -2.5]; $p < 0.001$) and a nonsignificant increase in triglyceride concentration (5.8 mg/dL; 95% CI = [-0.9, 12.6]; $p = 0.090$), compared with consumption of omnivorous diets [19]. A meta-analysis by Wang et al. of 11 RCTs utilizing vegetarian diet interventions similarly demonstrated significant reductions in LDL-C, non-HDL-C, and HDL-C, with nonsignificant changes in triglyceride levels [20].

HDL-C and Triglycerides

In addition to evidence supporting significant reductions in LDL-C, vegetarian/PBDs have also been associated with reductions of the "good cholesterol" HDL-C [19, 20, 55] without cardiovascular detriment. Overall, the mechanism of dietary factors on HDL-C levels is unclear;

replacing carbohydrates with polyunsaturated, monounsaturated, and saturated fat has been associated with greater HDL-C levels [57]. PBDs tend to be lower in fatty acid content and higher in carbohydrates, which could potentially contribute to lowering HDL-C.

The results from two meta-analyses [19, 20] found that PBDs might be ineffective in reducing serum triglycerides. In both analyses, studies were selected based on implementation of a PBD (including keywords "vegetarian" and "vegan") and did not stratify based on baseline triglyceride levels or caloric intake. The meta-analysis from Yokoyama et al. found nonsignificant changes in serum triglycerides in clinical trials (n = 19 studies; 5.8 mg/dL; 95% CI = [-0.9, 12.6]; $p = 0.090$) and observational studies (n = 30 studies; -6.5 mg/dL; 95% CI = [-14.0, 1.1]; $p = 0.092$) [19]. A meta-analysis by Wang et al. of 11 clinical trials of vegetarian diets also found a nonsignificant change in serum triglycerides (0.04 mmol/L; 95% CI = [-0.05, 0.13]; $p = 0.40$) [20]. Prior studies have found that replacing fat with carbohydrates might significantly increase serum triglycerides [58]. PBDs encompass a wide variation of carbohydrate consumption, with an emphasis on limiting refined carbohydrates and added sugars. One randomized parallel trial compared a low-carbohydrate PBD to a high-carbohydrate lacto-ovo-vegetarian diet and found that triglycerides were significantly lower in the low-carbohydrate diet compared to the high-carbohydrate (-29.2% vs. -17.8%; $p = 0.02$), with both groups demonstrating reductions in triglycerides over the study period [59]. Further studies are needed to elucidate the role of PBDs in affecting serum triglycerides, with emphasis on the role of carbohydrate consumption.

Biochemical Mechanisms

Aside from reductions in serum atherogenic lipids, PBDs exert their beneficial effects on cardiovascular health through several proposed mechanisms. Plant-based foods are associated with higher intake of certain vitamins and bioactive compounds that are anti-atherogenic while lacking pro-atherogenic compounds found in animal products.

Polyphenols and Fiber

Polyphenols, which can be further classified into flavonoids and phenolic acids, are found in higher amounts in many plant-based foods (fruits, vegetables, berries, nuts, tea, coffee) and are associated with a decreased risk of CAD [60]. Polyphenols have been implicated in reducing LDL-oxidation, inflammation, cell-adhesion, foam cell formation, and platelet adhesion [61]. They might also be involved in enhanced vascular endothelial nitric oxide (NO) release, which is protective against endothelial cell dysfunction and atherosclerosis [62]. A meta-analysis by Rienks et al. found that increased polyphenol biomarker levels were associated with decreased risk for all cause (0.70; 95% CI = [0.53, 0.93]) and CVD (0.55; 95% CI = [0.37, 0.82]) mortality [63].

The high amount of fiber found in a PBD might also contribute to its beneficial effects on cardiovascular health. Higher dietary fiber leads to more satiety and less caloric consumption [64]. Fiber has also been shown to alter cholesterol synthesis, increase bile-acid synthesis, and promote bile-acid excretion [65, 66]. This corroborates findings that increased fiber consumption can lower serum lipids [65] and subsequently reduce the risk for CVD [67]. Studies have also shown that fiber leads to better insulin responses and a lower risk of DM2 [68]. Plant-based foods are also rich in vitamin C, vitamin E, potassium, antioxidants, and magnesium [69].

Avoiding Pro-atherogenic Compounds

The benefits of a PBD are also derived from avoidance of certain compounds that are found in higher abundance within animal-based foods. Saturated fats are found in high abundance in many animal-based foods (beef, chicken, pork, cheese, butter) and are associated with elevated atherogenic lipid levels [5], particularly LDL-C [53]. Furthermore,

saturated fats might be involved in increasing inflammation via TLR4 (toll-like receptor 4) signaling, enhancing intestinal epithelium leakage via microbial changes and translocation of lipopolysaccharide, thereby increasing systemic inflammation [70]. Conversely, polyunsaturated fatty acids (PUFAs), such as omega-3 and omega-6 fatty acids, are associated with anti-inflammation and decreased CAD risk [71]. PUFAs are found mostly in fish but are also present in pine nuts, walnuts, sunflower seeds, flaxseed, and several vegetable oils [72]. In a meta-analysis by Farvid et al., consumption of linoleic acid, an omega-6 fatty acid, was associated with 15% lower CHD events (RR: 0.85; 95% CI = [0.78, 0.92]) and 21% lower CHD deaths (RR: 0.79; 95% CI = [0.71, 0.89]) in the highest consumption group compared to the lowest [73]. Dietary cholesterol, which is found predominantly in animal products, has been the subject of controversy with regard to its association with CVD [74]. Limiting intake of dietary cholesterol is included in some dietary recommendations for cardiovascular health, and heart-healthy dietary patterns, such as the Mediterranean Diet and the DASH diet, tend to be low in dietary cholesterol [74].

Trimethylamine-N-oxide (TMAO), a compound derived from gut microbiome metabolism of L-carnitine (present in red meat), is associated with increased risk of inflammation, atherosclerosis, myocardial infarction, stroke, and death [9]. Consumption of a PBD has been shown to reduce TMAO levels [75]. Other factors in meat that might contribute to CVD risk are heme-iron [6, 76] chemical contaminants (e.g., heterocyclic amines and hydrocarbons [77], and N-glycolylneuraminic acid (Neu5Gc) [10]).

Potential Shortfalls of a Plant-Based Diet

Protein

One concern which has been expressed with regard to PBDs is risk of protein deficiency. Although protein is found in higher quantities in animal products, protein can be sufficiently

Table 6.1 Plant-based dietary sources of nutritional elements

Protein	Iron	Zinc	Vitamin D	Vitamin B12
Beans	Leafy green	Grains[a]	Fortified cereals	Fortified cereals
Legumes	vegetables	Seeds[a]	Fortified plant-based milk (e.g.,	Nutritional yeast
Brown	Tomatoes	Legumes[a]	soy, almond)	Fortified plant-based milk (e.g.,
rice	Beans		Maitake/Portobello mushrooms	soy, almond)
Quinoa				
Soy				
Nuts				

Though the use of supplements is also a valid source of protein, iron, zinc, and vitamins D and B12, this table describes their plant-based sources for dietary consumption
[a]Also contains phytates which reduce the bioavailability of zinc

derived from plant products such as beans, legumes, brown rice, quinoa, and soy (Table 6.1). People who eat a PBD are not at risk for protein deficiency [78].

Iron

Iron, a mineral essential for hemoglobin production, is found in the form of heme-iron in animal products, which is more bioactive and easily absorbed, whereas plant-based iron is mostly less active non-heme-iron [79]. However, iron deficiency is not more prevalent amongst vegans compared to omnivores [80]. Iron is found sufficiently in several plant-based foods, including leafy green vegetables, tomatoes, and beans [81] (Table 6.1). Furthermore, increased consumption of ascorbic acid (vitamin C) in a PBD increases the absorption of iron [82]. Of note, heme-iron has been associated with poor cardiovascular health and outcomes [76].

Zinc

Zinc is essential for proper gastrointestinal, immune, skeletal, and nervous system function [83]. Individuals eating a PBD are considered to be at risk for zinc deficiency due to higher consumption of phytates, which make zinc less bioavailable. The same plant-based foods that are high in zinc (grains, seeds, and legumes) also contain phytates (Table 6.1) [84]. However, existing studies have shown that there might be no difference in zinc status between vegetarians

and omnivores, although this is not conclusive [85]. Furthermore, the effects of zinc deficiency are not well understood, and there seems to be no supporting evidence that a vegan/vegetarian diet is associated with zinc-related systemic deficiencies [85], including immunologic deficiencies [86].

Vitamin D

Vitamin D is a fat-soluble vitamin that is needed for proper calcium, phosphorus metabolism, and bone health [87]. Vitamin D2, which is the form found in plants, is less bioavailable than vitamin D3, which is found in animal products; thus, individuals adhering to a PBD might be at higher risk of vitamin D deficiencies. Vitamin D deficiency can manifest as muscle pain, fatigue, depression, and bone malformation if chronic (rickets). An analysis of the EPIC-Oxford study found that vegans have roughly one-fourth the dietary vitamin D intake compared to omnivores [4]. However, an analysis of participants from the Adventist Health Study-2 found no differences in serum vitamin D levels based on vegetarian status [88]. Vitamin D deficiency can be avoided by the consumption of fortified cereals or supplementation (Table 6.1).

Vitamin B12

Vitamin B12 (cobalamin) is necessary for proper neuronal function, cell division, and red blood cell formation [89]. Vitamin B12 is synthesized by microorganisms that are almost exclusively found in animal products. Thus, individuals eating a PBD are at risk for B12 deficiency [90]. Vitamin B12 deficiency (<150 pmol/L) [91] can result in an increase in red blood cell mean corpuscular volume and macrocytic anemia. It can also lead to myelin degeneration and neuronal dysfunction [92]. In a meta-analysis of 20 studies assessing B12 status in vegans and vegetarians, B12 deficiency rates were reported between 0% and 81% of individuals; the wide variation in deficiency could be attributable to differences in deficiency definition, consumption of fortified foods, or PBD constitution [3].

B12 deficiency has been associated with increased CVD risk through a buildup of homocysteine, a metabolic intermediate that is converted to the amino acid methionine in a B12 dependent process. Homocysteine, which may be elevated in vegetarian populations [93], is independently associated with an increased risk for ischemic heart disease and stroke [94]. Proposed mechanisms of the relationship between homocysteine and CVD are increased generation of atherogenic reactive oxygen species, lower vascular endothelial cell nitric oxide (NO) synthesis [95], and increased inflammation [96]. Vitamin B12 deficiency is treated through supplementation or fortification. Individuals ascribing to a lacto-ovo-vegetarian diet can obtain B12 through dairy products, particularly fortified milk and eggs. However, individuals ascribing to vegan diets that completely abstain from animal products may seek supplementation through over-the-counter B12 supplements or fortified cereal/plant-based milk (Table 6.1).

Specific Plant-Based Diets and Lifestyle Programs

Given the potential CV benefits of adopting a PBD style, there has been much interest in developing comprehensive diet and lifestyle programs based around a PBD. The following section considers the scientific evidence underlying several popular PBD and lifestyle programs: Pritikin, Ornish, Esselstyn, and Barnard. While the poten-

tial benefits of these PBD and lifestyle programs are clear, additional research is needed in order to fully determine their impact on CVD risk.

The Pritikin Diet

The Pritikin diet has been used since the late 1970s as a means of prevention and treatment of CVD as well as a mechanism of glucose control in those with prediabetes or DM2 [97]. The Pritikin diet and lifestyle program is also a component implemented in certain cardiac rehabilitation programs in the United States [98].

Dietary Components

The Pritikin diet is briefly defined as a low fat, high fiber predominantly PBD regimen, although certain animal products exist in the dietary recommendations (Fig. 6.1). The components of the Pritikin diet are broken into a three-category paradigm: the "go" foods, the "caution" foods, and the "stop" foods. The foods that are encouraged without restriction are fruits, vegetables, whole grains, starchy vegetables, legumes, lean calcium-rich foods (including nonfat dairy), fish, and lean protein such as tofu or white skinless poultry. The caution foods, or foods to be eaten in small quantities only on occasion, include oils, refined sweeteners, salt, and refined grains. The foods to be avoided completely include saturated fat-rich foods, organ meats, processed meats, cholesterol rich foods (e.g., egg yolks), and partially hydrogenated vegetable oils [99]. With the Pritikin diet, 75–80% of the calories consumed in a day are recommended to be from carbohydrates, 10–15% of calories should be from protein, and less than 10% from fat [97] (Table 6.2).

Potential Benefits

The Health, Aging, and Body Composition Study is a prospective cohort study of dietary patterns in 3075 older adults. Longevity and quality of life assessed over a 10-year period were found to be significantly higher in those following a Pritikin style diet (high in low-fat dairy products, fruit, whole grains, poultry, fish, and vegetables; lower in meat, fried foods, sweets, high-energy drinks,

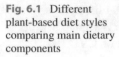

Fig. 6.1 Different plant-based diet styles comparing main dietary components

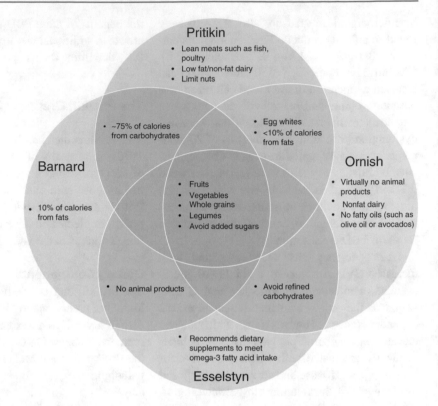

Table 6.2 Components of total caloric intake in representative plant-based diet styles

	Esselstyn	Ornish	Pritikin	Barnard
Fats	Avoid all added oils, avocado, and nuts. Supplement with flaxseed	<10%	<10%	10%
Carbohydrates	Avoid refined carbohydrates. Consume whole grains	Low refined carbohydrates	75–80%	75%
Protein	Avoid all fish, meat, poultry, and dairy. Consume legumes, lentils, vegetables	Egg whites and plant-based proteins	10–15%	15%
Sugars	Avoid added sugars, syrups, fructose, and fruit juices. Consume whole fruits	Avoid added sugars	Avoid added sugars	Avoid added sugars

and added fat) compared to those who reported high fat dairy and sweets and desserts as part of their diet [100]. A single arm study of 67 patients with metabolic syndrome was conducted as they attended the Pritikin Longevity Center for 12–15 days. After their time eating the Pritikin diet combined with regular exercise, the treated patients displayed a decrease in systolic (14.9% mean reduction, $p < 0.001$) and diastolic (8.9% mean reduction, $p < 0.001$) blood pressure, BMI (3% mean reduction, $p < 0.001$), blood glucose (11.6% mean reduction, $p < 0.001$), and LDL cholesterol (10.9% mean reduction, $p < 0.001$) [101]. A similar single arm study in overweight

children also showed promising results incorporating the high-fiber, low-fat diet in combination with aerobic exercise. In 2 weeks, this regimen led to the reversal of metabolic syndrome in all 7 of 16 participants who initially had it at baseline [102]. A 1991 study of 4587 participants who attended the Pritikin Longevity Center for 3 weeks revealed a significant average reduction ($p < 0.01$) in total cholesterol, LDL-cholesterol, non-HDL cholesterol, and triglycerides of 23%, 23%, 24%, and 33%, respectively [103]. Single arm studies of chronic inflammation in patients staying at the Pritikin Longevity Center show that CRP is reduced by 45% in postmenopausal females ($p < 0.01$) [104] and 39% in males with metabolic syndrome factors ($p < 0.05$) [105]. Because the Pritikin program is generally implemented as a comprehensive lifestyle change, more data are also needed on the use of the stand-alone PBD in reducing CVD risk (Table 6.3).

The Ornish Diet

The nutritional foundation of the Ornish Program consists of a low-fat, PBD with an emphasis on fruits, vegetables, whole grains, and legumes with an allowance of nonfat dairy and egg whites (Fig. 6.1). The Ornish diet is best known for its potential to improve several CVD risk factors including DM2, hypercholesterolemia, and HTN. The Ornish Program, which encompasses the Ornish Diet, is widely recognized and adopted as an authorized intensive cardiac rehabilitation program covered by Medicare [106, 107].

Dietary Components

This diet has no caloric restrictions; however, there are some general guidelines outlining daily intake of macronutrients. Small-portioned, frequent meals are encouraged. The diet limits highly processed carbohydrates such as sugar, concentrated sweeteners, white rice, and white flour to two servings/day. Alcohol is permitted but restricted to one serving/day classified as 1.5 oz. of liquor, 4 oz. of wine, or 12 oz. of beer. The low-fat component of this diet is defined as no more than 10% of daily calories from fat (Table 6.2). The 10% of fat intake should derive from naturally occurring fats in fruits, grains,

Table 6.3 Representative clinical studies and their outcomes for the Pritikin, Ornish, and Barnard diets

Study name	Sample size (n), patient characteristics	Intervention	Study type	Key outcomes	Magnitude of effect	p-Value
Effect of short-term Pritikin diet on the metabolic syndrome Sullivan, S. and Klein, S. 2006 [101]	67 patients with metabolic syndrome	Attended Pritikin Longevity Center and Spa for 12–15 days (single-arm study)	Cohort, single arm	BMI	−3.4%	$p < 0.001$
				Blood pressure	−14.9% (systolic) and − 8.9% (diastolic)	$p < 0.001$
				Glucose	−11.6%	$p < 0.001$
				LDL-C	−10.9%	$p < 0.001$
				HDL-C	−3.3%	$p < 0.05$
A low-fat vegan diet improves glycemic control and cardiovascular risk factors Barnard et al. 2006 [52]	99 individuals with type 2 diabetes	ADA diet ($n = 50$) or "Barnard" low fat vegan diet ($n = 49$) for 22 weeks	RCT	Vegan vs. ADA		
				LDL-C	−21.2% vs. −10.7%	$p = 0.02$
				Body weight	−6.5 kg vs. −3.1 kg	$p < 0.001$
				HbA1C	−1.23 vs. −0.38	$p = 0.01$
LIFESTYLE Heart Trial Ornish et al. 1990 [112]	48 individuals with CHD	Ornish diet (low-fat; plant-based; $n = 28$) or Usual care ($n = 20$) for 12 months	RCT	Ornish vs. usual care		
				Coronary artery diameter stenosis (by QCA)	−1.75% vs. 2.28%	$p = 0.02$
				Body weight	−10.1 kg vs. 1.4 kg	$p < 0.0001$
				LDL-C	−26.28 mg/dL vs. 4.5 mg/dL	$p < 0.0001$
				Apolipoprotein B	−24 mg/dL vs. 0.1 mg/dL	$p = 0.0104$

(continued)

Table 6.3 (continued)

Study name	Sample size (n), patient characteristics	Intervention	Study type	Key outcomes	Magnitude of effect	p-Value
Comparison of the Atkins, Ornish, Weight Watchers (WW), and Zone Diets for Weight Loss and Heart Disease Risk Reduction Dansinger et al. 2005 [111]	A total of 160 participants 4 groups; n = 40 per group	Participants randomized into one of four diets Atkins (carbohydrate restriction) Zone (macronutrient balance) WW (calorie restriction) Ornish (fat restriction) After 12 months of maximum effort, participants selected own levels of dietary adherence	RCT	Mean change in body weight	Atkins: −2.1 kg Zone: −3.2 kg WW: −3.0 kg Ornish: −3.3 kg	p value for trend across all diets (0.40)
				LDL:HDL cholesterol ratio	Atkins: −0.39 Zone: −0.40 WW: −0.55 Ornish: −0.31	p value for trend across all diets (0.92)
				Total fat intake baseline vs. end-of-study comparison	Baseline vs. 12 mos. Atkins: 78.0 g/day vs. 85.0 g/day Zone: 81.1 g/day vs. 71.5 g/day WW: 82.1 g/day vs. 64.0 g/day Ornish: 75.5 g/day vs. 64.0 g/day	p < 0.3 between groups

WW Weight Watchers, *QCA* Quantitative coronary angiography

vegetables, beans, and legumes, with minimal amounts of nuts and seeds. These fats can also come from supplements such as fish oil, flax-seed oil, and plankton-based omega-3 fatty acids. Some key sources of protein recommended for this diet are legumes, beans, nonfat dairy, tofu, and egg whites (Fig. 6.1) [107].

Adherence

The Alternate Healthy Eating Index (AHEI) was created as a modified version of the original Healthy Eating Index (HEI) to evaluate the adherence to Dietary Guidelines for Americans and assess the quality of food intake rather than just the macronutrient percentages [108]. Amongst eight of the most popular diet plans in the USA including Atkins, Weight Watchers, South Beach diet, and more, the Ornish plan had the highest AHEI score (score 6.9) due to its balanced integration of fruits, vegetables, and whole grains, all while maintaining low transfat intake [109]. This score was then developed to be used as a predictor for major chronic disease, with an emphasis in CVD risk. There was a significant 20% and 11% reduction in all major chronic diseases, encompassing CVD, of those in the top quintile when compared to the bottom in both male and female participants, respectively [110].

In a long-term randomized controlled trial, adherence to comprehensive diet and lifestyle change was observed via self-reported participant food logs where patterns of macronutrient intake as well as caloric reduction were assessed from baseline to 1 year. The mean caloric reduction was statistically significant in all groups ($p < 0.05$), and the Ornish group had a mean daily caloric intake reduction of 192 calories at 1 year [111]. Forty-eight participants were followed for 5 years with 28 participants in the arm that required comprehensive diet and lifestyle changes, including the Ornish diet, and the other 20 participants in a control group with only moderate diet and lifestyle changes. The results for the experimental group revealed that the percentage of energy intake composed of fat (percentage of fat intake) saw an exaggerated downward trend when compared to the control. The control group started at a 30.52% fat intake in baseline and decreased to 26.76% at the year mark. After 5 years, the control group finished with a 25.03% of the daily energy intake that consists of fat ($p < 0.001$). For the experimental group, the percentage of fat intake started at 29.71% at baseline and decreased to 6.22% at the year mark, and after 5 years, saw a slight increase to 8.51% ($p < 0.001$) (Table 6.3) [111].

Cardiovascular Risk Outcomes
The nature of the macronutrient intake and the high adherence for the Ornish diet likely contribute to improvements in CVD risk factors such as weight, LDL-C, and blood pressure [32, 107]. As discussed above, the Lifestyle Heart Trial of the Ornish lifestyle intervention exhibited reductions in serum atherogenic lipids in addition to evidence of reduction in average percent diameter stenosis in CAD by QCA (Table 6.3) [32, 112].
A study ($n = 120$) compared weight loss and cardiovascular outcomes from four popular diets:

Zone, Weight Watchers, Atkins, and Ornish. Individual's weights were evaluated at 2, 6, and 12 months. It was found that the individuals randomly assigned to the Ornish Diet ($n = 40$) experienced a mean weight loss of 3.3 kg which averaged the greatest weight loss of all four diet categories. The same study demonstrated that the Ornish Diet, as well as the other three diets, significantly lowered the LDL/HDL cholesterol ratio by 10% on average at 12 months (all $p < 0.05$) (Table 6.3) [113].

Dr. Esselstyn's Plant-Based Diet

Another PBD program for CVD prevention is the Esselstyn Diet (Dr. Caldwell Esselstyn Plant-Based Nutrition Program for the Reversal of CAD). The nutritional intake of this diet is vegetarian and consists mainly of fruits, vegetables, legumes, and whole grains. This diet completely prohibits animal products and therefore recommends organic dietary supplements such as flaxseed meal to meet recommended daily intake amounts of omega-3 fatty acids. In addition to meat, this diet also discourages foods with added amounts of salt as well as sugars such as sucrose and fructose (Table 6.2; Fig. 6.1) [114]. In a study conducted in 198 participants diagnosed with CVD, participants were counseled for a PBD with the aforementioned guidelines. The study revealed that of the 198 participants, 177 of them were able to adhere to the diet and that this group had a lower rate of major cardiac events compared with the 21 participants who were nonadherent [115]. A small pilot study conducted by Dr. Esselstyn and colleagues prescribed a plant-based nutritional program in addition to lipid-lowering drugs to 22 patients with CAD. The study revealed that all 17 adherent patients demonstrated evidence of potential, favorable changes in coronary artery plaque (by coronary angiography-based estimates of mean arterial stenosis and minimal lumen diameter)

[116]. While these findings are promising, additional research, including randomized-control trials, are needed to further examine the impact of this diet style on CVD risk.

Dr. Barnard's Vegan Diet

Dr. Neal Barnard is a psychiatrist and author in the field of diet and preventative medicine and has advocated for implementation of the "Barnard Diet": a low-fat vegan diet. In a 72-week clinical trial, Barnard et al. focused on the difference in outcomes when patients with DM2 eat the standard recommended diabetes diet versus a low-fat vegan diet. The prescribed vegan diet allowed 10% of calories from fat, 75% from carbohydrates, and 15% from protein. The conventional diabetes diet, following the 2004 American Diabetes Association (ADA) guidelines, consisted of 15–20% protein, <7% saturated fat, 60–70% carbohydrate and monounsaturated fats, and cholesterol ≤ 200 mg/day (Fig. 6.1; Table 6.2). While both groups did experience significant weight loss and improvement in plasma lipids, the vegan group showed more improvement than the standard diabetes diet [117]. After 22 weeks of the intervention diet and the ADA diet, it was found that in individuals with type 2 diabetes, the vegan diet resulted in a significantly greater reduction in LDL levels ($p = 0.02$), body weight ($p < 0.001$), hemoglobin A1C ($p = 0.01$), and urinary albumin levels ($p = 0.013$) compared to the ADA group (when controlling for baseline values and excluding those with medication changes) (Table 6.3) [52]. Interestingly, in the 22-week study of the vegan diet versus the ADA diet, adherence to the diet was found to be 67% for the vegan group and 44% for the ADA diet group. The authors attribute the limited adherence to the ADA diet to the fact that it limits portion sizes of foods rather than simply prohibiting certain foods as the vegan diet does.

This diet was also tested in postmenopausal women against a control diet recommended by the National Cholesterol Education Program, resulting in significantly greater weight loss in the vegan diet group [118]. A 2004 study was conducted in which overweight, postmenopausal women were randomized to either a low-fat vegan diet or the more moderate National Cholesterol Education Program Step II (NCEP) diet for 14 weeks. When adherence was assessed, the vegan diet acceptability was high and not significantly less than the NCEP diet, suggesting that adherence is possible [122].

Conclusion

A PBD is effective in lowering risk of CVD across several diseases and associated risk factors. Thus, consideration of a PBD in the armamentarium of cardiovascular risk-lowering strategies is highly warranted. Discussing the adoption of a PBD with patients can become complex given the varying PBD options, willingness to make dietary changes, and socioeconomic factors influencing access to plant-based food options [119]. In addition, many patients might find adherence to a PBD difficult, especially if it requires relinquishing a lifetime of habitual, familial, or cultural dietary practices [120]. Thus, a provider must closely consider the unique circumstances of each patient when attempting to prescribe a PBD regimen. An important facet of any therapeutic regimen is adherence [121], so constructing a PBD regimen for a patient must involve keen awareness of their willingness to incorporate it into their everyday life.

The Ornish, Pritikin, Barnard, and Esselstyn diets involve slight variations in their recommendations for a PBD, such as variations in fat versus carbohydrate consumption and varying leniency in incorporating animal products. However, cardiometabolic benefits have been shown for each diet in their study populations [32, 103, 116, 117], although further research into the effects of these diet patterns is warranted. Given that cardiovascular benefits are shown across a variety of healthy PBD profiles, the ideal PBD for reduction of CVD in an individual patient is one that ascribes closely to the preferences, motivations, values, and available food options for each individual patient such that adherence, quality of life, and cardiovascular benefits are maximized.

References

1. Tuso P, Stoll SR, Li WW. A plant-based diet, athero-genesis, and coronary artery disease prevention. Perm J. 2015 Winter;19(1):62–7.
2. Hever J, Cronise RJ. Plant-based nutrition for health-care professionals: implementing diet as a primary modality in the prevention and treatment of chronic disease. J Geriatr Cardiol. 2017;14(5):355–68.
3. Pawlak R, Lester SE, Babatunde T. The prevalence of cobalamin deficiency among vegetarians assessed by serum vitamin B12: a review of literature. Eur J Clin Nutr. 2014;68(5):541–8.
4. Davey GK, Spencer EA, Appleby PN, Allen NE, Knox KH, Key TJ. EPIC-Oxford: lifestyle character-istics and nutrient intakes in a cohort of 33 883 meat-eaters and 31 546 non meat-eaters in the UK. Public Health Nutr. 2003;6(3):259–69.
5. O'Sullivan TA, Hafekost K, Mitrou F, Lawrence D. Food sources of saturated fat and the association with mortality: a meta-analysis. Am J Public Health. 2013;103(9):e31–42.
6. Ahluwalia N, Genoux A, Ferrieres J, Perret B, Carayol M, Drouet L, et al. Iron status is associated with carotid atherosclerotic plaques in middle-aged adults. J Nutr. 2010;140(4):812–6.
7. Chemicals in meat cooked at high temperatures and cancer risk [Internet]. 2018 [cited 2020 Sep 5]. Available from: http://www.cancer.gov/cancertop-ics/causes-prevention/risk/diet/cooked-meats-fact-sheet
8. Uribarri J, Woodruff S, Goodman S, Cai W, Chen X, Pyzik R, et al. Advanced glycation end products in foods and a practical guide to their reduction in the diet. J Am Diet Assoc. 2010;110(6):911–6.e12.
9. Koeth RA, Wang Z, Levison BS, Buffa JA, Org E, Sheehy BT, et al. Intestinal microbiota metabolism of L-carnitine, a nutrient in red meat, promotes athero-sclerosis. Nat Med. 2013;19(5):576–85.
10. Martin PT, Camboni M, Xu R, Golden B, Chan-drasekharan K, Wang C-M, et al. N-Glycolylneur-aminic acid deficiency worsens cardiac and skeletal muscle pathophysiology in α-sarcoglycan-deficient mice. Glycobiology. 2013;23(7):833–43.
11. Estruch R, Ros E, Salas-Salvadó J, Covas M-I, Corella D, Arós F, et al. Primary prevention of cardiovascu-lar disease with a Mediterranean diet. N Engl J Med. 2013;368(14):1279–90.
12. Sacks FM, Svetkey LP, Vollmer WM, Appel LJ, Bray GA, Harsha D, et al. Effects on blood pressure of reduced dietary sodium and the dietary approaches to stop hypertension (DASH) diet. DASH-Sodium Collaborative Research Group. N Engl J Med. 2001;344(1):3–10.
13. Orlich MJ, Singh PN, Sabaté J, Jaceldo-Siegl K, Fan J, Knutsen S, et al. Vegetarian dietary patterns and mortality in Adventist Health Study 2. JAMA Intern Med. 2013;173(13):1230–8.
14. Satija A, Bhupathiraju SN, Spiegelman D, Chiuve SE, Manson JE, Willett W, et al. Healthful and unhealthful plant-based diets and the risk of coronary heart disease in U.S. adults. J Am Coll Cardiol. 2017;70(4):411–22.
15. Hyunju K, Caulfield Laura E, Vanessa G-L, Steffen Lyn M, Josef C, Rebholz Casey M. Plant-based diets are associated with a lower risk of incident cardio-vascular disease, cardiovascular disease mortality, and all-cause mortality in a general population of middle-aged adults. J Am Heart Assoc. 2019;8(16): e012865.
16. Martínez-González MA, Sánchez-Tainta A, Corella D, Salas-Salvadó J, Ros E, Arós F, et al. A proveg-etarian food pattern and reduction in total mortality in the Prevención con Dieta Mediterránea (PREDIMED) study. Am J Clin Nutr. 2014;100(Suppl 1):320S–8S.
17. Patel H, Chandra S, Alexander S, Soble J, Williams KA Sr. Plant-based nutrition: An essential component of cardiovascular disease prevention and manage-ment. Curr Cardiol Rep. 2017;19(10):104.
18. Kahleova H, Levin S, Barnard N. Cardio-metabolic benefits of plant-based diets. Nutrients [Internet]. 2017;9(8). Available from: https://doi.org/10.3390/nu9080848
19. Yokoyama Y, Levin SM, Barnard ND. Associa-tion between plant-based diets and plasma lipids: a systematic review and meta-analysis. Nutr Rev. 2017;75(9):683–98.
20. Wang F, Zheng J, Yang B, Jiang J, Fu Y, Li D. Effects of vegetarian diets on blood lipids: a systematic review and meta-analysis of randomized controlled trials. J Am Heart Assoc. 2015;4(10):e002408.
21. Yokoyama Y, Barnard ND, Levin SM, Watanabe M. Vegetarian diets and glycemic control in diabetes: a systematic review and meta-analysis. Cardiovasc Diagn Ther. 2014;4(5):373–82.
22. Kahleova H, Matoulek M, Malinska H, Oliyarnik O, Kazdova L, Neskudla T, et al. Vegetarian diet improves insulin resistance and oxidative stress mark-ers more than conventional diet in subjects with type 2 diabetes. Diabet Med. 2011;28(5):549–59.
23. Menzel J, Biemann R, Longree A, Isermann B, Mai K, Schulze MB, et al. Associations of a vegan diet with inflammatory biomarkers. Sci Rep. 2020;10(1):1933.
24. Melina V, Craig W, Levin S. Position of the academy of nutrition and dietetics: Vegetarian diets. J Acad Nutr Diet. 2016;116(12):1970–80.
25. Vegetarian, vegan and meals without meat [Inter-net]. [cited 2020 Sep 13]. Available from: https://www.heart.org/en/healthy-living/healthy-eating/eat-smart/nutrition-basics/vegetarian-vegan-and-meals-without-meat
26. Appendix 5. USDA Food Patterns: Healthy Vegetar-ian Eating Pattern [Internet]. [cited 2020 Sep 13]. Available from: https://health.gov/our-work/food-nutrition/2015-2020-dietary-guidelines/guidelines/appendix-5/
27. Leading Causes of Death [Internet]. 2020 [cited 2020 Sep 13]. Available from: https://www.cdc.gov/nchs/fastats/leading-causes-of-death.htm

28. Allen KE, Gumber D, Ostfeld RJ. Heart failure and a plant-based diet. a case-report and literature review [Internet]. Vol. 6, Front Nutr. 2019. Available from: https://doi.org/10.3389/fnut.2019.00082

29. Satija A, Hu FB. Plant-based diets and cardiovascular health [Internet]. Trends Cardiovasc Med. 2018;28:437–41. Available from: https://doi.org/10.1016/j.tcm.2018.02.004

30. Budoff MJ, Bhatt DL, Kinninger A, Lakshmanan S, Muhlestein JB, Le VT, et al. Effect of icosapent ethyl on progression of coronary atherosclerosis in patients with elevated triglycerides on statin therapy: final results of the EVAPORATE trial. Eur Heart J. 2020;41(40):3925–32.

31. Nicholls SJ, Puri R, Anderson T, Ballantyne CM, Cho L, Kastelein JJP, et al. Effect of Evolocumab on progression of coronary disease in statin-treated patients: the GLAGOV randomized clinical trial. JAMA. 2016;316(22):2373–84.

32. Ornish D, Scherwitz LW, Billings JH, Brown SE, Gould KL, Merritt TA, et al. Intensive lifestyle changes for reversal of coronary heart disease. JAMA. 1998;280(23):2001–7.

33. Beeson WL, Mills PK, Phillips RL, Andress M, Fraser GE. Chronic disease among seventh-day Adventists, a low-risk group. Rationale, methodology, and description of the population. Cancer. 1989;64(3):570–81.

34. Berkel J, de Waard F. Mortality pattern and life expectancy of seventh-day Adventists in the Netherlands. Int J Epidemiol. 1983;12(4):455–9.

35. Kwok CS, Umar S, Myint PK, Mamas MA, Loke YK. Vegetarian diet, seventh day Adventists and risk of cardiovascular mortality: a systematic review and meta-analysis. Int J Cardiol. 2014;176(3):680–6.

36. Borgi L, Curhan GC, Willett WC, Hu FB, Satija A, Forman JP. Long-term intake of animal flesh and risk of developing hypertension in three prospective cohort studies. J Hypertens. 2015;33(11):2231–8.

37. Yokoyama Y, Nishimura K, Barnard ND, Takegami M, Watanabe M, Sekikawa A, et al. Vegetarian Diets and Blood Pressure [Internet]. Vol. 174, JAMA Internal Medicine. 2014. p. 577. Available from: https://doi.org/10.1001/jamainternmed.2013.14547

38. Steffen LM, Kroenke CH, Yu X, Pereira MA, Slattery ML, Van Horn L, et al. Associations of plant food, dairy product, and meat intakes with 15-y incidence of elevated blood pressure in young black and white adults: the Coronary Artery Risk Development in Young Adults (CARDIA) Study. Am J Clin Nutr. 2005;82(6):1169–77; quiz 1363–4

39. Borgi L, Muraki I, Satija A, Willett WC, Rimm EB, Forman JP. Fruit and vegetable consumption and the incidence of hypertension in three prospective cohort studies [Internet]. Hypertension. 2016;67:288–93. Available from: https://doi.org/10.1161/hypertensionaha.115.06497

40. O'Donnell MJ, Chin SL, Rangarajan S, Xavier D, Liu L, Zhang H, et al. Global and regional effects of potentially modifiable risk factors associated with acute stroke in 32 countries (INTERSTROKE): a case-control study. Lancet. 2016;388(10046):761–75.

41. Hu D, Huang J, Wang Y, Zhang D, Qu Y. Fruits and vegetables consumption and risk of stroke: a meta-analysis of prospective cohort studies. Stroke. 2014;45(6):1613–9.

42. Larsson SC, Orsini N. Fish consumption and the risk of stroke [Internet]. Stroke. 2011;42:3621–3. Available from: https://doi.org/10.1161/strokeaha.111.630319

43. Wang C, Harris WS, Chung M, Lichtenstein AH, Balk EM, Kupelnick B. et al., n−3 Fatty acids from fish or fish-oil supplements, but not α-linolenic acid, benefit cardiovascular disease outcomes in primary- and secondary-prevention studies: a systematic review [Internet]. Am Clin Nutr. 2006;84:5–17. Available from: https://doi.org/10.1093/ajcn/84.1.5

44. Tonstad S, Stewart K, Oda K, Batech M, Herring RP, Fraser GE. Vegetarian diets and incidence of diabetes in the Adventist Health Study-2. Nutr Metab Cardiovasc Dis. 2013;23(4):292–9.

45. Lara KM, Levitan EB, Gutierrez OM, Shikany JM, Safford MM, Judd SE, et al. Dietary patterns and incident heart failure in U.S. adults without known coronary disease. J Am Coll Cardiol. 2019;73(16):2036–45.

46. Rautiainen S, Levitan EB, Mittleman MA, Wolk A. Fruit and vegetable intake and rate of heart failure: a population-based prospective cohort of women. Eur J Heart Fail. 2015;17(1):20–6.

47. Hicks KA, Mahaffey KW, Mehran R, Nissen SE, Wiviott SD, Dunn B, et al. 2017 cardiovascular and stroke endpoint definitions for clinical trials. J Am Coll Cardiol. 2018;71(9):1021–34.

48. Huang T, Yang B, Zheng J, Li G, Wahlqvist ML, Li D. Cardiovascular disease mortality and cancer incidence in vegetarians: a meta-analysis and systematic review. Ann Nutr Metab. 2012;60(4):233–40.

49. Satija A, Bhupathiraju SN, Rimm EB, Spiegelman D, Chiuve SE, Borgi L, et al. Plant-based dietary patterns and incidence of type 2 diabetes in US men and women: results from three prospective cohort studies. PLoS Med. 2016;13(6):e1002039.

50. Mishra S, Xu J, Agarwal U, Gonzales J, Levin S, Barnard ND. A multicenter randomized controlled trial of a plant-based nutrition program to reduce body weight and cardiovascular risk in the corporate setting: the GEICO study. Eur J Clin Nutr. 2013;67(7):718–24.

51. McMacken M, Shah S. A plant-based diet for the prevention and treatment of type 2 diabetes. J Geriatr Cardiol. 2017;14(5):342–54.

52. Barnard ND, Cohen J, Jenkins DJA, Turner-McGrievy G, Gloede L, Jaster B, et al. A Low-fat vegan diet improves glycemic control and cardiovascular risk factors in a randomized clinical trial in individuals with Type 2 diabetes [Internet]. Diabetes Care. 2006;29:1777–83. Available from: https://doi.org/10.2337/dc06-0606

53. Mensink RP, Katan MB. Effect of dietary trans fatty acids on high-density and low-density lipoprotein cholesterol levels in healthy subjects. N Engl J Med. 1990;323(7):439–45.

54. Gardner CD, Coulston A, Chatterjee L, Rigby A, Spiller G, Farquhar JW. The effect of a plant-based diet on plasma lipids in hypercholesterolemic adults: a randomized trial. Ann Intern Med. 2005;142(9): 725–33.
55. Ferdowsian HR, Barnard ND. Effects of plant-based diets on plasma lipids [Internet]. Am J Cardiol. 2009;104:947–56. Available from: https://doi.org/10.1016/j.amjcard.2009.05.032
56. Sacks FM, Carey VJ, Anderson CAM, Miller ER 3rd, Copeland T, Charleston J, et al. Effects of high vs low glycemic index of dietary carbohydrate on cardiovascular disease risk factors and insulin sensitivity: the OmniCarb randomized clinical trial. JAMA. 2014;312(23):2531–41.
57. Siri-Tarino PW. Effects of diet on high-density lipoprotein cholesterol [Internet]. Curr Atheroscler Rep. 2011;13:453–60. Available from: https://doi.org/10.1007/s11883-011-0207-y
58. Mensink RP, Zock PL, Kester ADM, Katan MB. Effects of dietary fatty acids and carbohydrates on the ratio of serum total to HDL cholesterol and on serum lipids and apolipoproteins: a meta-analysis of 60 controlled trials. Am J Clin Nutr. 2003;77(5): 1146–55.
59. Jenkins DJA, Wong JMW, Kendall CWC, Esfahani A, Ng VWY, Leong TCK, et al. The effect of a plant-based low-carbohydrate ("Eco-Atkins") diet on body weight and blood lipid concentrations in hyperlipidemic subjects [Internet]. Arch Intern Med. 2009;169:1046. Available from: https://doi.org/10.1001/archinternmed.2009.115
60. Manach C, Scalbert A, Morand C, Rémésy C, Jiménez L. Polyphenols: food sources and bioavailability [Internet]. Am J Clin Nutr. 2004;79:727–47. Available from: https://doi.org/10.1093/ajcn/79.5.727
61. Khurana S, Venkataraman K, Hollingsworth A, Piche M, Tai TC. Polyphenols: benefits to the cardiovascular system in health and in aging. Nutrients. 2013;5(10):3779–827.
62. Hollenberg NK. Red wine polyphenols enhance endothelial nitric oxide synthase expression and subsequent nitric oxide release from endothelial cells. Curr Hypertens Rep. 2003;5(4):287–8.
63. Rienks J, Barbaresko J, Nöthlings U. Association of polyphenol biomarkers with cardiovascular disease and mortality risk: a systematic review and meta-analysis of observational studies [Internet]. Nutrients. 2017;9:415. Available from: https://doi.org/10.3390/nu9040415
64. Rebello CJ, O'Neil CE, Greenway FL. Dietary fiber and satiety: the effects of oats on satiety. Nutr Rev. 2016;74(2):131–47.
65. Brown L, Rosner B, Willett WW, Sacks FM. Cholesterol-lowering effects of dietary fiber: a meta-analysis. Am J Clin Nutr. 1999;69(1):30–42.
66. Smith CE, Tucker KL. Health benefits of cereal fibre: a review of clinical trials. Nutr Res Rev. 2011;24(1):118–31.
67. Soliman GA. Dietary fiber, atherosclerosis, and cardiovascular disease. Nutrients [Internet]. 019;11(5):1155. Available from: https://doi.org/10.3390/nu11051155
68. Post RE, Mainous AG, King DE, Simpson KN. Dietary fiber for the treatment of Type 2 diabetes mellitus: a meta-analysis [Internet]. J Am Board Fam Med. 2012;25:16–23. Available from: https://doi.org/10.3122/jabfm.2012.01.110148
69. Quiñones M, Miguel M, Aleixandre A. Beneficial effects of polyphenols on cardiovascular disease [Internet]. Pharmacol Res. 2013;68:125–31. Available from: https://doi.org/10.1016/j.phrs.2012.10.018
70. Petersson H, Basu S, Cederholm T, Risérus U. Serum fatty acid composition and indices of stearoyl-CoA desaturase activity are associated with systemic inflammation: longitudinal analyses in middle-aged men. Br J Nutr. 2008;99(6):1186–9.
71. Lavie CJ, Milani RV, Mehra MR, Ventura HO. Omega-3 polyunsaturated fatty acids and cardiovascular diseases. J Am Coll Cardiol. 2009;54(7): 585–94.
72. Saini RK, Keum Y-S. Omega-3 and omega-6 polyunsaturated fatty acids: Dietary sources, metabolism, and significance — A review [Internet]. Vol. 203, Life Sci. 2018. p. 255–267. Available from: https://doi.org/10.1016/j.lfs.2018.04.049
73. Farvid MS, Ding M, Pan A, Sun Q, Chiuve SE, Steffen LM, et al. Dietary linoleic acid and risk of coronary heart disease: a systematic review and meta-analysis of prospective cohort studies. Circulation. 2014;130(18):1568–78.
74. Carson JAS, Lichtenstein AH, Anderson CAM, Appel LJ, Kris-Etherton PM, Meyer KA, et al. Dietary cholesterol and cardiovascular risk: a science advisory from the American Heart Association. Circulation. 2020;141(3):e39–53.
75. Janeiro M, Ramírez M, Milagro F, Martínez J, Solas M. Implication of Trimethylamine N-Oxide (TMAO) in disease: potential biomarker or new therapeutic target [Internet]. Nutrients. 2018;10:1398. Available from: https://doi.org/10.3390/nu10101398
76. Fang X, An P, Wang H, Wang X, Shen X, Li X, et al. Dietary intake of heme iron and risk of cardiovascular disease: a dose-response meta-analysis of prospective cohort studies. Nutr Metab Cardiovasc Dis. 2015;25(1):24–35.
77. Chemicals in meat cooked at high temperatures and cancer risk [Internet]. 2018 [cited 2020 Sep 16]. Available from: https://www.cancer.gov/about-cancer/causes-prevention/risk/diet/cooked-meats-fact-sheet
78. Young VR, Pellett PL. Plant proteins in relation to human protein and amino acid nutrition [Internet]. Am J Clin Nutr. 1994;59:1203S–12S. Available from: https://doi.org/10.1093/ajcn/59.5.1203s
79. Hunt JR. Bioavailability of iron, zinc, and other trace minerals from vegetarian diets. Am J Clin Nutr. 2003;78(3 Suppl):633S–9S.
80. Craig WJ, Mangels AR. American dietetic association. Position of the American dietetic association:

vegetarian diets. J Am Diet Assoc. 2009;109(7): 1266–82.

81. Saunders AV, Craig WJ, Baines SK, Posen JS. Iron and vegetarian diets. Med J Aust. 2013;199(S4): S11–6.

82. Hallberg L, Brune M, Rossander L. The role of vitamin C in iron absorption. Int J Vitam Nutr Res Suppl. 1989;30:103–8.

83. Roohani N, Hurrell R, Kelishadi R, Schulin R. Zinc and its importance for human health: An integrative review. J Res Med Sci. 2013;18(2):144–57.

84. Hunt JR. Moving toward a plant-based diet: Are Iron and Zinc at Risk? [Internet]. Nutr Rev. 2002;60:127–34. Available from: https://doi.org/10.1301/00296640260093788

85. Gibson RS, Heath A-LM, Szymlek-Gay EA. Is iron and zinc nutrition a concern for vegetarian infants and young children in industrialized countries? Am J Clin Nutr. 2014;100(Suppl 1):459S–68S.

86. Haddad EH, Berk LS, Kettering JD, Hubbard RW, Peters WR. Dietary intake and biochemical, hematologic, and immune status of vegans compared with nonvegetarians. Am J Clin Nutr. 1999;70(3 Suppl):586S–93S.

87. Quinn C. Vitamin D: the sunshine vitamin [Internet]. Br J Nurs. 2010;19:1160–3. Available from: https://doi.org/10.12968/bjon.2010.19.18.79048

88. Chan J, Jaceldo-Siegl K, Fraser GE. Serum 25-hydroxyvitamin D status of vegetarians, partial vegetarians, and nonvegetarians: the Adventist Health Study-2 [Internet]. Am J Clin Nutr. 2009;89:1686S–92S. Available from: https://doi.org/10.3945/ajcn.2009.26736x

89. Rizzo G, Laganà AS, Rapisarda AMC, La Ferrera GMG, Buscema M, Rossetti P, et al. Vitamin B12 among vegetarians: status, assessment and supplementation. Nutrients [Internet]. 2016;8(12). Available from: https://doi.org/10.3390/nu8120767

90. Allen LH. Causes of vitamin B12 and folate deficiency. Food Nutr Bull. 2008;(2 Suppl):29, S20–S34; discussion S35–7.

91. Langan RC, Goodbred AJ. Vitamin B12 deficiency: recognition and management. Am Fam Physician. 2017;96(6):384–9.

92. O'Leary F, Samman S. Vitamin B12 in Health and Disease [Internet]. Nutrients. 2010;2:299–316. Available from: https://doi.org/10.3390/nu2030299

93. Pawlak R. Is vitamin B12 deficiency a risk factor for cardiovascular disease in vegetarians? Am J Prev Med. 2015;48(6):e11–26.

94. Collaboration HS. Homocysteine studies collaboration. homocysteine and risk of ischemic heart disease and stroke [Internet]. JAMA. 2002;288:2015. Available from: https://doi.org/10.1001/jama.288.16.2015

95. Mechanisms of disease: Homocysteine and atherothrombosis [Internet]. Transfus Med Rev. 1998;12: 312. Available from: https://doi.org/10.1016/s0887-7963(98)80027-8

96. Basu A, Jenkins AJ, Stoner JA, Thorpe SR, Klein RL, Lopes-Virella MF, et al. Plasma total homocysteine and carotid intima-media thickness in type 1 diabetes: a prospective study. Atherosclerosis. 2014;236(1):188–95.

97. Li Z, Heber D. The pritikin diet. JAMA. 2020;323 (11):1104.

98. Pritikin ICR: Pritikin intensive cardiac rehab [Internet]. 2012 [cited 2020 Sep 5]. Available from: https://www.pritikin.com/your-health/health-benefits/reverse-heart-disease/pritikin-icr.html

99. Pritikin Diet [Internet]. 2018 [cited 2020 Sep 5]. Available from: https://www.pritikin.com/healthiest-diet/pritikin-eating-plan

100. Anderson AL, Harris TB, Tylavsky FA, Perry SE, Houston DK, Hue TF, et al. Dietary patterns and survival of older adults. J Am Diet Assoc 2011;111(1):84–91.

101. Sullivan S, Samuel S. Effect of short-term Pritikin diet therapy on the metabolic syndrome. J Cardiometab Syndr. 2006;1(5):308–12.

102. Chen AK, Roberts CK, Barnard RJ. Effect of a short-term diet and exercise intervention on metabolic syndrome in overweight children. Metabolism. 2006;55(7):871–8.

103. Barnard RJ. Effects of life-style modification on serum lipids. Arch Intern Med. 1991;151(7): 1389–94.

104. Wegge JK, Roberts CK, Ngo TH, Barnard RJ. Effect of diet and exercise intervention on inflammatory and adhesion molecules in postmenopausal women on hormone replacement therapy and at risk for coronary artery disease. Metabolism. 2004;53(3): 377–81.

105. Roberts CK, Won D, Pruthi S, Kurtovic S, Sindhu RK, Vaziri ND, et al. Effect of a short-term diet and exercise intervention on oxidative stress, inflammation, MMP-9, and monocyte chemotactic activity in men with metabolic syndrome factors. J Appl Physiol. 2006;100(5):1657–65.

106. Decision Memo for Intensive Cardiac Rehabilitation (ICR) Program – Dr. Ornish's Program for Reversing Heart Disease (CAG-00419N) [Internet]. [cited 2020 Sep 16]. Available from: https://www.cms.gov/medicare-coverage-database/details/nca-decision-memo.aspx?NCAId=240&ver=7&NcaName=Intensive+Cardiac+Rehabilitation+(ICR)+Program+-+Dr.+Ornish%2527s+Program+for+Reversing+Heart+Disease&bc=ACAAAAAAIA-AA&siteTool=Medic

107. Nutrition [Internet]. [cited 2020 Sep 16]. Available from: https://www.ornish.com/proven-program/nutrition/

108. Department of Health and Human Services, U.S. Department of Agriculture. Dietary Guidelines for Americans 2015-2020. Simon and Schuster; 2017. 146 p.

109. Ma Y, Pagoto SL, Griffith JA, Merriam PA, Ockene IS, Hafner AR, et al. A dietary quality comparison

of popular weight-loss plans. J Am Diet Assoc. 2007;107(10):1786–91.

110. McCullough ML, Willett WC. Evaluating adherence to recommended diets in adults: the alternate healthy eating index. Public Health Nutr. 2006;9(1A): 152–7.

111. Dansinger ML, Gleason JA, Griffith JL, Selker HP, Schaefer EJ. Comparison of the Atkins, Ornish, weight watchers, and zone diets for weight loss and heart disease risk reduction: a randomized trial. JAMA. 2005;293(1):43–53.

112. Ornish D, Brown SE, Scherwitz LW, Billings JH, Armstrong WT, Ports TA, et al. Can lifestyle changes reverse coronary heart disease? The Lifestyle Heart Trial. Lancet [Internet]. 1990 Jul 21 [cited 2021 Mar 16];336(8708). Available from: https://pubmed.ncbi.nlm.nih.gov/1973470/

113. Bessesen DH. Comparison of the Atkins, Ornish, Weight Watchers, and zone diets for weight loss and heart disease risk reduction: a randomized trial [Internet]. Yearbook Endocrinol. 2006;2006:151–3. Available from: https://doi.org/10.1016/s0084-3741(08)70337-8

114. Plant-Based Nutrition [Internet]. [cited 2020 Sep 16]. Available from: http://www.dresselstyn.com/site/plant-based-nutrition/

115. Esselstyn CB Jr, Gendy G, Doyle J, Golubic M, Roizen MF. A way to reverse CAD? J Fam Pract. 2014;63(7):356–64b.

116. Esselstyn CB Jr, Ellis SG, Medendorp SV, Crowe TD. A strategy to arrest and reverse coronary artery disease: a 5-year longitudinal study of a single physician's practice. J Fam Pract. 1995;41(6):560–8.

117. Barnard ND, Cohen J, Jenkins DJA, Turner-McGrievy G, Gloede L, Green A, et al. A low-fat vegan diet and a conventional diabetes diet in the treatment of type 2 diabetes: a randomized, controlled, 74-wk clinical trial. Am J Clin Nutr. 2009;89(5):1588S–96S.

118. Barnard ND, Scialli AR, Turner-McGrievy G, Lanou AJ, Glass J. The effects of a low-fat, plant-based dietary intervention on body weight, metabolism, and insulin sensitivity. Am J Med. 2005;118(9):991–7.

119. Pechey R, Monsivais P. Socioeconomic inequalities in the healthiness of food choices: exploring the contributions of food expenditures. Prev Med. 2016;88:203–9.

120. Marcone MF, Madan P, Grodzinski B. An overview of the sociological and environmental factors influencing eating food behavior in Canada. Front Nutr. 2020;7:77.

121. Brown MT, Bussell JK. Medication adherence: WHO cares? Mayo Clin Proc. 2011;86(4):304–14.

122. Neal D. Barnard, Anthony R. Scialli, Gabrielle Turner-McGrievy, Amy J. Lanou. Acceptability of a Low-fat Vegan Diet Compares Favorably to a Step II Diet in a Randomized, Controlled Trial. J Cardiopulm Rehab. 2004;24(4):229–235.

Plant-Based Oils

7

Katrina Han, Kelley Jo Willams,
and Anne Carol Goldberg

Introduction

Since 1961, the American Heart Association has recommended reducing dietary saturated fat to reduce atherosclerotic cardiovascular disease (ASCVD) risk. This is due to the effect of saturated fat on raising low-density lipoprotein (LDL) cholesterol, a major contributor to atherosclerosis [1]. Replacing saturated fat with polyunsaturated fat reduces the incidence of ASCVD in randomized control trials. Additionally, populations with diets low in saturated fat and high in unsaturated fat have lower rates of ASCVD [2, 3]. For the general population, the current Dietary Guidelines for Americans recommend consuming less than 10% of calories from saturated fat. However, most Americans continue to consume more saturated fat than is recommended [4].

Fatty Acids

Most fats have a hydrophobic center with fairly long carbon chains (Fig. 7.1). Lipids associate with each other and are not soluble in water. Fatty acids and cholesterol are simple lipids, whereas triglycerides and phospholipids are complex

Stearic acid: $CH_3—(CH_2)_{16}—COOH$
Oleic acid: $CH_3—(CH_2)_7—CH=CH—(CH_2)_7—COOH$
Linoleic acid: $CH_3—(CH_2)_4—CH=CH—CH_2-CH=CH—(CH_2)_7—COOH$

Fig. 7.1 Structure of Fatty Acids

lipids. Differences in the metabolic effects of fatty acids can be attributed to their distinct biochemical properties. Fatty acids are characterized by the number of carbon atoms and double bonds present in their chemical structures. Saturated fatty acids, such as stearic acid (C18:0), do not contain any double bonds. Monounsaturated fatty acids, such as oleic acid (C18:1), contain only one double bond. Polyunsaturated fatty acids, such as linoleic acid (C18:2), have at least two double bonds within their long hydrocarbon chains [5, 6].

The presence of only single bonds within saturated fatty acids creates a linear hydrocarbon chain that allows for these molecules to be packed together tightly, which causes them to be solid at room temperature. Double bonds in unsaturated fatty acids create kinks within the hydrocarbon tail which prevents tight packing of these molecules allowing them to remain liquid at room temperature [7].

Polyunsaturated fatty acids are further characterized based on the location of the first carbon double bond. For example, omega-3 fatty (n-3) acids are polyunsaturated fatty acids in which the first double bond is located at the third carbon from the end of the molecule farthest from the carboxy (–COOH)-terminal. Fish oils are rich

K. Han · K. J. Willams · A. C. Goldberg (✉)
Division of Endocrinology, Metabolism, and Lipid Research, Department of Medicine, Washington University School of Medicine, St. Louis, MO, USA
e-mail: agoldber@wustl.edu

© Springer Nature Switzerland AG 2021
M. J. Wilkinson et al. (eds.), *Prevention and Treatment of Cardiovascular Disease*, Contemporary Cardiology, https://doi.org/10.1007/978-3-030-78177-4_7

Table 7.1 Important fatty acids

Common name	Chemical structure	Sources
Saturated fatty acids		
Lauric	C12:0	Coconut oil, palm kernel oil
Myristic	C14:0	Butter fat, coconut oil
Palmitic	C16:0	Butter, cheese, beef, pork
Stearic	C18:0	Beef, pork, chocolate
Monounsaturated fatty acids		
Oleic	C18:1	Olive oil, canola oil, avocado, peanut oil
Polyunsaturated fatty acids		
Omega-6 fatty acids		
Linoleic	C18:2	Soybean oil, corn oil, walnut oil
Omega-3 fatty acids		
α-Linolenic acid	C18:3	Canola oil, flaxseed oil, soybean oil, walnut oil
Eicosapentaenoic	C20:5	Fatty fish: salmon, tuna, mackerel
Docosahexaenoic	C22:6	Fatty fish: salmon, tuna, mackerel

Fig. 7.2 Cis- and Trans-Configuration

in omega-3 fatty acids, and plant oils are rich in omega-6 (n-6) fatty acids, both of which lower lipids. Most omega-3 and omega-6 fatty acids are essential (i.e., humans cannot synthesize them). Saturated fatty acids and some unsaturated fatty acids are nonessential [8]. Table 7.1 lists common food sources of major fatty acids.

Trans-fatty acids are monounsaturated or polyunsaturated fatty acids containing at least one double bond with hydrogens on opposite sides of the double bond (trans-configuration). This is in contrast to the cis-configuration in which the two hydrogen atoms adjacent to the double bond are on the same side (Fig. 7.2) [9].

Oils High in Polyunsaturated Fatty Acids

Polyunsaturated fatty acids have two or more double bonds and exist in the n-3 or n-6 isomeric configurations (omega-3 or omega-6). Both of these forms are essential fatty acids. Overall, omega-6 fatty acids are more prevalent in the diet than omega-3 fatty acids. Walnuts, pine nuts, flaxseed, corn oil, and soybean oil are all high in polyunsaturated fatty acids. Fish oil contains very-long-chain omega-3 polyunsaturated fatty acids—eicosapentaenoic acid (EPA) and docosahexaenoic acid (DHA), which are found in salmon, trout, tuna, herring, and mackerel. The plant sources of omega-3 fatty acids include walnuts and flax seeds [10].

Soybean Oil

Background and Biochemistry

Soybeans are the greatest source of edible oil in the world, and soybean oil accounts for most of the vegetable oil produced in the USA [11]. Soybeans are processed to extract the oil, and the remaining products are mostly used for animal feed. This oil is commonly used in cooking oil, salad dressings, margarines, and frying fats.

Soybean oil is predominantly a polyunsaturated fat. Its content is 50% omega-6 polyunsaturated fatty acid, linoleic acid (C18:2; n-6), and 7% omega-3 polyunsaturated fatty acid, α-linolenic acid (C18:3; n-3). The monounsaturated fatty acid, oleic acid (C18:1), comprises 23%, and the remaining 16% is saturated fatty acids (predominately palmitic acid) [12].

Metabolic Effects and Cardiovascular Outcomes

Several studies show that replacing saturated fatty acids with soybean oil reduces cholesterol and decreases coronary heart disease [1]. One of these studies was the British Medical Research

Council study comparing a diet high in soybean oil with a diet high in saturated fat. Replacing saturated fat with soybean oil lowered total cholesterol by 16% [1, 13]. The Finnish Mental Hospital Study compared a diet high in polyunsaturated fat, mostly soybean oil, with one high in saturated fat and found lower risk of coronary heart death in the polyunsaturated fat group [1, 14, 15]. Meta-analyses show that replacing saturated fat with oils high in polyunsaturated fat, again primarily soybean oil, lowers coronary heart disease. Other observational studies have found that increased intake of α-linolenic acid is associated with decreased risk of cardiovascular disease [16]. The high α-linolenic acid compostion within soybean oil may contribute to its impact on decreasing coronary heart disease.

Corn Oil

Background and Biochemistry

Corn germ is the embryo of the corn kernel and the part from which corn oil is extracted. Various methods are used to extract oil from the germ, most frequently wet milling. [17] Corn oil has five times more plant phytosterols than extra virgin olive oil, which contributes to its cholesterol lowering properties [18]. Corn oil has a high smoking point, making it useful for deep frying foods. It has a light color and is thus popular for salad dressings, cooking oil, mayonnaise, and margarines [19].

Corn oil is predominantly a polyunsaturated fat. It is composed of 53% linoleic acid (C18:2; n-6), 27% oleic acid (C18:1), and 13% saturated fatty acids (predominately palmitic acid) [12].

Metabolic Effects and Cardiovascular Outcomes

Controlled feeding studies show that intake of corn oil results in a larger reduction in LDL-cholesterol compared to olive oil [18]. In one study, consumption of corn oil lowered LDL-cholesterol by 10.9% compared to the average American diet and by 3.5% compared to a diet supplemented with extra virgin olive oil [18]. Another study showed that diets using corn oil as the predominant fat had a reduction of LDL-

cholesterol by 17% compared to a Western diet (compared to 16% reduction with canola oil and 13% reduction with olive oil) [20]. Circulating apoliproprotein B levels were also lower in the corn oil group compared to the olive oil group. Apolipoprotein B is the primary protein in VLDL-cholesterol and LDL-cholesterol. Elevated levels of apolipoprotein B-containing lipoproteins are associated with increased risk of ASCVD, making apolipoprotein B a useful biomarker [21]. Wagner et al. showed that corn oil has more influence on lipoproteins compared to oils predominantly composed of monounsaturated fatty acids [22]. This study was a 2-week feeding trial and found that a diet with corn oil as the main fat had lower LDL-cholesterol, VLDL-cholesterol, and total cholesterol than diets using olive oil as the main fat. This is thought to be due to the high polyunsaturated fatty acid content, as well as the high phytosterol content of corn oil. The Wadsworth Hospital and Veterans Administration Center conducted a double-blind feeding trial comparing a conventional diet high in saturated fat to an experimental diet high in polyunsaturated fat (using corn oil along with soybean, high-linoleic safflower, and cottonseed oils). The experimental diet group had significantly reduced combined primary and secondary cardiovascular endpoints including myocardial infarction, ischemic stroke, or sudden death [23]. However, a much smaller study by Rose et al. did not show a benefit of a corn oil diet [24].

Walnut Oil

Background and Biochemistry

In general, tree nut oils are low in saturated fats (with the exception of Brazil nut and cashew oils) and high in unsaturated fats. Most contain higher amounts of monounsaturated fatty acids than polyunsaturated fatty acids, except for Brazil nut and walnut oils. The predominant monounsaturated fatty acid in tree nut oils is oleic acid (C18:1), while the predominant polyunsaturated fatty acid is linoleic acid (C18:2) [25].

Compared to other tree nut oils, walnut oil contains the greatest ratio of polyunsaturated-to-monounsaturated fatty acids, with a higher omega-3-

to-omega-6 ratio [25, 26]. Its fatty acid composition includes about 58% linoleic acid (C18:2; n-6), 14% linolenic acid (C18:3; n-3), 13% oleic acid (C18:1), and 9% saturated fatty acids [27].

Metabolic Effects and Cardiovascular Outcomes

There has been extensive research on the effects of walnut consumption on lipids and lipoproteins. One meta-analysis, which included 26 trials, compared walnut consumption of 15–108 g/day to control (Western) diets for periods of 4 weeks to 1 year. Of the 26 studies, 6 were randomized parallel trials, and 20 had a crossover design. The analyses showed that walnut consumption was associated with a significant reduction in total cholesterol by about 7 mg/dL ($p < 0.001$; 3.25% greater reduction compared to controls), LDL-cholesterol by 5.5 mg/dL ($p < 0.001$; 3.73% reduction), triglycerides by 4.7 mg/dL ($p = 0.03$; 5.5% reduction), and apolipoprotein B by nearly 4 mg/dL ($p = 0.008$) [28].

These findings were further supported by a randomized, controlled, crossover feeding trial demonstrating that replacement of saturated fatty acids with polyunsaturated fatty acids from walnuts significantly reduced total cholesterol, LDL-cholesterol, non-HDL-cholesterol, and diastolic blood pressure [29].

Another randomized, double-blind, placebo-controlled clinical trial demonstrated that adding 15 mL of walnut oil per day to the diet of patients with type 2 diabetes was associated with significant decreases in total cholesterol and LDL-cholesterol levels [30].

Summary of Oils High in Polyunsaturated Fatty Acids

Several controlled trials have examined replacing diets high in saturated fat with diets high in polyunsaturated fat. Prospective observational studies have shown that replacing carbohydrate or saturated fat intake with α-linoleic acid (the major polyunsaturated fatty acid in soybean and corn oil) lowers the risk of coronary heart disease and coronary heart disease-related deaths [2].

A recent meta-analysis examined four core trials that looked at replacing a diet high in saturated fat with one high in polyunsaturated fat (predominately soybean oil). The results showed that replacing saturated fat with oils high in polyunsaturated fat lowered coronary heart disease by 29% [4]. Other meta-analyses looking at the four core trials, along with other trials, have found reductions in CVD events by 19–27% [31–33]. The amount of reduction in saturated fat was significantly associated with the decrease in CVD events, which is felt to be due to lower LDL-cholesterol. Reducing LDL-cholesterol is a key focus in reducing CVD risk. In summary, replacing saturated fat with polyunsaturated fat lowers ASCVD risk more than replacing saturated fat with monounsaturated fat.

Oils High in Monounsaturated Fatty Acids

Monounsaturated fatty acids have one double bond. Oleic acid (C18:1) is an example of a monounsaturated fatty acid. Common sources of monounsaturated fatty acids include almonds, cashews, hazelnuts, pistachios, pecans, avocados, olive oil, canola oil, peanut oil, and high oleic sunflower and safflower oils. Monounsaturated fats are also part of animal fats like beef, chicken, and pork [10].

Canola and Rapeseed Oil

Background and Biochemistry

After palm oil and soybean oil, canola oil is the third major plant-based oil produced in the world [36]. Rapeseed oil is produced from the seed of the rape plant. Rapeseed oil naturally contains high levels of erucic acid (C22:1) which has been associated with myocardial lipidosis in rats. From selective plant breeding, rapeseed plants containing lower levels of erucic acid were cultivated. These plants and their oils were named canola since they were first produced in Canada [37]. For an oil to be labeled as canola, the FDA has mandated that no more than 2% of its fatty acid profile can come from erucic acid [38].

Canola oil consists of high levels of monounsaturated fatty acids and low levels of saturated fatty acids, including 60% oleic acid (C18:1; n-9), 20% linoleic acid (C18:2; n-6), 10% α-linolenic acid (C18:3; n-3), and < 7% saturated fatty acids [39]. It contains a 2:1 ratio of omega-6-to-omega-3 fatty acids, which some researchers suggest is a favorable balance that may have implications for lowering the risk of cardiovascular disease [40]. However, the ideal ratio has not been well defined, and there is greater consensus that increasing consumption of omega-3 fatty acids, including EPA and DHA, is more likely to improve cardiovascular outcomes than decreasing intake of omega-6 fatty acids, such as linoleic and arachidonic acid [41].

Selective plant breeding has also produced high-oleic canola oils, in which increased levels of monounsaturated fats replace a fraction of polyunsaturated fats. These varieties contain as much as 80–85% oleic acid, and this shift in fatty acid composition results in improved shelf-life and stability under high temperatures [42].

Metabolic Effects and Cardiovascular Outcomes

A limited number of high-quality trials have examined the effects of canola oil on cardiometabolic markers [43]. One meta-analysis that included two randomized, controlled crossover trials and three randomized, controlled, parallel studies comparing canola oil consumption to typical Western diets demonstrated that canola oil consumption was associated with a significant decrease in total cholesterol by an average of 12% and LDL-cholesterol by 17%. No significant changes were seen in HDL-cholesterol or triglyceride levels. This meta-analysis also examined four studies comparing the consumption of canola oil to sunflower oil. There was no significant difference in the reduction of total cholesterol and LDL-cholesterol. In three studies that compared canola oil to olive oil consumption, canola oil-based diets were associated with greater reductions in total cholesterol and LDL-cholesterol levels [44].

Sunflower and Safflower Oil

Background and Biochemistry

Safflower is a thistle-like annual plant predominantly grown in California. The seeds are occasionally used as a substitute for saffron and to make dyes. Seeds are also extracted to produce safflower oil, which is nutritionally similar to sunflower oil. The existence of two varieties of safflower creates the difference between the high-oleic versus high-linoleic compositions [45]. Safflower oil is commonly used for cooking oil, dressings, and margarines.

Sunflower oil is produced from the seeds of the sunflower. This oil has a mild flavor and is commonly used for frying foods and is used in cosmetics. It is also high in vitamin E. Different varieties of sunflower seeds exist, which leads to different fatty acid compositions [46].

High-oleic varieties of sunflower and safflower oil are much more common than the original high-linoleic varieties. *High-oleic* safflower oil is predominantly a monounsaturated fat. It is composed of 75% oleic acid (C18:1), 13% linoleic acid (C18:2; n-6), and 8% saturated fatty acids. *High-linoleic* safflower oil is predominantly a polyunsaturated fat. It is composed of 75% linoleic acid (C18:2; n-6), 14% oleic acid (C18:1), and 6% saturated fatty acids.

High-oleic sunflower oil is composed of 84% oleic acid (C18:1), 4% linoleic acid (C18:2; n-6), and 10% saturated fatty acids. *High-linoleic* sunflower oil is 66% linoleic acid (C18:2; n-6), 20% oleic acid (C18:1), and 10% saturated fatty acids [12].

Metabolic Effects and Cardiovascular Outcomes

High-linoleic acid safflower oil has been shown to lower LDL cholesterol by 15% compared to olive and peanut oils [47]. If the sunflower/safflower oil is predominantly composed of polyunsaturated fatty acids, it reduces LDL-cholesterol to a greater extent than olive oil [48]. As previously discussed, the Wadsworth Hospital and Veterans Administration Center conducted one of the core clinical trials looking at replacing saturated fat with unsaturated fat using high linoleic-acid safflower oil, in addition to corn, soybean, and cottonseed oils in the experimental group. The primary outcomes were sudden death due to coronary heart disease or myocardial infarction. One of the major secondary outcomes was cerebral infarction. No statistical difference was found between groups in regard to the two primary outcomes. However, when this was pooled with cerebral infarction and other secondary outcomes, the reduction was statistically significant with $p = 0.01$. Fatal atherosclerotic events were less in the experimental group with $p < 0.05$. Incidence for all combined primary and secondary endpoints was 31.3% for the experimental group versus 47.7% for the control group; $p = 0.02$ [1, 23].

Olive Oil

Background and Biochemistry

Different types of olive oil exist depending on the processing method. Virgin olive oil is obtained by purely mechanical processes without any alterations to the oil, and phenolic compounds are retained. Virgin olive oil has no more than 2.0% free fatty acid content. Extra virgin olive oil is the highest grade of olive oil and has no more than 0.8% free fatty acid content. Refined olive oil has altered acidity, and phenolic compounds are lost. Ordinary olive oil is a mixture of refined and virgin olive oil. [49, 50]

Olive oil is a popular cooking oil and a staple of the Mediterranean diet. The Mediterranean diet became of interest because of the low incidence of cardiovascular disease and higher life expectancy in parts of this geographic region [51]. It is thought that the diet in this area is a major contributor.

Olive oil is mostly a monounsaturated fat. It is composed of 71% of the monounsaturated fatty acid, oleic acid (C18:1). The remaining composition is 14% saturated fatty acids (predominately palmitic acid) and 10% of the omega-6 polyunsaturated fatty acid, linoleic acid (C18:2; n-6) [12].

Metabolic Effects and Cardiovascular Outcomes

Olive oil has a favorable effect on lipoproteins but not to the extent of oils composed of predominately polyunsaturated fatty acids do [52]. Some controlled feeding trials have shown that corn oil lowers LDL cholesterol to a greater extent than does olive oil [18]. However, compared to saturated fatty acids, olive oil does reduce LDL cholesterol [49]. Some of the phenol components are also thought to alter VLDL and to scavenge superoxide radicals [49, 53]. Some animal models have shown slowed development of coronary artery disease and regression of atherosclerosis with olive oil use [49].

The Seven Countries Study was one of the first epidemiology studies looking at diet and lifestyle and its relationship to cardiovascular risk. Its results led to interest in the Mediterranean diet. It showed that death rate differences between groups were positively related to the average percent of dietary energy intake from saturated fatty acids and negatively related to intake from monounsaturated fatty acids. Death rates were negatively related to the ratio of monounsaturated-to-saturated fatty acids. Oleic acid was the main monounsaturated fatty acid, reflecting olive oil use. All cause and coronary heart disease deaths were low in the group using olive oil as the main fat [1, 54]. However, other studies have not found an association between the use of olive oil and the reduction of cardiovascular disease. The PREDIMED study was a multicenter trial in Spain in which participants with high risk of cardiovascular disease were assigned to either a Mediterranean diet supplemented with extra virgin olive oil, a Mediterranean diet supplemented with mixed nuts (hazelnuts, almonds, walnuts), or a control diet with the advice to reduce dietary fat. The results showed protective effects with both experimental diets versus the control diet on major cardiovascular events, including myocardial infarction, stroke, or death from a cardiovascular cause. There was an absolute risk reduction of three major cardiovascular events per 1000 person-years and a relative risk reduction of 30%, but only stroke was significantly reduced among the individual components. The trial took place among very high-risk participants making generalizability uncertain, the control group had a much higher dropout rate; and there have been concerns regarding the ability to confirm randomization and adherence to the initial randomization group.

Peanut Oil

Background and Biochemistry

Peanuts are legumes but are often grouped with tree nuts. Peanut oil is intermediate in terms of composition between poly- and monounsaturated fatty acids. The monounsaturated fatty acid, oleic acid (C18:1), comprises 45% of this oil. The polyunsaturated fatty acid, linoleic acid (C18:2; n-6), comprises 32%. The remaining 17% is from saturated fatty acids (mostly palmitic acid) [12]. Phytosterols are also found in peanut oil. Peanut oil has a strong aroma and flavor and is commonly used in American, South Asian, Southeast Asian, and Chinese cuisines.

Metabolic Effects and Cardiovascular Outcomes

Studies are mixed regarding significant changes in LDL cholesterol or other lipoproteins after peanut oil intake [47]. The nuts themselves have been found to have lipid-lowering effects, though the translation to nut oils does not seem as clear. [47, 55]. This may be due to other components found in the nuts other than fatty acids. Most literature supports favorable effects of peanut oil when replacing saturated fat [56].

Summary of Oils High in Monounsaturated Fatty Acids

Prospective observational studies in many populations have demonstrated that reduced saturated fat intake coupled with higher intake of monounsaturated and polyunsaturated fat is associated with lower rates of CVD and all-cause mortality [1]. While replacing saturated fat with monounsaturated fat lowers ASCVD events, the effect is less than that of replacement with

polyunsaturated fat. Recommendations favoring replacement with polyunsaturated fat over monounsaturated fat stem from positive results of randomized clinical trials that used polyunsaturated fat compared with a lack of adequate trials that used monounsaturated fat [32]. It is further supported by greater relative risk reduction for polyunsaturated fats in observational studies [35], greater reduction in LDL with polyunsaturated fat [35, 57], and lower amounts of coronary artery atherosclerosis in nonhuman primates that were fed polyunsaturated fat rather than monounsaturated or saturated fat [34]. Nevertheless, replacement of saturated fat with either type of unsaturated fat results in reduction of CVD.

Oils High in Saturated Fatty Acids

Saturated fatty acids do not contain any double bonds. They occur naturally in many foods, primarily meats and dairy products and some plant oils. Major sources of saturated fatty acids include beef, pork, lamb, butter, cheese, and tropical plant oils (palm oil, palm kernel oil, and coconut oil).

Palm and Palm Kernel Oil

Background and Biochemistry

The production of palm oil has grown steadily worldwide leading to economic growth within rural communities but also resulting in negative environmental impacts, such as loss of habitats of endangered species. Palm oil is one of the most versatile plant-based oils. It functions as a natural preservative in processed foods, raises the melting point of ice cream, and provides the foaming agent in most shampoos and soaps. It is further used in cosmetic products and as a raw material for biofuels. It is naturally a semisolid at room temperature but can be processed to form a liquid oil for cooking [58].

Palm oil is high in saturated fat. It is composed of about 45% palmitic acid (C16:0), 39% oleic acid (C18:1), and 10% linoleic acid (C18:2). The low percentage of linoleic acid allows palm oil to be resistant to oxidative deterioration during food preparation [59].

While palm oil is extracted from the pulp of the oil palm fruit, palm kernel oil is extracted from the seed. Palm kernel oil has a higher saturated fat content than palm oil. The composition of palm kernel oil is similar to that of coconut oil with lauric acid (C12:0) comprising about 48%, myristic acid (C14:0) 16%, oleic acid (C18:1) 15%, and palmitic acid (C16:0) 8% [60].

Metabolic Effects and Cardiovascular Outcomes

The effect of palm oil on cardiovascular risk appears to be less favorable when compared to vegetable oils low in saturated fatty acids but more favorable when compared to oils rich in trans-fatty acids.

One meta-analysis included 27 trials that compared consumption of palm oil to vegetable oils low in saturated fatty acids (soybean, sunflower, canola, olive, or peanut oil). Twenty-four trials had a crossover feeding design, and three had a parallel design. Intake of palm oil varied across studies from 12% to 43% of total energy intake with duration ranging from 2 to 16 weeks. Compared to vegetable oils low in saturated fatty acids, palm oil intake was associated with significant increases in total cholesterol by 5.8 mg/dL and LDL-cholesterol by 3.6 mg/dL. This meta-analysis also examined nine trials that compared consumption of palm oil to partially hydrogenated oils (oils rich in trans-fatty acids). Palm oil intake was associated with a 1.26-mg/dL increase in HDL-cholesterol compared to partially hydrogenated oils [61]. Cardiovascluar outcomes from clinical trials have been variable partly due to differences in types of control oils used and levels of test oil used.

Coconut Oil

Background and Biochemistry

Coconut oil is commonly used as a cooking fat, body oil, and industrial oil. It is widely found in manufactured products, including margarines, ice creams, and confectionary items due to its low melting point, resistance to oxidative rancidity, and digestibility [62].

Coconut oil is composed primarily of saturated fat. Lauric acid (C12:0), often classified as a medium-chain (C6–12) saturated fatty acid, accounts for approximately 47% of the total fat content. Long-chain ($\geq$C14) saturated fatty acids, including myristic acid (C14:0) and palmitic acid (C16:0), make up about 25% [63, 64]. There is evidence from animal studies to suggest that medium-chain fatty acids have more favorable effects on metabolic profiles compared to long-chain fatty acids. This has been attributed to the unique pathways in which these fatty acids are metabolized [65, 66]. Medium-chain fatty acids are directly transported to the liver via absorption through the portal vein and demonstrate higher rates of mitochondrial oxidation, thus serving as a more efficient energy source compared to long-chain fatty acids, which require incorporation into chylomicrons and travel through the lymphatic circulation before reaching the bloodstream [67, 68]. This is one reason that coconut oil has been speculated to have beneficial effects on lipid profiles given its composition high in lauric acid. However, although lauric acid is chemically classified as a medium-chain fatty acid, it is largely absorbed and transported by chylomicrons, and thus behaves like the long-chain fatty acids. Thus, its biologic effects may be different from other medium-chain fatty acids [69, 70]. This may explain why clinical feeding trials comparing coconut oil to other plant-based oils have not demonstrated expected benefits of coconut oil.

Metabolic Effects and Cardiovascular Outcomes

Evidence suggests that coconut oil intake is associated with increased risk for ASCVD. This is supported by one meta-analysis of 16 crossover-randomized, parallel-randomized, and non-randomized sequential feeding trials in which coconut oil was compared to non-tropical vegetable oils (primarily soybean oil, safflower oil, canola oil, and olive oil) for a duration of

≥2 weeks. Coconut oil consumption was associated with significant increases in total cholesterol by 14.69 mg/dL, LDL-cholesterol by 10.47 mg/dL, and HDL-cholesterol by 4.00 mg/dL. There was no significant change in triglyceride levels, markers of glycemia (fasting plasma glucose), inflammation (C-reactive protein), or adiposity (body weight, waist circumference, % body fat). This analysis also demonstrated that compared to palm oil, coconut oil significantly increased total cholesterol and LDL-cholesterol [63].

Summary of Oils High in Saturated Fatty Acids

Human feeding trials have demonstrated that palm oil intake is associated with higher total cholesterol and LDL-cholesterol levels compared to vegetable oils low in saturated fatty acids. It may be preferable to trans-fat rich oils due to its effects on HDL-cholesterol, but the clinical significance of its effects on HDL-cholesterol remains unclear. Further studies are needed to better understand the effects of palm oil consumption on cardiovascular risk.

Similarly, feeding trials show that consumption of coconut oil is associated with significant increases in total cholesterol, LDL-cholesterol, and HDL-cholesterol. Again, the importance of the observed effect on HDL-cholesterol as it relates to cardiovascular risk remains uncertain.

Palm, palm kernel, and coconut oil are high in saturated fatty acids; thus, the consumption of these oils should be limited due to their adverse effects on lipid profiles and associated risk for ASCVD.

Reducing the intake of saturated fatty acids is associated with lower risk of ASCVD. One pooled analysis of 11 cohort studies (344,696 participants with 5249 CHD events) and one meta-analysis of 8 randomized controlled trials (13,614 participants with 1042 CHD events) showed that replacing 5% of energy intake from saturated fat with polyunsaturated fat was associated with a 10–13% decrease in risk of ASCVD [33, 71].

Oils Enriched in Trans-Fatty Acids

Trans-fatty acids contain at least one double bond in the trans-configuration. Naturally occurring trans-fatty acids are found primarily in meats and dairy products. They are produced in the stomachs of ruminant animals (cattle, sheep, goats, etc.) through bacterial transformation of unsaturated fatty acids to trans-fatty acids. Artificial trans-fatty acids are primarily found in partially hydrogenated vegetable oils.

Partially Hydrogenated Vegetable Oils

Background and Biochemistry

Hydrogenation is a process in which a liquid oil is heated in the presence of hydrogen atoms and a catalyst to produce a semisolid or solid fat. This process leads to the transformation of some polyunsaturated fatty acids to monounsaturated and saturated fatty acids as well as monounsaturated to saturated fatty acids. Some fatty acids are converted from a cis- to a trans-configuration, thus leading to the production of trans-fatty acids. Partially hydrogenated vegetable oils are appealing to the food service industry due to their increased shelf-life, stability during deep-frying, and flavor quality [72]. Fully hydrogenated oils contain essentially no trans-fats, but they do contain saturated fatty acids [73].

Metabolic Effects and Cardiovascular Outcomes

The effect of trans-fatty acids on cardiovascular risk has been evaluated in controlled dietary trials. One meta-analysis of 12 randomized controlled trials that examined isocaloric replacement of saturated or cis-unsaturated fatty acids by trans-fatty acids demonstrated that consumption of trans-fatty acids raised LDL-cholesterol, decreased HDL-cholesterol, and increased triglyceride levels. It also raised lipoprotein(a) levels [74].

Lipoprotein(a) is a particle that contains LDL and apolipoprotein(a)—a glycoprotein that is covalently linked to apolipoprotein B, the principal apolipoprotein of LDL-cholesterol. Lipoprotein(a) is a causal, independent risk factor for ASCVD [75, 76]. Data from seven placebo-controlled, randomized statin trials demonstrated that the risk of ASCVD events increased linearly with lipoprotein(a) concentrations [77].

The consumption of trans-fatty acids has been linked directly to an increase in incidence of coronary artery disease. In a meta-analysis of four prospective cohort studies involving nearly 140,000 subjects, a 2% increase in energy intake from trans-fatty acids was associated with a 23% increase in incidence of coronary artery disease [74, 78–81]. Due to the harmful effects that trans-fatty acids have on cardiovascular health, the FDA has banned the use of trans-fats in all foods sold in American grocery stores and restaurants [82].

Summary of Trans-Fatty Acids

Data from controlled feeding trials and prospective observational studies have demonstrated that consumption of trans-fatty acids from partially hydrogenated vegetable oils results in significant risk for atherosclerotic cardiovascular disease. It is strongly recommended that consumers avoid products containing trans-fatty acids and that food manufacturers use alternative fatty acids, ideally cis-unsaturated fatty acids, in food production.

Summary of Plant-Based Oils

Randomized controlled trials have consistently demonstrated that the risk and incidence of coronary heart disease are significantly reduced by replacing saturated fats with unsaturated fats.

In general, replacing saturated with polyunsaturated fats results in greater benefit compared to the replacement with monounsaturated fats. Due to the heterogeneity of human feeding trials, including differences in control diets, control oils, and quantity and frequency of study oil intake, it is difficult to discern which oils within

each of these categories provide the greatest benefit in regard to cardiovascular health.

The favorable effects of polyunsaturated and monounsaturated fats on cardiovascular outcomes are related to their associations with LDL-cholesterol reduction. Diets high in plant-based oils composed primarily of polyunsaturated fatty acids (soybean and corn oils) have been consistently shown to reduce LDL-cholesterol levels and coronary heart disease rates [1, 22]. Intake of oils high in monounsaturated fatty acids (olive, peanut, walnut, canola, and high-oleic safflower/sunflower oils) is also associated with LDL-cholesterol reduction, with some studies demonstrating improved cardiovascular outcomes [54]. However, the evidence demonstrating a direct correlation between the intake of monounsaturated fatty acids and decreased incidence of coronary heart disease is less clear compared to the data supporting the effects of polyunsaturated fatty acids.

The recommendation to limit saturated fat in the diet stems from its effect on raising LDL-cholesterol levels, which is a major cause of atherosclerosis [1]. Coconut, palm, and palm kernel oils are high in saturated fatty acids. Consumption of these oils is associated with increased LDL-cholesterol levels and cardiovascular risk and thus should be limited in the diet [61, 63]. Trans-fatty acids, including partially hydrogenated vegetable oils, are associated with even greater increase in risk and incidence of coronary heart disease and should be eliminated from the diet [74].

References

1. Sacks FM, et al. Dietary fats and cardiovascular disease: a presidential advisory from the American Heart Association. Circulation. 2017;136:e1–e23.
2. Farvid MS, et al. Dietary linoleic acid and risk of coronary heart disease: a systematic review and meta-analysis of prospective cohort studies. Circulation. 2014;130:1568–78.
3. Keys A. Seven countries. A multivariate analysis of death and coronary heart disease. Cambridge, MA: Harvard University Press; 1980.
4. Dietary Guidelines Advisory Committee. Advisory Report | health.gov. https://health.gov/our-work/food-nutrition/2015-2020-dietary-guidelines/advisory-report (2015).

5. The Editors of Encyclopaedia Britannica. Fatty acid: definition, structure, functions, properties, & examples. Encyclopedia Britannica https://www.britannica.com/science/fatty-acid (2020).

6. Bhagavan NV. Chapter 18 – lipids i: fatty acids and eicosanoids. In: Bhagavan NV, editor. Medical biochemistry. 4th ed. London: Academic Press; 2002. p. 365–99. https://doi.org/10.1016/B978-012095440-7/50020-2.

7. Gunstone FD. Fatty acids — Nomenclature, structure, isolation and structure determination, biosynthesis and chemical synthesis. In: Gunstone FD, editor. Fatty acid and lipid chemistry. Springer US; 1996. p. 1–34. https://doi.org/10.1007/978-1-4615-4131-8_1.

8. Williams R. Williams textbook of endocrinology. Philadelphia: Elsevier; 2016.

9. Cole AS, Eastoe JE. Chapter 8 - Lipids. In: Cole AS, Eastoe JE, editors. Biochemistry and oral biology. 2nd ed. Butterworth: Heinemann; 1988. p. 100–8. https://doi.org/10.1016/B978-0-7236-1751-8.50015-6.

10. U.S. Department of Health and Human Services. 2015–2020 dietary guidelines for Americans. https://health.gov/our-work/food-nutrition/2015-2020-dietary-guidelines/guidelines/chapter-1/a-closer-look-inside-healthy-eating-patterns/#callout-dietary-fats (2020).

11. Fan L, Eskin NAM. 15 - The use of antioxidants in the preservation of edible oils. In: Shahidi F, editor. Handbook of antioxidants for food preservation. Cambridge, UK: Woodhead Publishing; 2015. p. 373–88. https://doi.org/10.1016/B978-1-78242-089-7.00015-4.

12. U.S. Department of Agriculture: FoodData Central. https://fdc.nal.usda.gov/index.html (2020).

13. Morris JNEA. Controlled trial of soyabean oil in myocardial infarction. Lancet. 1968;2:693–700.

14. Miettinen M, et al. Dietary prevention of coronary heart disease in women: The Finnish Mental Hospital Study. Int J Epidemiol. 1983;12:17–25.

15. Turpeinen O, et al. Dietary prevention of coronary heart disease: The Finnish Mental Hospital Study. Int J Epidemiol. 1979;8:99–118.

16. Pan A, et al. α-Linolenic acid and risk of cardiovascular disease: a systematic review and meta-analysis. Am J Clin Nutr. 2012;96:1262–73.

17. Moreau RA, Johnston DB, Hicks KB, Haas MJ. 3 - aqueous extraction of corn oil after fermentation in the dry grind ethanol process. In: Farr WE, Proctor A, editors. Green vegetable oil processing. Urbana: AOCS Press; 2014. p. 53–72. https://doi.org/10.1016/B978-0-9888565-3-0.50006-6.

18. Maki KC, et al. Corn oil intake favorably impacts lipoprotein cholesterol, apolipoprotein and lipoprotein particle levels compared with extra-virgin olive oil. Eur J Clin Nutr. 2017;71:33–8.

19. Smithers GW. Reference module in food science. Amsterdam: Elsevier; 2015.

20. Lichtenstein AH, et al. Effects of canola, corn, and olive oils on fasting and postprandial plasma lipoproteins in humans as part of a National Cholesterol Education Program Step 2 diet. Arterioscler Thromb J Vasc Biol. 1993;13:1533–42.

21. Walldius G, et al. High apolipoprotein B, low apolipoprotein A-I, and improvement in the prediction of fatal myocardial infarction (AMORIS study): a prospective study. Lancet Lond Engl. 2001;358:2026–33.

22. Wagner K-H, Tomasch R, Elmadfa I. Impact of diets containing corn oil or olive/sunflower oil mixture on the human plasma and lipoprotein lipid metabolism. Eur J Nutr. 2001;40:161–7.

23. Seymour D, Lee PM, Sam H, Dixon Wilfrid J, Uwamie T. A controlled clinical trial of a diet high in unsaturated fat in preventing complications of atherosclerosis. Circulation. 1969;40:II–1–II-63.

24. Rose GA, Thomson WB, Williams RT. Corn oil in treatment of Ischaemic heart disease. Br Med J. 1965;1:1531–3.

25. Gong Y, Pegg RB. 3 - Tree nut oils: Properties and processing for use in food. In: Talbot G, editor. Specialty oils and fats in food and nutrition. Cambridge, UK: Woodhead Publishing; 2015. p. 65–86. https://doi.org/10.1016/B978-1-78242-376-8.00003-X.

26. Hayes D, Angove MJ, Tucci J, Dennis C. Walnuts (Juglans regia) chemical composition and research in human health. Crit Rev Food Sci Nutr. 2016;56:1231–41.

27. U.S. Department of Agriculture: National Nutrient Database for Standard Reference, Release 28. USDA https://fdc.nal.usda.gov/fdc-app.html#/food-details/171030/nutrients (2017).

28. Guasch-Ferré M, Li J, Hu FB, Salas-Salvadó J, Tobias DK. Effects of walnut consumption on blood lipids and other cardiovascular risk factors: an updated meta-analysis and systematic review of controlled trials. Am J Clin Nutr. 2018;108:174–87.

29. Tindall AM, et al. Replacing saturated fat with walnuts or vegetable oils improves central blood pressure and serum lipids in adults at risk for cardiovascular disease: a randomized controlled-feeding trial. J Am Heart Assoc. 2019;8:e011512.

30. Zibaeenezhad MJ, et al. Effects of walnut oil on lipid profiles in hyperlipidemic type 2 diabetic patients: a randomized, double-blind, placebo-controlled trial. Nutr Diabetes. 2017;7:e259.

31. Chowdhury R, et al. Association of dietary, circulating, and supplement fatty acids with coronary risk: a systematic review and meta-analysis. Ann Intern Med. 2014;160:398.

32. Hooper L, Martin N, Abdelhamid A, Smith GD. Reduction in saturated fat intake for cardiovascular disease. Cochrane Database Syst Rev. 2015; https://doi.org/10.1002/14651858.CD011737.

33. Mozaffarian D, Micha R, Wallace S. Effects on coronary heart disease of increasing polyunsaturated fat in place of saturated fat: a systematic review and meta-analysis of randomized controlled trials. PLoS Med. 2010;7

34. Rudel LL, Parks JS, Sawyer JK. Compared with dietary monounsaturated and saturated fat, polyun-

saturated fat protects African Green Monkeys from coronary artery atherosclerosis. Arterioscler Thromb Vasc Biol. 1995;15:2101–10.

35. Heyden S. Polyunsaturated and monounsaturated fatty acids in the diet to prevent coronary heart disease via cholesterol reduction. Ann Nutr Metab. 1994;38:117–22.

36. Ghazani SM, Marangoni AG. Healthy fats and oils. in reference module in food science. Elsevier; 2016. https://doi.org/10.1016/B978-0-08-100596-5.00100-1.

37. Logan A, Fagan P. Chapter 15 - strategies to prevent oxidative deterioration in oil-in-water emulsion systems: canola-based phenolic applications. In: Logan A, Nienaber U, Pan X, editors. Lipid Oxidation. AOCS Press; 2013. p. 457–83. https://doi.org/10.1016/B978-0-9830791-6-3.50018-7.

38. U.S. Food & Drug Administration. Code of Federal Regulations Title 21. https://www.accessdata. fda.gov/scripts/cdrh/cfdocs/cfCFR/CFRSearch. cfm?fr=184.1555 (2019).

39. Barthet V, Canola J. Overview. in reference module in food science. Elsevier; 2016. https://doi.org/10.1016/B978-0-08-100596-5.00029-9.

40. Simopoulos A, The P. Importance of the Omega-6/Omega-3 fatty acid ratio in cardiovascular disease and other chronic diseases. Exp Biol Med. 2008;233:674–88.

41. Wang, C. et al. Effects of Omega-3 Fatty Acids on Cardiovascular Disease: Summary. AHRQ Evidence Report Summaries (Agency for Healthcare Research and Quality (US), 2004).

42. Liu, L. & Iassonova, D. High-oleic canola oils and their food applications. American Oil Chemists' Society https://www.aocs.org/stay-informed/inform-magazine/featured-articles/high-oleic-canola-oils-and-their-food-applications-september-2012?SSO=True (2012).

43. Amiri M, et al. The effect of canola oil compared with sesame and sesame-canola oil on cardio-metabolic biomarkers in patients with type 2 diabetes: design and research protocol of a randomized, triple-blind, three-way, crossover clinical trial. ARYA Atheroscler. 2019;15:168–78.

44. Lin L, et al. Evidence of health benefits of canola oil. Nutr Rev. 2013;71:370–85.

45. Oelke, E. A. et al. Safflower. Purdue University Center for New Crops & Plant Products https://hort.purdue.edu/newcrop/afcm/safflower.html (2020).

46. Putnam, D. H. et al. Sunflower. https://hort.purdue.edu/newcrop/afcm/sunflower.html (2020).

47. Sales RL, et al. The effects of peanut oil on lipid profile of normolipidemic adults: a three-country collaborative study. J Appl Res. 2008;8:216–25.

48. Binkoski AE, Kris-Etherton PM, Wilson TA, Mountain ML, Nicolosi RJ. Balance of unsaturated fatty acids is important to a cholesterol-lowering diet: comparison of mid-oleic sunflower oil and olive oil on cardiovascular disease risk factors. J Am Diet Assoc. 2005;105:1080–6.

49. Ruiz-Canela M, Martínez-González MA. Olive oil in the primary prevention of cardiovascular disease. Maturitas. 2011;68:245–50.

50. U.S. Department of Agriculture. Olive Oil and Olive-Pomace Oil Grades and Standards. Agricultural marketing service. https://www.ams.usda.gov/grades--standards/olive-oil-and-olive-pomace-oil-grades-and-standards (2020).

51. Keys A. Coronary heart disease in seven countries. Circulation. 1970;41:186–95.

52. Berry EM, et al. Effects of diets rich in monounsaturated fatty acids on plasma lipoproteins—the Jerusalem Nutrition Study: high MUFAs vs high PUFAs. Am J Clin Nutr. 1991;53:899–907.

53. Fitó M, et al. Protective effect of olive oil and its phenolic compounds against low density lipoprotein oxidation. Lipids. 2000;35:633–8.

54. Keys A, et al. The diet and 15-year death rate in the seven countries study. Am J Epidemiol. 1986;124:903–15.

55. Chisholm A, Mc Auley K, Mann J, Williams S, Skeaff M. Cholesterol lowering effects of nuts compared with a Canola oil enriched cereal of similar fat composition. Nutr Metab Cardiovasc Dis. 2005;15:284–92.

56. Stephens AM, Dean LL, Davis JP, Osborne JA, Sanders TH. Peanuts, Peanut oil, and fat free peanut flour reduced cardiovascular disease risk factors and the development of atherosclerosis in Syrian Golden Hamsters. J Food Sci. 2010;75:H116–22.

57. Clarke R, Frost C, Collins R, Appleby P, Peto R. Dietary lipids and blood cholesterol: quantitative meta-analysis of metabolic ward studies. BMJ. 1997;314:112.

58. Lai O-M, Tan C-P, Akoh CC. Palm oil: production, processing, characterization, and uses. Champaign: Elsevier Science; 2015.

59. Voon PT, et al. Intake of palm Olein and lipid status in healthy adults: a meta-analysis. Adv Nutr. 2019;10:647–59.

60. Berger KG. Palm kernel oil. In: Caballero B, editor. Encyclopedia of food sciences and nutrition. 2nd ed. London: Academic Press; 2003. p. 4322–4. https://doi.org/10.1016/B0-12-227055-X/01379-1.

61. Sun Y, et al. Palm oil consumption increases LDL cholesterol compared with vegetable oils low in saturated fat in a meta-analysis of clinical trials. J Nutr. 2015;145:1549–58.

62. Lal, J. J., Sreeranjit Kumar, C. V. & Indira, M. Coconut palm. in Encyclopedia of food sciences and nutrition (2nd Edition) (ed. Caballero, B.) 1464–1475 (Academic Press, 2003). doi:https://doi.org/10.1016/B0-12-227055-X/00263-7.

63. Nithya N, Hoong SJY, van Dam Rob M. The effect of coconut oil consumption on cardiovascular risk factors. Circulation. 2020;141:803–14.

64. Eyres L, Eyres MF, Chisholm A, Brown RC. Coconut oil consumption and cardiovascular risk factors in humans. Nutr Rev. 2016;74:267–80.

65. Montgomery MK, et al. Contrasting metabolic effects of medium- versus long-chain fatty acids in skeletal muscle. J Lipid Res. 2013;54:3322–33.
66. Arunima S, Rajamohan T. Virgin coconut oil improves hepatic lipid metabolism in rats--compared with copra oil, olive oil and sunflower oil. Indian J Exp Biol. 2012;50:802–9.
67. Bach AC, Babayan VK. Medium-chain triglycerides: an update. Am J Clin Nutr. 1982;36:950–62.
68. Marten B, Pfeuffer M, Schrezenmeir J. Medium-chain triglycerides. Int Dairy J. 2006;16:1374–82.
69. Denke MA, Grundy SM. Comparison of effects of lauric acid and palmitic acid on plasma lipids and lipoproteins. Am J Clin Nutr. 1992;56:895–8.
70. Bloom B, Chaikoff IL, Reinhardt WO. Intestinal lymph as pathway for transport of absorbed fatty acids of different chain lengths. Am J Physiol-Leg Content. 1951;166:451–5.
71. Jakobsen MU, et al. Major types of dietary fat and risk of coronary heart disease: a pooled analysis of 11 cohort studies. Am J Clin Nutr. 2009;89:1425–32.
72. Mirmiran P, Hosseini S, Hosseinpour-Niazi S. Chapter 2 - hydrogenated vegetable oils and trans fatty acids: profile and application to diabetes. In: Watson RR, Preedy VR, editors. Bioactive food as dietary interventions for diabetes. 2nd ed. London: Academic Press; 2019. p. 19–32. https://doi.org/10.1016/B978-0-12-813822-9.00002-3.
73. Crupkin M, Zambelli A. Detrimental impact of trans fats on human health: stearic acid-rich fats as possible substitutes. Compr Rev Food Sci Food Saf. 2008;7:271–9.
74. Mozaffarian D, Katan MB, Ascherio A, Stampfer MJ, Willett WC. Trans fatty acids and cardiovascular disease. N Engl J Med. 2006;354:1601–13.
75. Kamstrup PR, Tybjærg-Hansen A, Steffensen R, Nordestgaard BG. Genetically elevated lipoprotein(a) and increased risk of myocardial infarction. JAMA. 2009;301:2331–9.
76. Clarke R, et al. Genetic variants associated with Lp(a) lipoprotein level and coronary disease. N Engl J Med. 2009;361:2518–28.
77. Willeit P, et al. Baseline and on-statin treatment lipoprotein(a) levels for prediction of cardiovascular events: individual patient-data meta-analysis of statin outcome trials. Lancet Lond Engl. 2018;392:1311–20.
78. Pietinen P, et al. Intake of fatty acids and risk of coronary heart disease in a cohort of Finnish men. The Alpha-Tocopherol, Beta-Carotene Cancer Prevention Study. Am J Epidemiol. 1997;145:876–87.
79. Oomen CM, et al. Association between trans fatty acid intake and 10-year risk of coronary heart disease in the Zutphen Elderly Study: a prospective population-based study. Lancet Lond Engl. 2001;357:746–51.
80. Oh K, Hu FB, Manson JE, Stampfer MJ, Willett WC. Dietary fat intake and risk of coronary heart disease in women: 20 years of follow-up of the nurses' health study. Am J Epidemiol. 2005;161:672–9.
81. Ascherio A, et al. Dietary fat and risk of coronary heart disease in men: cohort follow up study in the United States. BMJ. 1996;313:84–90.
82. U.S. Food & Drug Administration. Trans Fat. FDA http://www.fda.gov/food/food-additives-petitions/trans-fat (2018).

Prevention and Treatment of Obesity for Cardiovascular Risk Mitigation: Dietary and Pharmacologic Approaches

8

Joanne Bruno, David Carruthers, and José O. Alemán

Introduction

Obesity has become the most important preventable cause of cardiovascular disease (CVD) in the USA, with one in three adults afflicted by this disease. The World Health Organization describes obesity as an abnormal accumulation of fat that presents health consequences. As previously outlined in several chapters in this book, dietary and lifestyle intervention conform the foundation through which obesity is treated clinically. Over the last 30 years, surgical and most recently medical treatment of obesity demonstrated weight loss and maintenance effects that improve type 2 diabetes and directly impact the incidence of CVD. We focus this chapter on dietary strategies that reduce food quantity or improve food quality and are used in combination with pharmacotherapy or surgical strategies for weight loss. Lastly, we describe current medical and surgical therapies for obesity that are increasingly important in the prevention of CVD.

Dietary Approaches

Dietary and lifestyle modifications have long been the mainstay of treatment for obesity; it is only in recent years that safe and effective medical and surgical therapies have become available for the management of weight loss, and even these treatment modalities require concurrent comprehensive lifestyle interventions to maximize their effectiveness. As such, current American consensus guidelines for the treatment of obesity stress the importance of dietary and lifestyle change in promoting weight loss [1], especially in those patients with additional cardiovascular risk factors and obesity-related comorbidities. The American Association of Clinical Endocrinology (AACE) guidelines are largely in agreement with these and specify the importance of a ≥10% weight loss in preventing the progression to diabetes in obese patients [2]. This recommendation is based on the findings from a series of studies that utilized either lifestyle intervention, weight loss medications, or bariatric surgery to provoke weight loss, each of which showed that an 80% reduction in progression to type 2 diabetes can be achieved with a ≥10% weight loss. In the Look AHEAD trial comparing intensive lifestyle intervention to diabetes support and education in obese and overweight patients, those subjects who achieved a ≥10% weight loss had a >20% reduction in the hazard ratio for cardiovascular events [3].

J. Bruno · D. Carruthers · J. O. Alemán (✉)
Division of Endocrinology, Department of Medicine,
New York University Langone Health,
New York, NY, USA
e-mail: joanne.bruno@nyulangone.org;
dcarruther@montefiore.org;
jose.aleman@nyulangone.org

© Springer Nature Switzerland AG 2021
M. J. Wilkinson et al. (eds.), *Prevention and Treatment of Cardiovascular Disease*, Contemporary
Cardiology, https://doi.org/10.1007/978-3-030-78177-4_8

Despite overwhelming evidence that dietary modifications are a critical component of any effective weight loss strategy, no clear guidelines exist to aid health-care providers in counseling patients on how to eat in order to lose weight. Based on conservation of energy, the most straightforward way to lose weight is through caloric restriction (CR), as a calorie deficit will inevitably result in the breakdown of fat stores in order to fuel energy output. All dietary interventions rely on this principle to some degree, whether they do so overtly by tracking calorie consumption, or more subtly by emphasizing changes in the quality of one's diet and intake of low calorie density foods (and thus fewer calories).

Food Quantity or Caloric Restriction

Caloric Restriction

CR is linked to increased longevity in diverse model organisms, including yeast, flies, worms, fish, and rodents [4] primarily via a delay in the deterioration in biological function that occurs through aging alone. In more complex species such as rodents, there is also an effect of CR on secondary aging due to the prevention of chronic diseases such as CVD. These beneficial effects appear to be a direct result of the metabolic adaptations from CR itself and are independent of weight changes or body mass index (BMI), as leanness achieved via other mechanisms such as exercise does not result in a similar increase in longevity in these animals [5, 6]. In humans, a reduction in body weight by surgical removal of adipose tissue, such as liposuction, does not decrease metabolic risk [7], whereas weight loss induced by a negative calorie balance does, suggesting that the journey may be just as important as the destination when it comes to achieving healthy weight loss and garnering the metabolic benefits that accompany it.

Proving a link between CR and aging in humans while controlling for the innumerable factors that affect the aging process has been difficult. Long-term cross-sectional diet-controlled studies have been done comparing cohorts of indi-

viduals who practice self-imposed CR, defined as eating ~30% fewer calories than would be found in a typical Western diet (roughly 1800 kcal/day v 2600 kcal/day), to healthy age-matched individuals eating ad libitum. These showed that individuals on a calorie-restricted diet exhibit significant beneficial metabolic phenotypes, including lower body fat percentage, lower blood pressure (BP), improved lipid profiles, increased insulin sensitivity, decreased ectopic lipid deposition, and increased HDL levels [8, 9]. More recently, the CALERIE trial examined the effects of 25% CR versus an ad-libitum control diet on the metabolic profiles of young and middle-aged healthy non-obese men and women in the USA for 2 years. In this randomized controlled trial, they found that modest CR produces widespread reduction in cardiometabolic risk factors, including decreases in systolic and diastolic BP, LDL-C, waist circumference, and markers of inflammation, while improving insulin sensitivity and metabolic syndrome scores [10]. These dramatic improvements in healthy individuals suggest that CR may not only be an effective strategy in the treatment of established cardiometabolic disease but in its prevention as well.

Intermittent Fasting

While calorie reduction is necessary for weight loss to occur, newer evidence suggests that timing of caloric intake may also play a role in promoting weight loss. Intermittent fasting is a widely studied dietary strategy that restricts food consumption to a specific number of hours in a day or days within the week, with the remaining time spent fasting. The fasting-to-eating ratios can differ significantly, with the most common being the 16/8 method of time-restricted feeding, which specifies a 16-h fast followed by an 8-h eating period. While it does not set constraints on calorie consumption outright, intermittent fasting may inadvertently result in reduced caloric intake purely by limiting the amount of time that people spend eating. In support of this, the majority of human and animal studies on intermittent fasting have reported weight loss, suggesting that some reduction in energy intake must be occurring. Intermittent fasting has also been linked to cardiovascular benefits [11], some of which may even be independent of weight loss [12], and is discussed in further detail in Chap. 9 of this compendium.

Meal Replacements

Meal replacements are another popular means of achieving weight loss in the community as they remove the onus of having to grapple with food choice from the dieter while still effecting a calorie deficit. These programs replace one or more meals with discrete food products or drinks in order to reduce daily calorie intake and thus achieve weight loss or weight maintenance. While such strategies are used to effect short-term weight loss, the durability on achieving and maintaining weight loss over longer periods of time is controversial [13, 14]. These regimens can be inflexible and expensive, resulting in decreased adherence over time and a return to previous eating habits. However, meal replacements can serve as a bridge to more definitive therapy such as bariatric surgery, or in conjunction with a more comprehensive weight loss strategy with lifestyle change so that these guiding principles can be maintained even after the meal replacement program is stopped.

Food Quality

Food Processing

Tracking calorie consumption may appear to be the most straightforward means of achieving a negative calorie balance, but in practice, it can be time-consuming and difficult to adhere to as a long-term weight loss solution. Thus, many dietary interventions stray from this approach and focus instead on changes in the quality of calories consumed rather than the quantity. A recent study from Hall et al. [15] investigated the effects of food quality on the eating habits of 20 weight-stable adults. The participants were admitted to an inpatient research facility and randomized to receive either ultraprocessed or unprocessed ad-libitum diets for 2 weeks, followed by crossover to the alternate diet for 2 weeks. While on the ultraprocessed diet, participants consumed

approximately 500 calories more per day than those on the unprocessed diet and gained, on average, 0.9 kg over the 2-week period, whereas those on the unprocessed diet lost 0.9 kg. The reason for these differences in energy intake remains unclear. However, it is interesting to note that there was no change in the perceived pleasantness of the food, hunger, or satiety between the two groups. These results suggest that minimizing ultraprocessed foods in the diet may be an effective strategy for obesity prevention and/or treatment, and dietary strategies rich in whole, unprocessed foods should be encouraged.

Mediterranean Diet

The Mediterranean diet is based on the dietary habits of "blue zones" in Italy and Greece with a high concentration of centenarians, where rates of CVD and diabetes are among the lowest in the world. This diet is characterized by plentiful consumption of plant-based foods (fruits, vegetables, breads, legumes, nuts, and seeds) with dairy products, meat (mostly poultry), and fish consumed in low-to-moderate amounts [16]. Olive oil is the primary source of dietary fat, which results in a low saturated fat diet despite overall fat intake within the normal recommended range of 25–35% for the average adult [16]. The DIRECT study showed that the Mediterranean and low carbohydrate diets were equally successful in provoking weight loss as well as in promoting long-term weight maintenance and glycemia and were superior to a low-fat diet in both of these endpoints [17]. Observational cohort studies show that adherence to a Mediterranean diet is associated with lower cardiovascular risk [18, 19]. The Lyon Diet Heart Study, a randomized secondary prevention trial of the Mediterranean diet to reduce the rate of recurrence after a first myocardial infarction, showed a protective effect of the Mediterranean diet that was maintained up to 4 years after the initial cardiac event [20]. However, in this study, classical modifiable CVD risk factors such as cholesterol levels and BP were independently associated with recurrent MI, suggesting that dietary intervention alone is not enough to achieve maximal cardiac protection in high-risk patients and that a comprehensive strategy including pharmacologic intervention is likely needed in these individuals [20]. The cardiovascular benefits of the Mediterranean diet have been studied in the context of primary prevention as well, most prominently in the PREDIMED trial [21]. The Mediterranean diet groups had a lower rate of major cardiovascular events over the 5-year study period compared to the control low-fat diet group, with a greater magnitude of cardiovascular risk reduction seen in those study participants with increased dietary adherence. Surprisingly there was no description of weight gain or loss associated with these Mediterranean dietary interventions in either of these two trials. Therefore, it is still unclear what role, if any, weight loss has in the Mediterranean diet's mitigation of cardiovascular risk or whether it is an independent effect.

Plant-Based Diets

Further along the spectrum of emphasizing a diet rich in whole, unprocessed foods is the plant-based diet plan described in Chap. 6. There are various flavors of plant-based diets, including vegetarianism, which omits all meat and fish intake, and veganism, which prohibits the ingestion of the above animal proteins as well as any animal-derived product, including dairy and eggs. Observational studies of cohorts which adhere to these eating habits for cultural and theistic reasons, including Seventh-Day Adventists and Taiwanese Buddhists, show a decreased prevalence of type 2 diabetes [22–24]. Additionally, these studies show that increasing BMI appears to be inversely correlated with level of adherence to a plant-based diet such that those with the lowest BMIs tended to consume the highest percentage of plant-based foods.

That is not to say that all plant-based diets are created equal or that all plant-based foods are beneficial for metabolic health. Post-hoc analysis of the Nurses' Health Study, the Nurses' Health Study 2, and the Health Professionals Follow-Up Study stratified those participants who were adherent to a plant-based diet into either a "healthy" plant-based diet group or an "unhealthy" plant-based diet group [25]. Those in the healthy diet group tended more toward a

diet that was rich in unprocessed foods, including whole grains, nuts, fruits, vegetables, and legumes. When adjusted for BMI, the healthy plant-based diet group had a decreased incidence of type 2 diabetes (HR 0.66, 95% CI 0.61–0.72, p trend <0.001) [26]. In contrast, consumption of an unhealthy plant-based diet was positively associated with type 2 diabetes (HR 1.16, 95% CI 1.08–1.25, p trend <0.001) [25]. Therefore, even within the dietary restrictions of a plant-based diet, it is still important to emphasize enriched consumption of whole, unprocessed foods to achieve optimal metabolic health. Finally, while processed foods and red meats are the worst offenders regarding risk of metabolic disease [26], we do not yet fully understand where highly processed plant-based proteins will fall on this spectrum. Therefore, the focus of dietary recommendations should still be grounded in promoting intake of unprocessed fruits, vegetables, and whole grains.

In addition to diabetes prevention, plant-based diets are also shown to be helpful in the treatment of type 2 diabetes and reducing cardiometabolic risk in these already high-risk patients. When compared to a typical diabetic diet as recommended by American Diabetes Association guidelines, those following a low-fat vegan diet had more significant reductions in their hemoglobin A1c, increased weight loss, and more improvement in their lipid control [27]. In both groups, hemoglobin A1c improvement was mediated primarily by weight loss, and participants ate on average 425 kcal less per day [28]. In the conventional diabetic diet group, this occurred via explicit CR, whereas in the vegan group, the caloric deficit was incidental to increased intake of lower calorie density foods.

Even in nondiabetic patients, eating a vegetarian diet is associated with decreased incidence and mortality from ischemic heart disease [29–31]. This holds true after adjustment for confounders such as age, total calorie intake, smoking, physical activity, alcohol use, lipids, and BMI [31]. For example, the Lifestyle Heart Trial demonstrated that intensive lifestyle interventions, including adherence to a 10% fat whole foods vegetarian diet, led to regression of coronary atherosclerosis and a 50% reduction in cardiac events as compared to control subjects who made more moderate lifestyle changes [32].

For some patients switching to a plant-based diet may seem overwhelming, but even small changes in dietary habits toward a more plant-based framework can yield cardiometabolic benefits. Assessment of dietary data from the Nurses' Health Study and Health Professionals Follow-Up Study showed that when subjects substituted just 3% of energy from animal protein with plant protein, all-cause mortality was significantly decreased [33]. Similar beneficial effects of a moderate reduction of animal protein intake were shown in a randomized, controlled, crossover trial in which individuals with type 2 diabetes were randomly assigned either to consume a control legume-free diabetic diet or a legume-based diabetic diet [34]. The legume-based diet significantly reduced fasting blood glucose, fasting insulin, triglyceride concentrations, and LDL concentrations independent of any changes in BMI [34], indicating that even modest reductions in the consumption of animal protein can be beneficial for cardiometabolic health.

Pharmacologic Approaches

The aforementioned dietary strategies form the foundation of lifestyle interventions for treatment of obesity, focusing on reducing food quantity and improving food quality. While there has been evidence that weight loss is beneficial in improving risk factors for CVD such as improved glycemic control in people with type 2 diabetes mellitus (DM) [35–40], evidence that weight loss improves cardiovascular health has been mixed, possibly due to the difficulty of maintaining sustained sufficient weight loss with lifestyle interventions alone to see long-term cardiovascular benefits [36]. Interventions with more substantial weight loss such as bariatric surgery and glucagon-like peptide (GLP-1) agonist medications, which are approved by the Food and Drug Administration (FDA) for the treatment of obesity and type 2 DM,

have repeatedly shown cardiovascular benefits [41–45]. This evidence is in line with AACE's recommendation of ≥10% weight loss for preventative health in obesity (source page 5) and summarized in Table 8.1.

Achieving sustained weight loss of ≥10% of baseline weight is challenging, and only 20% of participants in the Look AHEAD intensive lifestyle intervention arm reached this mark. Given the difficulty of reaching and maintaining clinical meaningful weight loss, many patients would benefit from further intervention with pharmacotherapy or bariatric surgery, though this is a vastly underused resource, with approximately 1% of eligible patients undergoing bariatric surgery or filling a weight loss medication prescription annually [46, 47]. The aim of the following section is to review the evidence for the current pharmacotherapies and surgical interventions for weight loss, to improve physician awareness of these options to treat obesity.

There are currently four medications approved by the US FDA to treat obesity: orlistat, phentermine-extended release topiramate, bupropion–naltrexone, and high-dose liraglutide. Lorcaserin (Belviq), a 5-HT serotonin receptor agonist appetite suppressant, was recently pulled from the market by the FDA in February 2020, after a cardiovascular safety trial showed an increased risk of cancer [48, 49].

Orlistat

Orlistat is a pancreatic lipase inhibitor, which works completely within the gastrointestinal (GI) tract by inhibiting lipases in the lumen of the stomach and small intestine, thereby blocking dietary triglyceride hydrolysis. This decreases intraluminal micelle formation, resulting in reduced triglyceride, long-chain fatty acid, and fat-soluble vitamin absorption. It is recommended to take orlistat as part of a low-fat reduced-calorie diet, with no more than 30% of calories coming from fat in a meal. Therapeutic dosing is 120 mg three times daily with meals. At this dose, orlistat inhibits dietary fat by approximately 30% [50]. As fat is not absorbed in the GI tract, the

Table 8.1 Summary of pharmacotherapy for management of obesity and its CVD risk effects

Medication	Mechanism of action	Therapeutic dose	Contraindications	Percentage weight loss vs. placebo	CV outcome trial	Effect on CV risk factors
Orlistat	Pancreatic lipase inhibitor	120 mg three times daily with meals	Gall stones or cholecystitis. Kidney stones, pregnancy	3%	No	Improve BP and glycemic control. Decrease LDL-C [52, 53]
Phentermine–topiramate	Sympathomimetic/GABA modulation	7.5 mg/46 mg orally daily	CVD, pregnancy, glaucoma, hyperthyroidism, psychotic disorder, uncontrolled hypertension	7.5–9.3%	No	Improve glycemic control, increase HDL, and decrease triglycerides [56, 58]
Naltrexone SR–bupropion SR	Dopamine and norepinephrine reuptake inhibitor/opioid inhibitor	32 mg/360 mg orally daily	Opioid use, manic depression, psychotic disorders, suicidal thoughts, seizure disorder, uncontrolled hypertension	2.5–5.2%	Terminated early, unable to assess for noninferiority	Modest improvements in lipid panel and glycemic control. Increase in systolic BP [61, 66]
Liraglutide	GLP-1 receptor agonist	3.0 mg subcutaneously daily	Pancreatitis, MEN type 2, medullary thyroid carcinoma, risk of hypoglycemia with other glucose-lowering medications	5.5%	LEADER trial showing cardiovascular superiority	Decreased systolic and diastolic BP, improved glycemic control, decrease in LDL-C and triglycerides, increase in HDL-C. reduced inflammation, improved endothelial function, and ischemic conditioning [66]

most common side effects from orlistat are fatty or oily loose stools/diarrhea, excessive gas, and bloating. Fat-soluble vitamin deficiencies can also occur while taking orlistat. Other side effects include an increased risk of kidney stone or gall stone formation [51]. Weight loss is achieved by a caloric deficit of unabsorbed dietary fat. In the XENDOS trial, patients taking orlistat 120 mg 3 times daily lost an average of 5.8 kg, compared to 3.0 kg in the placebo arm [52].

Treatment with orlistat leads to improvements in cardiovascular risk factors, including reduction in systolic and diastolic BP, and glycemic control, but cardiovascular outcome trials are lacking [53]. Orlistat also improves the lipid profile with decreased LDL-C levels, likely due to decreased GI fat absorption [54].

Phentermine-Extended Release Topiramate

Phentermine is a sympathomimetic similar to amphetamines, which acts as a nervous system stimulant that increases neuronal catecholamine (primarily norepinephrine) release in the hypothalamus, which decreases appetite. Topiramate, initially approved for seizure disorders, modifies γ-aminobutyric acid (GABA)-mediated pathways. The exact mechanism for weight loss is unknown, but it is thought that increased energy expenditure and appetite suppression contribute [55]. The combination phentermine–topiramate (Qsymia) was approved by the FDA for use as a weight loss drug in 2012 and has shown 7.5–9.3% weight loss in phase 3 clinical trials versus placebo [56, 57].

Given the neurostimulating properties of phentermine, it is contraindicated in use with any patient with underlying CVD. However, in the above trials, use did result in improved glycemic control, increased HDL-C, and decreased triglycerides, with no significant effect on LDL-C. Despite the theoretical risk of worsened hypertension, systolic BP decreased in the above trials, but less than expected for similar weight loss through other means, and diastolic BP was neutral. Furthermore, a retrospective cohort study showed no increase in cardiovascular risk, but no prospective cardiovascular trials have been performed [58].

Naltrexone SR–Bupropion SR

Bupropion is an antidepressant approved for the treatment of depression and smoking-cessation, which inhibits neuronal dopamine and norepinephrine reuptake. Naltrexone is an opioid antagonist. The combination bupropion–naltrexone was approved for weight loss in 2014, and is believed to affect the mesolimbic dopamine reward pathway, which can modulate behaviors like food intake, and the hypothalamus circuit by proopiomelancortin (POMC) stimulation, which promotes anorectic energy balance and satiety [59, 60]. Together, the medication targets the brain's satiety and behavioral pathways to improve control of feeding behavior.

In phase 3 trials, bupropion–naltrexone showed 2.5–5.2% weight loss versus placebo [61]. Within these trials, naltrexone SR + bupropion SR showed modest improvements in lipid panel with decreases in LDL-C and triglycerides and an increase in HDL-C. Changes in HbA1c were neutral to slightly favorable and systolic BP increased compared to placebo [61, 62]. Though the FDA requested a cardiovascular outcomes trial, it was stopped prematurely due to the inappropriate release of data by the study sponsor [63].

Liraglutide

Liraglutide is a human GLP-1 receptor agonist, given subcutaneously. It was first developed and used for glycemic control in type 2 DM (Victoza,

1.8 mg daily) but now is also FDA-approved for the treatment of obesity (Saxenda 3.0 mg daily). GLP-1 is an incretin-like peptide released by the epithelial cells of the small intestine in response to a food bolus. GLP-1 acts on the liver to reduce gluconeogenesis, and on pancreatic islet cells increasing β-cell sensitivity for insulin secretion and decreasing α-cell glucagon secretion, promoting glucose control in patients with type 2 DM. GLP-1 promotes weight loss both centrally in the mesolimbic neurons as well as the arcuate nucleus of the hypothalamus decreasing appetite, and peripherally by slowing gut motility increasing satiety [64]. Common side effects are related to effects on the GI tract and include nausea, vomiting, constipation, diarrhea, and dyspepsia.

The SCALE trial was a 56-week randomized, controlled trial comparing liraglutide 3.0 mg daily against placebo in nondiabetic patients. The treatment arm showed a weight loss of 8.4 kg (8.1%) versus 2.8 kg (2.6%) in the placebo arm. Patients treated with liraglutide showed improvements in cardiometabolic risk factors, with significant decrease in systolic and diastolic BP, decrease in LDL-C, triglycerides, and increases in HDL-C, and decrease in glycated hemoglobin [65]. Subsequently, the LEADER trial was a 3.8-year cardiovascular outcomes trial comparing liraglutide 1.8 mg daily to placebo, which was landmark in showing superiority in the treatment arm for the primary outcome of death from cardiovascular causes, nonfatal myocardial infarction, or nonfatal stroke [66]. This appears to be a class effect, with multiple other GLP-1 medications showing decreased cardiovascular events and mortality [42]. In addition to improving traditional cardiovascular risk factors, GLP-1 agonists could have direct cardiovascular benefits from increased nitric oxide synthase activity, improved coronary flow velocity, and myocardial ischemic conditioning [62]. Semaglutide, another GLP-1 agonist available in once-weekly injectable and now a daily oral form, is approved for use in diabetes. It has shown promise for use in weight loss, is currently under investigation for weight-loss specific approval [62], and may be available for weight loss practitioners in the near future.

Bariatric Surgery

Bariatric surgery is shown to be the most effective and lasting treatment for obesity with long-term metabolic improvements and decreased cardiovascular events including mortality. While initial benefits for bariatric surgery were thought to be due to restrictive and malabsorptive effects, it is now recognized that there are metabolic changes that directly contribute to weight loss and confer cardiovascular benefits (Fig. 8.1) [41]. In this section, we will review three most common bariatric procedures: laparoscopic adjustable gastric banding (LAGB), sleeve gastrectomy (SG), and Roux-en-Y gastric bypass (RYGB).

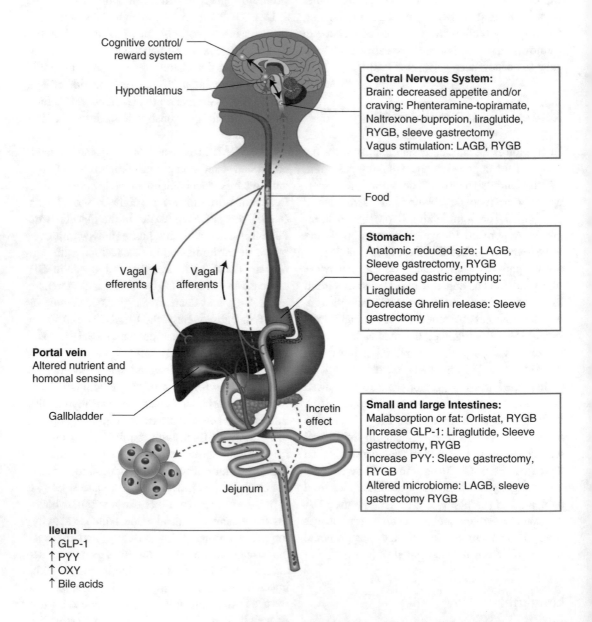

Fig. 8.1 Mechanisms of weight loss from pharmacologic or surgical intervention. *RYGB* Roux-en-Y Gastric Bypass, *LAGB* laparoscopic adjustable gastric banding, *GLP-1* Glucagon-Like-Peptide 1, *PYY* Peptide YY, *OXY* oxyntomodulin. (Adapted from Miras and Leroux [73])

Gastric Banding

LAGB is a reversible procedure that places an adjustable band around the fundus of the stomach, forming a restricted gastric pouch limiting the amount of food that can be consumed in a meal. The band also increases esophageal and gastric peristaltic activity, leading to vagus nerve stimulation and increased satiety [70]. At 7-year follow-up, patients who underwent LAGB had sustained 14.9% mean weight loss from baseline [71]. In that study, it found that LAGB had initial modest improvements in diabetes, hypertension, and dyslipidemia, but at 7 years, only changes in HDL and triglycerides were statistically significant [67]. In recent years, gastric banding has fallen out of favor as it hasn't been shown to be an effective long-term weight loss strategy, with many patients regaining weight in long-term follow-up [68].

Sleeve Gastrectomy

SG is a nonreversible procedure generally performed laparoscopically that removes 70–80% of the stomach, including the fundal and antral portions, leaving the patient with a tube-like remnant gastric "sleeve." SG is an effective and durable weight loss intervention, with a mean 25–30% weight loss sustained at 5 years postoperatively [69, 70]. Along with weight loss, SG purports sizable improvements in BP, HbA1c, dyslipidemia, and decreased inflammatory markers [69–71].

Weight loss and improved metabolic profile following SG are driven by anatomic restriction of the stomach, vagal nerve stimulation, and through GI hormonal and intestinal microbiome changes which promote weight loss [72]. With the removal of 70–80% of the stomach, there is a decrease in the release of ghrelin, a hormone that acts in the hypothalamus to promote hunger. Post-SG there is also increased secretion of peptide-YY (PYY) and GLP-1, which are anorectic and promote satiety and glycemic control in patients with type 2 DM [72, 73].

Roux-en-Y Gastric Bypass

RYGB is a nonreversible procedure that reduces the size of the stomach to a small pouch and then is reattached to the small intestine, bypassing the majority of the stomach and a portion of the small intestine. Of all weight loss interventions, RYGB and SG have the greatest amount of weight loss, with a mean weight loss of ~25–30% maintained over 5 years postoperatively, and like SG, RYGB improvements in BP, diabetes, and dyslipidemia that remain for >5 years [67, 69, 70]. Due to the altered anatomy, more undigested lipids go through the intestine unabsorbed, which lead to greater reductions in LDL-C than seen by other weight loss methods [71]. Like SG, increases in GI hormones GLP-1 and PYY, along with positively altering the microbiome, are implicated in the long-term weight loss and metabolic benefits seen in RYGB [72]. Improvements in diabetes control are rapid in both SG and RYGB, with patients showing large improvements in glycemic control immediately after the weight loss procedure, with many patients who previously on insulin either having large reductions in insulin requirement or coming off of insulin entirely postoperatively.

In 2012, the Swedish Obese Subjects (SOS) study evaluated cardiovascular outcomes in patients who underwent bariatric surgery (LAGB, SG, or RYGB) with mean follow-up of 14.7 years and found patients who underwent bariatric surgery had significantly reduced cardiovascular events (9.9% vs. 11.5%) and mortality (1.4% vs. 2.4%) versus the control group [44].

In selecting between RYGB and SG, one must consider patient preferences, baseline weight, metabolic profile, and comorbidities. RYGB is a more complex surgery and leads to an increased risk of postoperative dumping syndrome; for this reason, we often recommend SG for many of our patients. However, RYGB has been shown to be slightly more effective than SG for weight loss and DM improvement, and in patients with BMI >45 or more severe insulin resistance, RYGB may be a better option [74, 75].

Fig. 8.2 Overall CV
risk reduction with
treatment of obesity

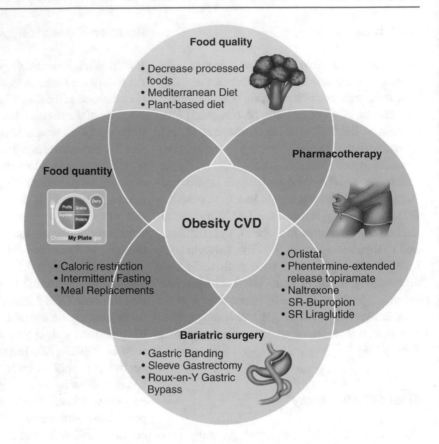

Conclusions

We summarize our framework for treatment of
obesity for the prevention of CVD in Fig. 8.2.
It is in line with multiple professional society
guidelines and includes implementing lifestyle
interventions that decrease food quantity consumption, thereby restricting calories, while
also improving diet quality. These dietary interventions, along with exercise, are then attempted
for periods of 3–6 months before determining
if clinically meaningful weight loss occurs and
before augmentation with pharmacotherapy of
surgery. The continuum of lifestyle intervention and pharmacotherapy followed by invasive
interventions will expand as our armamentarium for CVD prevention grows in subsequent
chapters of this book.

References

1. Jensen MD, Ryan DH, Apovian CM, Ard JD,
   Comuzzie AG, Donato KA, et al. 2013 AHA/ACC/
   TOS guideline for the management of overweight and
   obesity in adults: a report of the American College of
   Cardiology/American Heart Association Task Force
   on Practice Guidelines and The Obesity Society. J Am
   Coll Cardiol. 2014;63(25 Pt B):2985–3023.
2. Garvey WT, Mechanick JI, Brett EM, Garber AJ,
   Hurley DL, Jastreboff AM, et al. American Association
   of Clinical Endocrinologists and American College of
   Endocrinology comprehensive clinical practice guidelines for medical care of patients with obesity. Endocr
   Pract. 2016;22 Suppl 3:1–203.
3. Look ARG, Gregg EW, Jakicic JM, Blackburn G,
   Bloomquist P, Bray GA, et al. Association of the
   magnitude of weight loss and changes in physical
   fitness with long-term cardiovascular disease outcomes in overweight or obese people with type 2
   diabetes: a post-hoc analysis of the Look AHEAD
   randomised clinical trial. Lancet Diabetes Endocrinol.
   2016;4(11):913–21.

4. Guarente L. Calorie restriction and sirtuins revisited. Genes Dev. 2013;27(19):2072–85.
5. Holloszy JO. Mortality rate and longevity of food-restricted exercising male rats: a reevaluation. J Appl Physiol (1985). 1997;82(2):399–403.
6. Harrison DE, Archer JR, Astle CM. Effects of food restriction on aging: separation of food intake and adiposity. Proc Natl Acad Sci U S A. 1984;81(6):1835–8.
7. Klein S, Fontana L, Young VL, Coggan AR, Kilo C, Patterson BW, et al. Absence of an effect of liposuction on insulin action and risk factors for coronary heart disease. N Engl J Med. 2004;350(25):2549–57.
8. Fontana L, Meyer TE, Klein S, Holloszy JO. Long-term calorie restriction is highly effective in reducing the risk for atherosclerosis in humans. Proc Natl Acad Sci U S A. 2004;101(17):6659–63.
9. Larson-Meyer DE, Heilbronn LK, Redman LM, Newcomer BR, Frisard MI, Anton S, et al. Effect of calorie restriction with or without exercise on insulin sensitivity, beta-cell function, fat cell size, and ectopic lipid in overweight subjects. Diabetes Care. 2006;29(6):1337–44.
10. Kraus WE, Bhapkar M, Huffman KM, Pieper CF, Krupa Das S, Redman LM, et al. 2 years of calorie restriction and cardiometabolic risk (CALERIE): exploratory outcomes of a multicentre, phase 2, randomised controlled trial. Lancet Diabetes Endocrinol. 2019;7(9):673–83.
11. Malinowski B, Zalewska K, Wesierska A, Sokolowska MM, Socha M, Liczner G, et al. Intermittent fasting in cardiovascular disorders-an overview. Nutrients. 2019;11(3):673.
12. Sutton EF, Beyl R, Early KS, Cefalu WT, Ravussin E, Peterson CM. Early time-restricted feeding improves insulin sensitivity, blood pressure, and oxidative stress even without weight loss in men with prediabetes. Cell Metab. 2018;27(6):1212–21 e3.
13. Heymsfield SB, van Mierlo CA, van der Knaap HC, Heo M, Frier HI. Weight management using a meal replacement strategy: meta and pooling analysis from six studies. Int J Obes Relat Metab Disord. 2003;27(5):537–49.
14. Astbury NM, Piernas C, Hartmann-Boyce J, Lapworth S, Aveyard P, Jebb SA. A systematic review and meta-analysis of the effectiveness of meal replacements for weight loss. Obes Rev. 2019;20(4):569–87.
15. Hall KD, Ayuketah A, Brychta R, Cai H, Cassimatis T, Chen KY, et al. Ultra-processed diets cause excess calorie intake and weight gain: an inpatient randomized controlled trial of ad libitum food intake. Cell Metab. 2019;30(1):226.
16. Willett WC, Sacks F, Trichopoulou A, Drescher G, Ferro-Luzzi A, Helsing E, et al. Mediterranean diet pyramid: a cultural model for healthy eating. Am J Clin Nutr. 1995;61(6 Suppl):1402S–6S.
17. Shai I, Schwarzfuchs D, Henkin Y, Shahar DR, Witkow S, Greenberg I, et al. Weight loss with a low-carbohydrate, Mediterranean, or low-fat diet. N Engl J Med. 2008;359(3):229–41.
18. Trichopoulou A, Costacou T, Bamia C, Trichopoulos D. Adherence to a Mediterranean diet and survival in a Greek population. N Engl J Med. 2003;348(26):2599–608.
19. Sofi F, Abbate R, Gensini GF, Casini A. Accruing evidence on benefits of adherence to the Mediterranean diet on health: an updated systematic review and meta-analysis. Am J Clin Nutr. 2010;92(5):1189–96.
20. de Lorgeril M, Salen P, Martin JL, Monjaud I, Delaye J, Mamelle N. Mediterranean diet, traditional risk factors, and the rate of cardiovascular complications after myocardial infarction: final report of the Lyon Diet Heart Study. Circulation. 1999;99(6):779–85.
21. Estruch R, Ros E, Salas-Salvado J, Covas MI, Corella D, Aros F, et al. Primary prevention of cardiovascular disease with a Mediterranean diet supplemented with extra-virgin olive oil or nuts. N Engl J Med. 2018;378(25):e34.
22. Tonstad S, Butler T, Yan R, Fraser GE. Type of vegetarian diet, body weight, and prevalence of type 2 diabetes. Diabetes Care. 2009;32(5):791–6.
23. Vang A, Singh PN, Lee JW, Haddad EH, Brinegar CH. Meats, processed meats, obesity, weight gain and occurrence of diabetes among adults: findings from Adventist Health Studies. Ann Nutr Metab. 2008;52(2):96 104.
24. Chiu TH, Huang HY, Chiu YF, Pan WH, Kao HY, Chiu JP, et al. Taiwanese vegetarians and omnivores: dietary composition, prevalence of diabetes and IFG. PLoS One. 2014;9(2):e88547.
25. Satija A, Bhupathiraju SN, Rimm EB, Spiegelman D, Chiuve SE, Borgi L, et al. Plant-based dietary patterns and incidence of type 2 diabetes in US men and women: results from three prospective cohort studies. PLoS Med. 2016;13(6):e1002039.
26. Schwingshackl L, Hoffmann G, Lampousi AM, Knuppel S, Iqbal K, Schwedhelm C, et al. Food groups and risk of type 2 diabetes mellitus: a systematic review and meta-analysis of prospective studies. Eur J Epidemiol. 2017;32(5):363–75.
27. Barnard ND, Cohen J, Jenkins DJ, Turner-McGrievy G, Gloede L, Jaster B, et al. A low-fat vegan diet improves glycemic control and cardiovascular risk factors in a randomized clinical trial in individuals with type 2 diabetes. Diabetes Care. 2006;29(8):1777–83.
28. Barnard ND, Cohen J, Jenkins DJ, Turner-McGrievy G, Gloede L, Green A, et al. A low-fat vegan diet and a conventional diabetes diet in the treatment of type 2 diabetes: a randomized, controlled, 74-wk clinical trial. Am J Clin Nutr. 2009;89(5):1588S–96S.
29. Crowe FL, Appleby PN, Travis RC, Key TJ. Risk of hospitalization or death from ischemic heart disease among British vegetarians and nonvegetarians: results from the EPIC-Oxford cohort study. Am J Clin Nutr. 2013;97(3):597–603.
30. Huang T, Yang B, Zheng J, Li G, Wahlqvist ML, Li D. Cardiovascular disease mortality and cancer incidence in vegetarians: a meta-analysis and systematic review. Ann Nutr Metab. 2012;60(4):233–40.

31. Kim H, Caulfield LE, Garcia-Larsen V, Steffen LM, Coresh J, Rebholz CM. Plant-based diets are associated with a lower risk of incident cardiovascular disease, cardiovascular disease mortality, and all-cause mortality in a general population of middle-aged adults. J Am Heart Assoc. 2019;8(16):e012865.

32. Ornish D, Scherwitz LW, Billings JH, Brown SE, Gould KL, Merritt TA, et al. Intensive lifestyle changes for reversal of coronary heart disease. JAMA. 1998;280(23):2001–7.

33. Song M, Fung TT, Hu FB, Willett WC, Longo VD, Chan AT, et al. Association of animal and plant protein intake with all-cause and cause-specific mortality. JAMA Intern Med. 2016;176(10):1453–63.

34. Hosseinpour-Niazi S, Mirmiran P, Hedayati M, Azizi F. Substitution of red meat with legumes in the therapeutic lifestyle change diet based on dietary advice improves cardiometabolic risk factors in overweight type 2 diabetes patients: a cross-over randomized clinical trial. Eur J Clin Nutr. 2015;69(5): 592–7.

35. Gummesson A, Nyman E, Knutsson M, Karpefors M. Effect of weight reduction on glycated haemoglobin in weight loss trials in patients with type 2 diabetes. Diabetes Obes Metab. 2017;19(9):1295–305.

36. Look ARG, Wing RR, Bolin P, Brancati FL, Bray GA, Clark JM, et al. Cardiovascular effects of intensive lifestyle intervention in type 2 diabetes. N Engl J Med. 2013;369(2):145–54.

37. Shantha GP, Kumar AA, Kahan S, Cheskin LJ. Association between glycosylated hemoglobin and intentional weight loss in overweight and obese patients with type 2 diabetes mellitus: a retrospective cohort study. Diabetes Educ. 2012;38(3):417–26.

38. The effects of nonpharmacologic interventions on blood pressure of persons with high normal levels. Results of the trials of hypertension prevention, phase I. JAMA. 1992;267(9):1213–20.

39. Ebrahim S, Smith GD. Lowering blood pressure: a systematic review of sustained effects of non-pharmacological interventions. J Public Health Med. 1998;20(4):441–8.

40. Neter JE, Stam BE, Kok FJ, Grobbee DE, Geleijnse JM. Influence of weight reduction on blood pressure: a meta-analysis of randomized controlled trials. Hypertension. 2003;42(5):878–84.

41. Aminian A, Zajichek A, Arterburn DE, Wolski KE, Brethauer SA, Schauer PR, et al. Association of metabolic surgery with major adverse cardiovascular outcomes in patients with type 2 diabetes and obesity. JAMA. 2019;322:1271–82.

42. Kristensen SL, Rorth R, Jhund PS, Docherty KF, Sattar N, Preiss D, et al. Cardiovascular, mortality, and kidney outcomes with GLP-1 receptor agonists in patients with type 2 diabetes: a systematic review and meta-analysis of cardiovascular outcome trials. Lancet Diabetes Endocrinol. 2019;7(10):776–85.

43. Benotti PN, Wood GC, Carey DJ, Mehra VC, Mirshahi T, Lent MR, et al. Gastric bypass surgery produces a durable reduction in cardiovascular disease risk factors and reduces the long-term risks of congestive heart failure. J Am Heart Assoc. 2017;6(5):e005126.

44. Sjostrom L, Peltonen M, Jacobson P, Sjostrom CD, Karason K, Wedel H, et al. Bariatric surgery and long-term cardiovascular events. JAMA. 2012;307(1):56–65.

45. Sundstrom J, Bruze G, Ottosson J, Marcus C, Naslund I, Neovius M. Weight loss and heart failure: a nationwide study of gastric bypass surgery versus intensive lifestyle treatment. Circulation. 2017;135(17):1577–85.

46. Martin M, Beekley A, Kjorstad R, Sebesta J. Socioeconomic disparities in eligibility and access to bariatric surgery: a national population-based analysis. Surg Obes Relat Dis. 2010;6(1):8–15.

47. Saxon DR, Iwamoto SJ, Mettenbrink CJ, McCormick E, Arterburn D, Daley MF, et al. Antiobesity medication use in 2.2 million adults across eight large health care organizations: 2009–2015. Obesity (Silver Spring). 2019;27(12):1975–81.

48. Administration FaD. FDA requests the withdrawal of the weight-loss drug Belviq, Belviq XR (lorcaserin) from the market February 13, 2020. Available from: https://www.fda.gov/drugs/drug-safety-and-availability/fda-requests-withdrawal-weight-loss-drug-belviq-belviq-xr-lorcaserin-market.

49. Bohula EA, Wiviott SD, McGuire DK, Inzucchi SE, Kuder J, Im K, et al. Cardiovascular safety of lorcaserin in overweight or obese patients. N Engl J Med. 2018;379(12):1107–17.

50. Zhi J, Melia AT, Guerciolini R, Chung J, Kinberg J, Hauptman JB, et al. Retrospective population-based analysis of the dose-response (fecal fat excretion) relationship of orlistat in normal and obese volunteers. Clin Pharmacol Ther. 1994;56(1):82–5.

51. FDA. Xenical (orlistat) Capsules. 2010. Available from: https://www.accessdata.fda.gov/drugsatfda_docs/label/2010/020766s028lbl.pdf.

52. Torgerson JS, Hauptman J, Boldrin MN, Sjostrom L. XENical in the prevention of diabetes in obese subjects (XENDOS) study: a randomized study of orlistat as an adjunct to lifestyle changes for the prevention of type 2 diabetes in obese patients. Diabetes Care. 2004;27(1):155–61.

53. Broom I, Wilding J, Stott P, Myers N, Group UKMS. Randomised trial of the effect of orlistat on body weight and cardiovascular disease risk profile in obese patients: UK Multimorbidity Study. Int J Clin Pract. 2002;56(7):494–9.

54. Sjostrom L, Rissanen A, Andersen T, Boldrin M, Golay A, Koppeschaar HP, et al. Randomised placebo-controlled trial of orlistat for weight loss and prevention of weight regain in obese patients. European Multicentre Orlistat Study Group. Lancet. 1998;352(9123):167–72.

55. Richard D, Ferland J, Lalonde J, Samson P, Deshaies Y. Influence of topiramate in the regulation of energy balance. Nutrition. 2000;16(10):961–6.

56. Aronne LJ, Wadden TA, Peterson C, Winslow D, Odeh S, Gadde KM. Evaluation of phentermine and

topiramate versus phentermine/topiramate extended-release in obese adults. Obesity (Silver Spring). 2013;21(11):2163–71.

57. Gadde KM, Allison DB, Ryan DH, Peterson CA, Troupin B, Schwiers ML, et al. Effects of low-dose, controlled-release, phentermine plus topiramate combination on weight and associated comorbidities in overweight and obese adults (CONQUER): a randomised, placebo-controlled, phase 3 trial. Lancet. 2011;377(9774):1341–52.

58. Ritchey ME, Harding A, Hunter S, Peterson C, Sager PT, Kowey PR, et al. Cardiovascular safety during and after use of phentermine and topiramate. J Clin Endocrinol Metab. 2019;104(2):513–22.

59. Morton GJ, Cummings DE, Baskin DG, Barsh GS, Schwartz MW. Central nervous system control of food intake and body weight. Nature. 2006;443(7109):289–95.

60. Andrew CA, Saunders KH, Shukla AP, Aronne LJ. Treating obesity in patients with cardiovascular disease: the pharmacotherapeutic options. Expert Opin Pharmacother. 2019;20(5):585–93.

61. Apovian CM, Aronne L, Rubino D, Still C, Wyatt H, Burns C, et al. A randomized, phase 3 trial of naltrexone SR/bupropion SR on weight and obesity-related risk factors (COR-II). Obesity (Silver Spring). 2013;21(5):935–43.

62. Heffron SP, Parham J, Pendse J, Aleman JO. Treatment of obesity in mitigating metabolic risk. Circ Res. 2020;126:1646–65.

63. Nissen SE, Wolski KE, Prcela L, Wadden T, Buse JB, Bakris G, et al. Effect of naltrexone-bupropion on major adverse cardiovascular events in overweight and obese patients with cardiovascular risk factors: a randomized clinical trial. JAMA. 2016;315(10):990–1004.

64. Pannacciulli N, Le DS, Salbe AD, Chen K, Reiman EM, Tataranni PA, et al. Postprandial glucagon-like peptide-1 (GLP-1) response is positively associated with changes in neuronal activity of brain areas implicated in satiety and food intake regulation in humans. Neuroimage. 2007;35(2):511–7.

65. Pi-Sunyer X, Astrup A, Fujioka K, Greenway F, Halpern A, Krempf M, et al. A randomized, controlled trial of 3.0 mg of liraglutide in weight management. N Engl J Med. 2015;373(1):11–22.

66. Marso SP, Daniels GH, Brown-Frandsen K, Kristensen P, Mann JF, Nauck MA, et al. Liraglutide and cardiovascular outcomes in type 2 diabetes. N Engl J Med. 2016;375(4):311–22.

67. Courcoulas AP, King WC, Belle SH, Berk P, Flum DR, Garcia L, et al. Seven-year weight trajectories and health outcomes in the longitudinal assessment of bariatric surgery (LABS) study. JAMA Surg. 2018;153(5):427–34.

68. Kowalewski PK, Olszewski R, Kwiatkowski A, Galazka-Swiderek N, Cichon K, Pasnik K. Life with a gastric band. Long-term outcomes of laparoscopic adjustable gastric banding-a retrospective study. Obes Surg. 2017;27(5):1250–3.

69. Peterli R, Wolnerhanssen BK, Peters T, Vetter D, Kroll D, Borbely Y, et al. Effect of laparoscopic sleeve gastrectomy vs laparoscopic Roux-en-Y gastric bypass on weight loss in patients with morbid obesity: the SM-BOSS randomized clinical trial. JAMA. 2018;319(3):255–65.

70. Salminen P, Helmio M, Ovaska J, Juuti A, Leivonen M, Peromaa-Haavisto P, et al. Effect of laparoscopic sleeve gastrectomy vs laparoscopic Roux-en-Y gastric bypass on weight loss at 5 years among patients with morbid obesity: the SLEEVEPASS randomized clinical trial. JAMA. 2018;319(3):241–54.

71. Heffron SP, Parikh A, Volodarskiy A, Ren-Fielding C, Schwartzbard A, Nicholson J, et al. Changes in lipid profile of obese patients following contemporary bariatric surgery: a meta-analysis. Am J Med. 2016;129(9):952–9.

72. Wang Y, Guo X, Lu X, Mattar S, Kassab G. Mechanisms of weight loss after sleeve gastrectomy and adjustable gastric banding: far more than just restriction. Obesity (Silver Spring). 2019;27(11):1776–83.

73. Miras AD, le Roux CW. Mechanisms underlying weight loss after bariatric surgery. Nat Rev Gastroenterol Hepatol. 2013;10(10):575–84.

74. Yu J, Zhou X, Li L, Li S, Tan J, Li Y, et al. The long-term effects of bariatric surgery for type 2 diabetes: systematic review and meta-analysis of randomized and non-randomized evidence. Obes Surg. 2015;25(1):143–58.

75. Shoar S, Saber AA. Long-term and midterm outcomes of laparoscopic sleeve gastrectomy versus Roux-en-Y gastric bypass: a systematic review and meta-analysis of comparative studies. Surg Obes Relat Dis. 2017;13(2):170–80.

Fasting for Cardiovascular Health

9

Elizabeth S. Epstein, Kathryn Maysent,
and Michael J. Wilkinson

Introduction

Fasting Throughout History

The practice of depriving oneself from food has long been recognized as having profound physical, mental, and spiritual effects. Since antiquity, fasting has been utilized in not just medical, but also religious, cultural, and political settings. In ancient Greece, fasting was integrated into religious practices and was done prior to visiting deities in temples. Similarly in ancient Peru, fasting was practiced following confession at temples [1]. Some Native American tribes incorporated fasting during vision quests or seasonal ceremonies. Siberian Shamans used fasting to prompt visions and control spirits. In modern times, fasting is used to enhance spirituality in Jainism, Buddhism, Hinduism, Judaism, Christianity, and Islam. Throughout history, fasting has also served as an expression of social and political views. Mahatma Gandhi famously fasted in peaceful protest of British rule in India as a part of *satyagraha*, or nonviolence [1].

E. S. Epstein · K. Maysent · M. J. Wilkinson (✉)
Division of Cardiovascular Medicine, Department of Medicine, University of California San Diego, San Diego, CA, USA
e-mail: esepstein@health.ucsd.edu;
mjwilkinson@health.ucsd.edu

In the 5th century BCE, Hippocrates introduced fasting to the medical community by prescribing it to patients as a treatment for certain illnesses [1]. He wrote: "Our food should be our medicine. Our medicine should be our food. But to eat when you are sick is to feed your sickness." Since then, animal and human studies have examined the role of fasting as a tool for the treatment and prevention of chronic disease.

Physiology of Fasting

Benefits of fasting are hypothesized to occur at least in part via a metabolic switch from glucose as an energy source to fatty acids and ketone bodies (Fig. 9.1) [2]. During the fed state, glucose is used for energy production, while fat is stored in the form of triglycerides in adipose tissue. During fasting after liver glycogen stores are depleted, triglycerides are broken down to fatty acids and glycerol for energy production. The liver then converts fatty acids to ketone bodies, which can be used for energy by certain metabolically active tissues such as the brain and skeletal muscle.

Beyond their role as an energy source, ketone bodies influence the expression of genes and proteins involved in health and longevity [3]. By activating extracellular G-protein coupled receptors such as HCAR2 and FFAR3, ketone bodies modulate lipolysis, metabolic rate, and sympathetic tone. Ketone bodies also inhibit

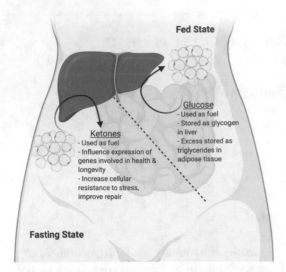

Fig. 9.1 Fasting and the metabolic switch. During times of fasting, use of ketones as a source of energy may contribute to some of the health benefits observed with IF

histone deacetylases to beneficially influence expression of genes involved in regulation of lifespan [3]. When this pathway is activated, cells become more resistant to oxidative and metabolic stress and are better able to remove and repair cellular damage, a process called autophagy [2]. Fasting ultimately leads to a reduction in inflammation which is a key component of the pathophysiology of cardiovascular disease in addition to diabetes, cancer, and neurodegenerative diseases [4].

Preclinical Data on Caloric Restriction and Fasting

The primary types of intermittent fasting (IF) include alternate-day fasting (ADF), 5:2, time-restricted eating (TRE), and periodic fasting (PF) (Fig. 9.2). All of these involve *temporal* reduction of food intake, limiting consumption of food or caloric beverages for a period of 12 h to 3 or more weeks. This is in opposition to caloric restriction (CR), which involves *quantitative* reduction of food intake, decreasing daily caloric intake by 20–40% [4]. The Fasting-

Mimicking Diet (FMD) is a hybrid method which involves eating a low-calorie, plant-based diet for 4–5 days per month. For the last 85 years, studies have repeatedly demonstrated that CR increases the lifespan of rodents [5, 6]. These studies have since been replicated in rhesus monkeys [7, 8]. The effect has been shown to be dose-dependent, with increased degree and duration of CR producing longer lifespans [9]. IF has also been shown to increase lifespan in animal models even without a decrease in overall caloric intake [10, 11]. This effect on longevity is thought to be related to decreased oxidative stress or improved responses to stress, including cellular autophagy [12–14].

Animal studies have also shown that CR and fasting have a mitigating effect on cardiovascular risk and atherosclerosis. In mice, rats, and rhesus monkeys, CR and fasting have been shown to improve heart rate (HR) and blood pressure (BP) response to stress, decrease low-density lipoprotein cholesterol (LDL-C), increase high-density lipoprotein cholesterol (HDL-C), and improve insulin sensitivity, all of which are risk factors for cardiovascular disease [8, 11, 15–18].

Beyond risk factor reduction, animal studies have suggested that CR and fasting may have an inhibitory effect on atherosclerosis and can prevent ischemic injury. Inflammation is a key contributor to the pathophysiology of atherosclerosis. In mice, CR has been shown to reduce several markers of inflammation, including leukocytes, tumor necrosis factor, and other inflammatory cytokines such as TNF-alpha and IL-6 [19, 20]. Further, rats maintained on a CR diet exhibit less oxidative damage to heart cells and reduced inflammation in the ischemic zone in response to left anterior descending (LAD) occlusion [21]. Similarly, rats on an IF diet exhibit significantly less damage in response to LAD ligation compared to control [22]. Rats on a CR diet have reduced mortality and better outcomes following myocardial infarction [23].

The animal studies evaluating TRE (referred to as time-restricted feeding (TRF) in animal studies) in particular are also compelling. The

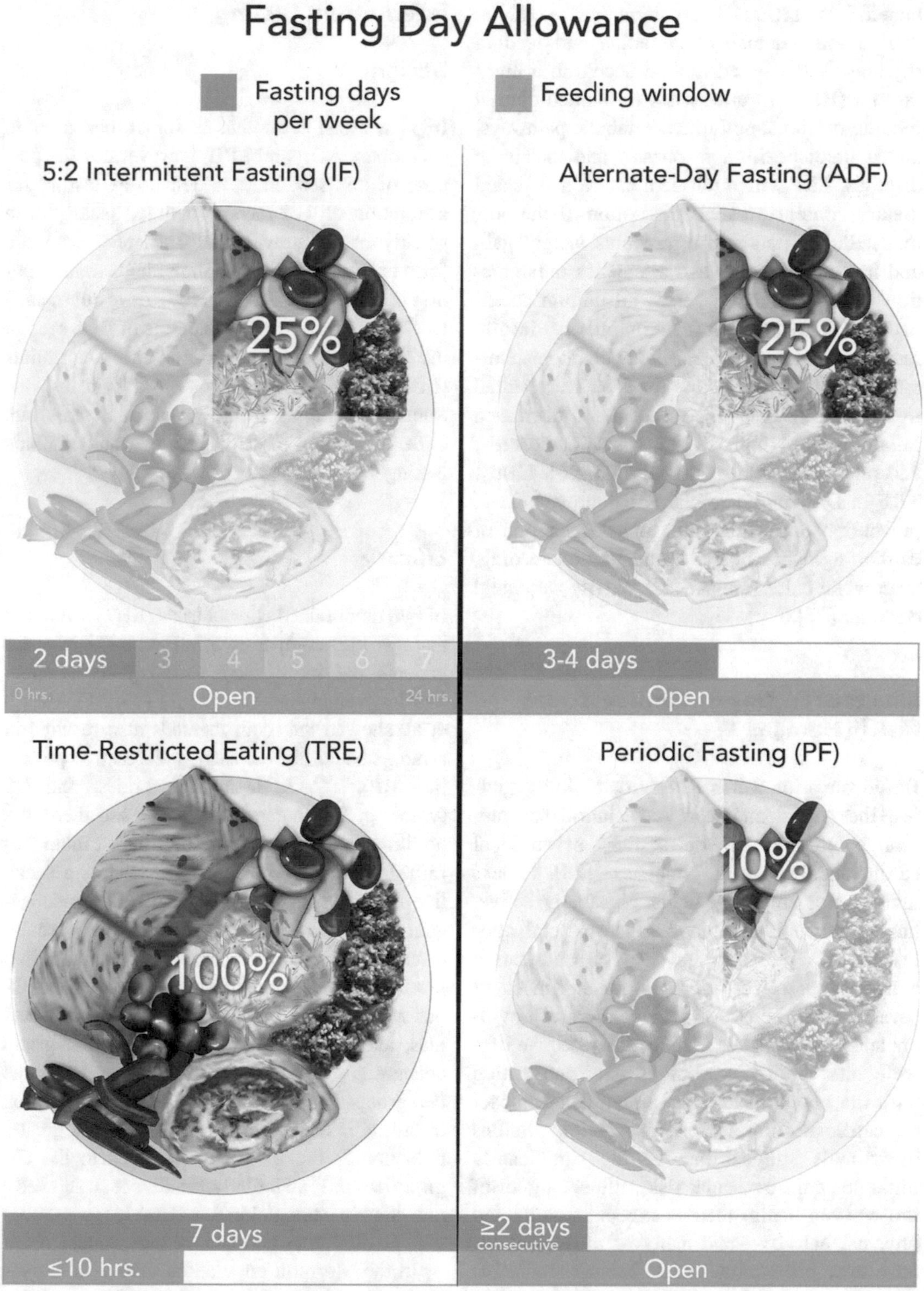

Fasting Day Allowance

Fig. 9.2 Fasting day allowance for different fasting protocols, including the number of days fasting per week and percent of non-fasting allowance on fasting days. Fading scale for 5:2 intermittent fasting reflects the heterogeneity in number of fasting days per week with this regimen. Note that different study protocols have slight variations on these general patterns

benefits of TRE/TRF are hypothesized to be due to maintenance of circadian and feeding rhythms. Whereas ad libitum access to a high-fat diet (HFD) in mice leads to blunted diurnal feeding rhythms, perturbed metabolic pathways, and a predisposition to obesity and metabolic diseases, TRF with equivalent caloric intake and dietary content prevents disruption of the normal cellular metabolism, prevents weight gain and hepatic steatosis, and attenuates inflammation [24]. Similarly, whereas ad libitum access to a HFD in mice results in obesity, insulin resistance, hepatic steatosis, hypercholesterolemia, and dyslipidemia, 8- to 9-h TRF resulted in weight loss and reduced fat mass, decreased inflammation, improved glucose homeostasis, and reduced insulin resistance [25, 26]. Lastly, TRF in *Drosophila* resulted in improved sleep, prevention of weight gain, and deceleration of cardiac aging compared to ad libitum feeding, even when caloric intake and activity were held constant [27].

Effects of Fasting on Cardiovascular Risk in Humans

Based on prior RCTs and epidemiologic studies, the American Heart Association has recommended that Americans meet seven ideal cardiovascular health metrics [28]. These include not smoking, being physically active, having normal BP, blood glucose, total cholesterol (TC) levels, and weight, and eating a healthy diet. Yet, <2% of patients meet all seven health metrics [29]. Health-care providers and patients seek realistic and effective lifestyle intervention. Fasting is one intervention with the potential to make a significant impact on cardiovascular disease prevention. Studies in animals suggest that fasting significantly mitigates cardiovascular risk, influencing all of those seven health metrics except smoking and physical activity—and many of those findings have now been translated to human studies as well. Each type of fasting has accumulated data in humans suggesting that fasting can mitigate cardiovascular risk.

Intermittent Fasting

Design

IF is a broad term that is sometimes used to encompass ADF and TRE; however, for the purpose of this section, it is defined as fasting for a duration of 1–2 days at a time, usually on a weekly or monthly basis. The most common form of IF is 5:2 in which individuals reduce calorie intake to 500–600 kcal for 2 days out of each week (Fig. 9.2). Another example of IF is seen in the Church of Jesus Christ of Latter-Day Saints (LDS), who typically engage in a 24-h fast one Sunday per month from the age of 8 years old. Other examples of IF schedules could include fasting for 1 or 3 days per week.

Efficacy

In two randomized clinical trials (RCTs) ($n = 107$ and $n = 112$) comparing 5:2 IF with CR in obese patients, the two methods were equally as effective for weight loss (Table 9.1) [30, 31]. Harvie et al. showed that both methods also resulted in a reduction in high-sensitivity C-reactive protein (hs-CRP), TC, LDL-C, triglycerides, and BP (within group changes, $p < 0.05$), and there was no difference between the two groups (Table 9.2) [30]. Inflammation, of which hs-CRP is a sensitive marker, has been shown to be an independent risk factor for atherosclerotic cardiovascular disease (ASCVD) regardless of atherogenic lipid levels [32]. Sundfør et al. showed that both methods resulted in a reduction of BP and triglycerides, and an increase in HDL-C (within group changes, $p < 0.05$) with no difference between the two groups [31]. Harvie et al. showed a reduction in fasting insulin levels ($p < 0.05$) with a greater reduction in the IF group compared to the CR group ($p = 0.04$). Similarly, Sundfør et al. showed a reduction in hemoglobin A1c (HbA1c) ($p < 0.001$) with no difference between the two groups.

In the Mormon population, fasting is associated with a decreased risk of ASCVD even after adjusting for traditional risk factors [33]. Utah consistently has one of the lowest rates of death

Table 9.1 Effect of 5:2 Intermittent fasting on weight

Author	Year	Trial design	Cohort, sample size	Intervention	Duration	Weight loss end-point(s)
Harvie et al. [30]	2011	RCT	Overweight and obese, $n = 107$	5:2 intermittent fasting (IF) ($n = 53$) vs continuous energy restriction (CER) ($n = 54$)	6 months	**Weight (kg) (95% CI):** *5:2 IF* Baseline: 81.5 (77.5–85.4) 6 months: 75.8 (73–81.8) *CER* Baseline 84.4 (79.7–89.1) 6 months: 79.9 (74.6–85.2) $P = 0.26$
Sundfør et al. [31]	2018	RCT	Obese, $n = 112$	5:2 intermittent fasting (IF) ($n = 54$) vs continuous energy restriction (CER) ($n = 58$)	6 months weight loss phase, 6 months weight maintenance	**Change in weight after 1 year (kg) (SD):** 5:2 IF: −8 (6.5) CER: −9 (7.1) $P = 0.6$
Carter et al. [35]	2018	RCT	Type 2 diabetes, $n = 137$	5:2 intermittent fasting (IF) ($n = 70$) vs continuous energy restriction (CER) ($n = 67$)	12 months	**Mean change in weight (kg) (SEM) [95% CI]:** All participants: −5.9 (0.6) [−7.1 to −4.8] $P < 0.001$ 5:2 IF: −6.8 (0.8) [−8.5 to −5.1] CER: −5 (0.8) [−6.6 to −3.5] $P = 0.25$

Table 9.2 Effect of 5:2 intermittent fasting on systolic and diastolic blood pressure (SBP and DBP)

Author	Year	Trial design	Cohort, sample size	Intervention	Duration	BP end-point(s)
Harvie et al. [30]	2011	RCT	Overweight and obese, $n = 107$	5:2 intermittent fasting (IF) ($n = 53$) vs continuous energy restriction (CER) ($n = 54$)	6 months	**SBP (mmHg) (95% CI):** *5:2 IF* Baseline: 115.2 (111.2–119.2) 6 months: 111.5 (107.7–115.2) *CER* Baseline: 116.8 (116.8 (113.1–120.4) 6 months: 109.3 (105.3–113.2) P-value between groups 0.99 *(Similar findings for DBP)*
Sundfør et al. [31]	2018	RCT	Obese, $n = 112$	5:2 intermittent fasting (IF) ($n = 54$) vs continuous energy restriction (CER) ($n = 58$)	6 months weight loss phase, 6 months weight maintenance	**Mean change in SBP (mmHg) (SD):** *5:2 IF* Baseline: 129 (13.4) 6 months: −4.9 (14.2) 12 months: −1.9 (12.3) *CER* Baseline: 128 (13.2) 6 months: −5.8 (10.6) 12 months: −3.6 (11.8) P-value between groups: 0.6 *(Similar findings for DBP)*

from CVD in the USA, and members of the Church of Jesus Christ of LDS have even lower CVD mortality than other Utah residents [33]. Further, fasting in this population is associated with decreased prevalence of diabetes [34]. This population demonstrates the potential preventive benefit of fasting even when carried out relatively infrequently.

IF (5:2) has been specifically studied in patients with type 2 diabetes mellitus (T2DM). In a paired RCT, 137 patients with T2DM followed either a 5:2 IF or CR diet [35]. The study showed that the two interventions were equivalent in terms of reduction of HbA1c (−0.5% [0.2%] vs −0.3% [0.1%]; $p = 0.65$), with a between-group difference of 0.2% (90% CI, −0.2% to 0.5%). Although mean weight change was similar between the CR and 5:2 IF groups, the two interventions did not meet the criteria for equivalence (−1.8 kg; 90% CI, −3.7 to 0.07 kg), with 5:2 IF tending to produce greater reduction of weight (−5.0 [0.8] kg vs −6.8 [0.8] kg; $p = 0.25$) and fat mass (−3.4 [0.6] kg vs −4.7 [0.7] kg; $p = 0.20$). The study involved an evidence-based protocol for medication management in these patients with the intention to minimize hypoglycemic events. Nevertheless, 17% of patients experienced hypoglycemic events during the study with no difference between groups; however, many of these patients also reported experiencing hypoglycemic events prior to starting the study.

The effect of IF on glucose regulation was investigated on a smaller scale in a case series carried out in three patients with T2DM requiring at least 70 units of insulin daily [36]. One patient completed a 24-h fast 3 times per week, while two patients completed 24-h fasts every other day for 7–11 months. On fasting days, the patients only consumed dinner, whereas on non-fasting days the patients consumed lunch and dinner. Low-carbohydrate meals were encouraged. In all three patients, fasting resulted in rapid elimination of the need for insulin as well as decreased body weight, waist circumference, and HbA1c. The minimum number of days to discontinuation of insulin was 5 and the maximum was 18. Importantly, these patients did not

experience any episodes of hypoglycemia and the intervention included twice weekly clinic visits up until discontinuation of insulin and strict instruction to stop fasting if participants felt unwell at any point. Subjectively, participants tolerated fasting well and even reported enjoying taking an active role in managing their diabetes.

Safety

The safety of 5:2 IF and other methods of fasting in patients with T2DM has been called into question given the risk of hypoglycemia and glycemic variability [34]. There is a potential for hypoglycemia in patients who are on antidiabetic medications known to be associated with hypoglycemia, including insulin (both prandial and bolus) and sulfonylureas. One RCT showed that 5:2 IF increased the rate of hypoglycemia despite reduction of hypoglycemic medications [37]. In addition, higher day-to-day glucose variability, which could in theory occur with IF, increases the risk of microvascular and macrovascular complications [38]. Guidelines for medication management in patients with T2DM have been recently proposed [39]; however, this patient population represents a group that should be more carefully monitored with the assistance of a multidisciplinary team in order to avoid complications.

Alternate-Day Fasting

Design

ADF involves 36-h periods of 0–30% energy allowance followed by 12-h periods of ad libitum food intake (100% energy allowance) (Fig. 9.2). ADF is considered "modified" when patients are allowed to consume 25–30% of usual energy needs on fast days (the more common scenario), while classic ADF involves 0% energy allowance. Non-fasting days can potentially involve consuming greater than 100% of energy needs [40].

Efficacy

ADF has been studied in a variety of patient populations and appears to be beneficial in reducing risk factors for CVD. In obese patients, ADF has consistently been shown to promote weight loss (with an average reduction of 4.2–7.1% total body weight) (Table 9.3) [40–44]. When compared to CR, ADF was equivalent in terms of weight loss [40]. In particular, one study

Table 9.3 Effect of alternate-day fasting on weight

Author	Year	Trial Design	Cohort, sample size	Intervention	Duration	Weight loss end-point(s)
Varady et al. [47]	2017	RCT	Normal weight and overweight, $n = 32$	Alternate day fasting (ADF) vs control	12 weeks	**Mean change in weight (kg) SEM:** ADF: -5.2 ± 0.9 $P < 0.001$
Klempel et al. [42]	2013	RCT	Obese, $n = 32$	Alternate day fasting high fat (ADF-HF) vs alternate-day fasting low fat (ADF-LF)	8 weeks	**Mean change in weight (kg) SEM:** ADF-HF: -4.3 ± 1 ADF-LF: -3.7 ± 0.7 $P < 0.0001$ *No differences between groups for weight loss at any point.*
Bhutani et al. [43]	2013	RCT	Obese, $n = 64$	Alternate day fasting (ADF) + exercise, ADF alone, exercise alone, or control	12 weeks	**Mean change in weight (kg) SEM:** ADF + exercise: -6 ± 4 ADF: -3 ± 1 Exercise: -1 ± 0 $P < 0.05$
Trepanowski et al. [40]	2017	RCT	Obese, $n = 100$	Alternate-day fasting (ADF) ($n = 34$) vs calorie restriction (CR) ($n = 35$) vs control ($n = 31$)	6 months weight loss, 6 months weight maintenance	**Body weight (% change) (95% CI):** *ADF* 6 months: -6.8 (-9.1 to -4.5) 12 months: -6 (-8.5 to -3.6) *CR* 6 months: -6.8 (-9.1 to -4.6) 12 months: -5.3 (-7.6 to -3)
Eshginia and Mohammadzadeh [44]	2013	Cohort	Overweight and obese, $n = 15$	Alternate-day fasting (ADF)	6 weeks	**Mean weight (kg) SEM:** Before: 84.3 ± 11.44 After: 78.3 ± 10.18 $P < 0.001$
Cai et al. [45]	2019	RCT	Non-alcoholic fatty liver disease (NAFLD), $n = 271$	Alternate-day fasting (ADF) vs time-restricted eating (TRE) vs control	12 weeks	**Mean change in weight (kg) SEM:** *ADF* 4 weeks: -4.56 ± 0.41 12 weeks: -4.04 ± 0.54 $P < 0.001$ *TRF* 4 weeks: -3.62 ± 0.65 12 weeks: -3.25 ± 0.67 $P < 0.001$ *No difference between ADF and TRF groups at either time point.*

Table 9.4 Effect of alternate-day fasting on systolic and diastolic blood pressure (SBP and DBP)

Author	Year	Trial design	Cohort, sample size	Intervention	Duration	BP end-point(s)
Eshginia and Mohammadzadeh [44]	2013	Cohort	Overweight and obese, $n = 15$	Alternate-day fasting (ADF)	6 weeks	**SBP (mmHg)** **SEM:** Before: 114.8 ± 9.16 After: 105.13 ± 10.19 $P < 0.001$ **DBP (mmHg)** **SEM:** Before: 82.86 ± 10.6 After: 74.5 ± 10.8 $P < 0.05$

($n = 32$) demonstrated a reduction in waist circumference (-7.2 ± 1.5 cm and -7.3 ± 0.9 cm in high fat and low fat ADF groups, $p < 0.001$) and visceral fat mass (from $45 +/-2\%$ to $42 +/-2\%$, $p < 0.01$) [42]. Another study ($n = 15$) demonstrated similar findings, with a decrease in waist circumference from 87.87 ± 9.74 cm to 82.86 ± 9.68 cm ($p < 0.001$) and a reduction in visceral fat mass by 5.7% ($p < 0.001$) [44]. ADF has resulted in improvements in the lipid profile, including decreased TC, LDL-C, and triglycerides ($p < 0.01$), as well as increased LDL particle size ($p < 0.001$) [41–43]. In addition, it has been shown to decrease systolic blood pressure (SBP) by $4.4–9.7\%$ ($p < 0.05$) (Table 9.4) [41, 44]. When combined with a moderate-intensity exercise program, the positive effects on weight, body composition, and the lipid profile were augmented [43]. Interestingly, when ADF with a HFD was compared to ADF with a low-fat diet, the content of the diet had no impact on the eating pattern's beneficial effects [42].

One RCT investigated the effect of ADF on 270 patients with non-alcoholic fatty liver disease (NAFLD). Around 12 weeks of ADF resulted in a reduction in body weight (-4.56 ± 0.41 kg ($6.1 \pm 0.5\%$), $p < 0.001$), fat mass (-3.49 ± 0.37 kg; $11 \pm 1.2\%$, $p < 0.001$), TC ($p < 0.001$), and triglycerides ($p < 0.001$) [45]. Changes in liver stiffness (a marker of liver fibrosis) as measured by transient elastography did not differ significantly between groups. NAFLD poses a risk of cardiovascular disease, and lifestyle modification is the first step in treatment. Longer trials are needed to evaluate whether any form of IF can reduce the risk of progression from NAFLD to non-alcoholic steatohepatitis (NASH) and liver fibrosis.

Importantly, ADF also has been found to be beneficial in normal weight or overweight, nonobese patients, suggesting that the preventive effects of ADF do not stem from weight loss alone [46–48]. In these patients, ADF decreased fat mass (-2.112 kg (-3.119 to -1.352), $p < 0.0001$), particularly trunk fat mass ($p < 0.0001$) and improved fat to lean ratio without a significant reduction in bone mineral density (BMD) [46, 47]. It again improved the metabolic profile, reducing TC ($p = 0.004$), LDL-C ($p = 0.011$), and triglycerides ($p = 0.01$) and increasing LDL particle size ($p < 0.01$) [46, 47]. Further, ADF resulted in decreased CRP ($p < 0.05$) and the age-related inflammation marker sICAM-1 ($p = 0.048$) [47, 48], suggesting decreased total body inflammation.

Safety

Studies have suggested that ADF is safe in terms of physical and mental health. ADF has been shown to cause mild adverse effects in similar frequency to CR, including gastrointestinal issues, occasional problems staying asleep, and minor dizziness or weakness [49]. There is concern that longer periods of continuous CR cause decreased BMD, white blood cell (WBC) count, and energy levels [50–52]. Another study found that more than 6 months of ADF did not cause a decline in BMD or WBC [46]. Similarly, greater than 6 months of ADF did not result in decreased resting or activity energy expenditure [46].

Another concern that has been raised is the potential for ADF to perpetuate disordered eating habits. One cohort study in 59 patients specifically examined the mental health effects of 8 weeks of ADF [49]. Reassuringly, ADF was shown to decrease depression and binge eating and improve body image perception. It did not increase purgative behavior or fear of being overweight, nor did it create an aversion to "forbidden" foods.

Time-Restricted Eating

Design

TRE or time-restricted feeding (TRF) is defined by a daily 6–10-h window of eating followed by a 14- to 18-h fast with zero calorie intake (Fig. 9.2). Similar to other fasting methods, it has been shown to promote weight loss and improve the metabolic profile. However, it is unique in that it follows the body's natural circadian rhythm and therefore harnesses the benefits of circadian physiology.

Modern humans tend to eat sporadically throughout the day for an average of more than 14 h and fast only while sleeping, regardless of the presence or absence of sunlight [53]. This stands in contrast to earlier mammals and *Homo sapiens* whose days closely followed the sun and who worked to obtain food during daylight hours. As a result, most mammalian genes have evolved variable expression throughout the course of a 24-h day based upon the influence of light and food [54]. This cyclical variation in gene expression serves to optimize energy metabolism when food is available as well as to optimize cellular repair during times of limited food availability [55]. The individual is therefore able to efficiently process fuels and initiate repair mechanisms in order to increase overall fitness. Studies have shown that disruption of the natural circadian rhythm (such as through shiftwork and time-zone changes) increases the risk of metabolic diseases, while TRE sustains daily rhythms and decreases the risk of metabolic diseases [54].

Efficacy

Similar to ADF, TRE has been shown to be beneficial across multiple patient populations. In obese patients, TRE with an 8-h feeding window resulted in decreased body weight and energy intake ($-2.6\% \pm 0.5$; -341 ± 53 kcal/d, $p < 0.05$) as well as decreased SBP (-7 ± 2 mm Hg, $p < 0.05$) [56] (Tables 9.5 and 9.6). Similarly, 4- to 6-h feeding windows resulted in a reduction in body weight ($p < 0.001$), fat mass ($p = 0.002$), oxidative stress ($p = 0.02$), fasting insulin ($p = 0.02$), and insulin resistance ($p = 0.03$) versus control, and there was no difference between the 4- and 6-h groups [57]. One RCT including 15 overweight patients at risk for T2DM demonstrated improved glucose tolerance assessed by a reduction in glucose incremental area under the curve ($p = 0.001$) and decreased fasting triglycerides ($p = 0.003$) within just 1 week of TRE [58]. Interestingly, a reduction in mean fasting glucose was significant only in the early TRE (8 am–5 pm, $p = 0.02$) group, not the delayed TRE group (12 pm–9 pm) or control.

Table 9.5 Effect of time-restricted eating on weight

Author	Year	Trial design	Cohort, sample size	Intervention	Duration	Weight loss end-point(s)
Gabel et al. [56]	2018	Single arm, paired sample	Obese, $n = 46$	8-h time-restricted eating (TRE) ($n = 23$) vs control ($n = 23$)	12 weeks	**Mean weight (kg) SEM:** *TRE* Baseline: 95 ± 3 Week 12: 92 ± 3 *Controls* Baseline: 92 ± 3 Week 12: 92 ± 3 $P < 0.001$
Cienfuegos et al. [57]	2020	RCT	Obese, $n = 58$	4-h time-restricted eating (TRE) ($n = 19$), 6-h TRE ($n = 20$), vs control ($n = 19$)	8 weeks	**Body weight (% change) SEM:** 4-h TRF: −3.2 ± 0.4 $P < 0.001$ 6-h TRF: −3.2 ± 0.4 $P < 0.001$ Control: +0.1 ± 0.4 *No significant difference between 4-h and 6-h groups.*
Wilkinson et al. [60]	2020	Single arm, paired sample	Metabolic syndrome, $n = 19$	10-h time-restricted eating (TRE) ($n = 19$)	12 weeks	**Weight (kg) (mean SD):** Baseline: 97.84 (19.73) TRE: 94.54 (13.38) Mean change in weight: −3.30 (3.2) $P = 0.00028$

Table 9.6 Effect of time-restricted eating on systolic and diastolic blood pressure (SBP and DBP)

Author	Year	Trial design	Cohort, sample size	Intervention	Duration	BP end-point(s)
Gabel et al. [56]	2018	Single arm, paired sample	Obese, $n = 46$	8-h time-restricted eating (TRE) ($n = 23$) vs control ($n = 23$)	12 weeks	**SBP (mmHg) SEM:** *TRE* Baseline: 128 ± 4 Week 12: 121 ± 3 *Controls* Baseline: 123 ± 4 Week 12: 124 ± 3 $P < 0.05$
Wilkinson et al. [60]	2020	Single arm, paired sample	Metabolic syndrome, $n = 19$	10-h time-restricted eating (TRE) ($n = 19$)	12 weeks	**SBP (mmHg) (mean SD):** *TRE* Baseline: 127.88 (8.89) TRE: 122.76 (13.35) $P = 0.041$ **DBP (mmHg) (mean SD):** Baseline: 78.47 (8.74) TRE: 72 (10.75) $P = 0.004$
Sutton et al. [61]	2018	RCT	Prediabetes, $n = 12$	Early time-restricted eating (eTRE) ($n = 5$) vs control ($n = 7$)	5 weeks	**Mean change in BP (mmHg) SEM:** SBP: −11 ± 4 $P = 0.03$ DBP: −10 ± 4 $P = 0.03$

In contrast, the only RCT to date which showed no significant benefit to TRE was the TREAT trial ($n = 116$) comparing delayed TRE (12 pm to 8 pm) with a standard 3-meal eating plan. In this study, there was minimal but statistically significant weight loss in the TRE group, but no difference between groups [59].There were no significant changes in fasting insulin, fasting glucose, estimated energy intake , total energy expenditure, or resting energy expenditure within or between groups. However, the level of patient adherence in this trial has been called into question. Although the reported adherence is 83.5% in the TRE group, only about 37% of participants responded to adherence surveys, and likely those that were engaged enough to respond to those surveys were also more likely to be adherent to the diet. There was a significant difference in appendicular lean mass index between groups by DEXA (-0.16 kg/m^2; 95% CI, -0.27 to -0.05; $p = 0.005$), which deserves further examination in future studies.

TRE is also beneficial in metabolic syndrome. In a single arm, paired sample trial involving 19 patients with metabolic syndrome who were already receiving standard of care medical therapy, including statins and antihypertensives, 10-h TRE (i.e., 14 h of nightly fasting) resulted in reductions in body weight (-3.30 (3.20); -3%, $p = 0.00028$), waist circumference (-4.46 (6.72); -4%, 0.0097), BMI (-1.09 (0.91); -3%, $p = 0.00011$), percent body fat (-1.01 (0.91); -3%, $p = 0.00013$), and visceral fat rating (-0.58 (0.77); -3%, $p = 0.004$) [60]. Further, the intervention resulted in a reduction of SBP (-5.12 (9.51); -4%, 0.041) and DBP (-6.47 (7.94; -8%, $p = 0.004$) as well as improvement in the metabolic profile, including reductions in LDL-C (-11.94 (19.01; -11%, $p = 0.016$) and non-HDL-C (-11.94 (19.01); -11%, $p = 0.040$). Further, TRE reduced HbA1c in patients with baseline elevated fasting glucose and/or HbA1c (-0.22% $\pm$ 0.32% [3.7%], $p = 0.04$). All of these cardiometabolic outcomes were independent of change in weight. There was also no significant change in physical activity during the study. Although weight loss is an important, preven-

tive effect of TRE that is conserved across most human studies, this study highlights that the cardiometabolic benefits of TRE are likely not solely due to weight loss.

Patients with prediabetes (defined as a HbA1c of 5.5–6.4% and impaired glucose tolerance, defined as a glucose level between 140–199 mg/dL at the end of a 2-h oral glucose tolerance test) also benefit from TRE compared to a 12-h feeding window, even when weight and food intake are held constant. A randomized, crossover, isocaloric, and eucaloric controlled feeding trial (with food intake precisely matched and monitored such that no weight loss occurs) examined the effect of 5 weeks of early, 6-h TRE in 12 patients with prediabetes. Early TRE (eTRE) necessitates dinner to occur before 15:00. The study demonstrated a significant decrease in fasting insulin ($p = 0.05$), insulin resistance ($p = 0.005$), and pancreatic beta-cell responsiveness ($p \leq 0.01$) [61]. In addition, the intervention resulted in a dramatic improvement in SBP and DBP by 11 ± 4 mm Hg ($p = 0.03$) and 10 ± 4 mm Hg ($p = 0.03$), respectively, an effect size unusual for dietary interventions alone and similar to that of angiotensin-converting enzyme (ACE) inhibitors. Relative to control, TRE also resulted in a decrease in 8-isoprostane, a marker of oxidative stress to lipids (-11 ± 5 pg/mL; -14%, $p = 0.05$); however, there was no difference in inflammatory markers between the two groups. Lastly, early TRE resulted in dramatically increased sensations of fullness in the evening ($p < 0.0001$). All of these findings occurred without a reduction in caloric intake or weight loss in the TRE group compared to control, reinforcing that the cardiometabolic benefits of TRE are distinct from the benefits of CR and weight loss alone. Long-term adherence to eTRE may also be more challenging because the timing of daily dietary intake becomes potentially very different from that of friends and family members.

The aforementioned study raises the possibility that preferential consumption of calories earlier in the day during TRE could have an additional positive impact on cardiometabolic risk, a concept which is in keeping with current understanding of circadian variation in gene expression related to metabolism. Human studies have shown that insulin sensitivity, pancreatic beta-cell responsiveness, and the thermic effect of food are higher in the morning [62–64]. Correspondingly, several studies have demonstrated that preferential food intake earlier in the day results in improved glycemic control as well as a reduction in weight, lipid levels, and hunger [53, 65–70]. An RCT comparing eTRE and TRE with a feeding window of the same duration shifted later in the day is needed to investigate whether additional benefit can be obtained from eTRE beyond TRE alone.

Safety

Studies examining the effects of TRE have not shown any major adverse effects. While studies with a 6-h feeding window reported minor adverse effects such as vomiting, headaches, increased thirst, and diarrhea, these effects were not observed in TRE with a 10-h feeding window [60, 61]. In one study that specifically evaluated the safety of TRE, 12 weeks of 8-h TRE in obese patients elicited no change in self-reported adverse events, body image perception, complete blood count, or disordered eating patterns from baseline to week 12 [71].

Periodic Fasting

Design

Periodic fasting is defined as restricted caloric intake for 2 or more days in succession (Fig. 9.2). This is the most widely variable type of fasting and the least studied, likely because it poses a greater challenge for patients to tolerate and greater safety risk. Nonetheless, several studies have evaluated the effect of periodic fasting of various durations and found it to have positive effects on weight and metabolic profile. A recent study evaluating the mechanism underlying periodic fasting found that 58 h of continuous fasting ramped up metabolism such that 44 of ~130 evaluated metabolites increased by 1.5 to 60-fold [72].

Efficacy

The Buchinger fasting method was developed and studied in Germany and involves consuming a specified regimen of water, tea, honey, fresh-squeezed juice, and vegetable soup with a total caloric value of 200–250 kcal for various periods of time. One observational study ($n = 1422$) demonstrated that 4–21 days of Buchinger fasting results in a significant reduction in weight, abdominal circumference, SBP, and DBP ($p < 0.001$) (Tables 9.7 and 9.8) [73]. Reduction in weight and BP increased with increased duration of fasting [73]. One small cohort study ($n = 30$) also demonstrated reductions in LDL-C ($p < 0.001$) and fasting insulin ($p = 0.001$) [74]. Interestingly, the positive effects on BP, LDL-C, and triglycerides were amplified in patients with metabolic syndrome [74]. In an RCT ($n = 32$), 1 week of Buchinger fasting in patients with T2DM resulted in a reduction in weight ($p = 0.03$), abdominal circumference ($p = 0.001$), SBP and DBP ($p = 0.01$ and $p = 0.003$), and improved quality of life ($p = 0.04$) [75]. Mental health benefits were also observed in patients participating in Buchinger fasting, including decreased anxiety, depression, and fatigue as well as increased emotional and physical well-being and improved sleep quality [73, 74]. Overall the prospective studies that have evaluated Buchinger fasting are small, and more RCTs are needed to further investigate the method (Tables 9.7 and 9.8).

Two small, early cohort studies investigated the effect of 0 caloric intake over extended periods of time in obese patients. Both studies demonstrated significant effects on weight loss (up to –44 kg) [76, 77]. In particular, one study in obese patients undergoing 30 days of strict fasting demonstrated that weight loss occurred in a predictable pattern following the start of fasting, with rapid weight loss at the outset followed by a decreased, yet steady rate of weight loss [77]. Initial rapid weight loss coincided with breakdown of lean tissue, utilization of body fat, and elimination of body fluid, while subsequent loss was solely due to catabolism of lean tissue and fat. Although these drastic fasting regimens would no longer be a feasible or

Table 9.7 Effect of Buchinger fasting on weight

Author	Year	Trial design	Cohort, sample size	Intervention	Duration	Weight loss end-point(s)
De Toledo et al. [73]	2019	Cohort	N = 1422	Buchinger fasting (n = 1422)	Buchinger fasting for 5, 10, 15, and 10 todays	**Mean weight (kg) SEM:** *All* Baseline: 82 ± 0.5 After fasting 5, 10, 15, or 20 days: 77.9 ± 0.5 *5-day fast* Baseline: 79.3 ± 0.8 After fasting: 76.1 ± 0.7 *10-day fast* Baseline: 82.7 ± 0.9 After fasting: 78.3 ± 0.8 *15-day fast* Baseline: 86.6 ± 1.6 After fasting: 80.5 ± 1.4 *20-day fast* Baseline: 96.7 ± 4 After fasting: 89.6 ± 3.7 P < 0.001 (fasting intervention) P < 0.001 (between fasting duration groups)
Li et al. [74]	2013	RCT	Type 2 diabetes and metabolic syndrome, n = 32	Buchinger fasting (n = 16) vs control	Buchinger fasting for 7 days	**Mean weight (kg) SEM:** *Fasting* Baseline: 89.3 ± 12.6 Follow-up: 85.8 ± 13.4 Mean change: −3.5 ± 4.5 P = 0.01 *Control* Baseline: 95.3 ± 17.9 Follow-up: 93.3 ± 15.6 Mean change: −2 ± 4.8 P = 0.83 **Between-group difference of change (95% CI):** −3 (−6 to −0.4) P = 0.03

safe regimen for modern patients, the two studies serve as a demonstration of the predictable effect of strict, long-term fasting on weight loss.

Safety

The Bunchinger fasting method appears to be safe in terms of physical and mental health. In a cohort study involving 1422 patients, mild symptoms such as fatigue, dry mouth, back pain, and hunger were reported, with sleep disturbances being the most common symptom [73]. Most symptoms occurred early in the fast and improved with continued fasting. Although no deaths or permanent adverse effects were observed, 2 patients out of 1422 (0.01%) had to be hospitalized; however, both ultimately returned to fasting after a brief hospital stay. Patients reported significantly improved emotional well-being throughout the course of the fast. Another study demonstrated significant improvements in anxiety, depression, and sleep quality [74].

Longer term, 0-calorie periodic fasting resulted in several mild side effects, including headache, lightheadedness, and nervousness, worst at the start of the fast [76]. One patient developed severe oliguria and edema (unknown cause) and required

Table 9.8 Effect of Buchinger fasting on systolic and diastolic blood pressure (SBP and DBP)

Author	Year	Trial design	Cohort, sample size	Intervention	Duration	BP end-point(s)
De Toledo et al. [73]	2019	Cohort	N = 1422	Buchinger fasting (n = 1422)	5, 10, 15, and 20 todays	**Mean SBP (mmHg) SEM:** Baseline: 131.6 ± 0.7 After fasting: 120.7 ± 0.4 P < 0.001 **Mean DBP (mmHg) SEM:** Baseline: 83.7 ± 0.4 After fasting: 77.9 ± 0.3 P < 0.001
Li et al. [74]	2013	RCT	Type 2 diabetes and metabolic syndrome, n = 32	Buchinger fasting (n = 16) vs control	7 days	**Mean SBP (mmHg) SEM:** *Fasting* Baseline: 141.9 ± 16 Follow-up: 128 ± 17 P = 0.04 *Control* Baseline: 136.3 ± 26.9 Follow-up: 136.7 ± 19.5 P = 0.25 **Between-group difference of change (95% CI):** −15 (−25 to −2) P = 0.01 *(Similar findings for DBP)*

treatment with daily furosemide. The investigators specifically avoided questioning patients about hunger, so it is unclear how this affected patients throughout the fast; however, the investigators did report that prolonged fasting was surprisingly tolerated with ease. Vitamin supplementation was essential to prevent vitamin deficiency.

Importantly, all of the studies in PF were carried out in a controlled environment, suggesting a need for heightened supervision in order to prevent harm.

The Fasting Mimicking Diet

Designed as an alternative to traditional fasting methods, the fasting mimicking diet (FMD) is meant to function similarly to fasting through a very low-calorie, plant-based diet that is followed for 4–5 days per month, with the majority of calories derived from fat and the minority from protein [78, 79]. While allowing a limited intake during the fasting days, a FMD is meant to provide similar benefits to fasting through the greatly reduced amount of calories and protein. Because the FMD is a relatively short time commitment each month, it may be more feasible compared to other fasting patterns.

Early studies suggest that the FMD may offer similar benefits to other forms of fasting. In a pilot clinical trial (n = 38), three cycles of the FMD resulted in a significant reduction in fasting glucose (p < 0.001) and total body weight (p < 0.001) [78]. A similar RCT (n = 100) comparing the FMD to an unrestricted control diet also found that three FMD cycles resulted in a significant reduction in body weight (p < 0.0001), waist circumference (p < 0.0001), SBP and DBP (p < 0.0001, p < 0.0004), and TC (p = 0.004) [79]. Both studies reported low rates of adverse events, suggesting that the FMD may be safe and effective, especially for those who cannot or prefer not to sustain longer periods of fasting. More studies in different patient populations are still needed to understand the effects of the FMD.

Conclusion and Recommendations

With evidence pointing to fasting as an effective method to reduce cardiovascular risk, one question becomes whether or not these regimens are feasible and sustainable for patients in the long term. Although they do not involve the cumbersome calorie-counting of CR diets, some studies in ADF, TRE, and PF have demonstrated high attrition rates of 27–40% in fasting groups [35, 40, 75, 80]. However, other studies have demonstrated excellent adherence. For example, one RCT in early TRE with a 6-h feeding window had 100% adherence [61]. Because TRE is closest to patients' baseline eating pattern, it might be the easiest fasting regimen to adopt, particularly in TRE with a 10-h feeding window. In addition, evidence that patients can choose the timing of their feeding window without significantly affecting the results suggests that TRE may be more easily integrated into patients' lives [60].

Recognizing the challenges that fasting poses, there is ongoing research into ways to achieve the benefits of fasting without actually refraining from eating. Fasting-mimicking diets low in calories, sugars, and protein, but high in unsaturated fats have yielded similar results to fasting diets, including reduced weight, BP, and insulin-like growth factor in a small number of initial studies [79]. In addition, pharmaceutical CR mimetics are sought with the goal of mitigating the need for patient commitment to lifestyle changes [14].

Research in animal and human studies is incredibly promising in terms of the potential of fasting to reduce the risk of CVD. Ongoing human studies still aim to elucidate some of the dramatic effects seen in animal studies. Overall, more large-scale randomized, controlled, clinical trials are needed in order to integrate these fasting regimens into clinical practice. In particular, more studies are needed in older patients and those with diabetes mellitus, and more specific guidelines are needed to manage antidiabetic medications during fasting and these groups likely require close monitoring and the assistance of a multidisciplinary team in order to ensure safety. However, based on current data, it is appropriate to use patient-centered decision-making to raise the possibility of fasting as an intervention in obese or normal weight patients at risk for CVD.

Acknowledgment Figure 9.1 was created with BioRender. com.
Figure 9.2 was created by Christina Pecora, MSMI.

References

1. The Editors of Encyclopædia Britannica. Fasting. Encyclopædia Britannica; 2020.
2. de Cabo R, Mattson MP. Effects of intermittent fasting on health, aging, and disease. N Engl J Med. 2019;381:2541–51.
3. Newman JC, Verdin E. Ketone bodies as signaling metabolites. Trends Endocrinol Metab. 2014;25:42–52.
4. Longo VD, Mattson MP. Fasting: molecular mechanisms and clinical applications. Cell Metab. 2014;19: 181–92.
5. McCay CM, Crowell MF, Maynard LA. The effect of retarded growth upon the length of life span and upon the ultimate body size. J Nutr. 1935;10:63–79.
6. Weindruch R, Sohal RS. Caloric intake and aging. N Engl J Med. 1997;337:986–94.
7. Bodkin NL, Alexander TM, Ortmeyer HK, Johnson E, Hansen BC. Mortality and morbidity in laboratory-maintained Rhesus monkeys and effects of long-term dietary restriction. J Gerontol A Biol Sci Med Sci. 2003;58:212–9.
8. Mattison JA, Lane MA, Roth GS, Ingram DK. Calorie restriction in rhesus monkeys. Exp Gerontol. 2003;38:35–46.
9. Mattson MP, Wan R. Beneficial effects of intermittent fasting and caloric restriction on the cardiovascular and cerebrovascular systems. J Nutr Biochem. 2005;16:129–37.
10. Goodrick CL, Ingram DK, Reynolds MA, Freeman JR, Cider N. Effects of intermittent feeding upon body weight and lifespan in inbred mice: interaction of genotype and age. Mech Ageing Dev. 1990;55: 69–87.
11. Anson RM, et al. Intermittent fasting dissociates beneficial effects of dietary restriction on glucose metabolism and neuronal resistance to injury from calorie intake. Proc Natl Acad Sci U S A. 2003;100: 6216–20.
12. Mattson MP, Chan SL, Duan W. Modification of brain aging and neurodegenerative disorders by genes, diet, and behavior. Physiol Rev. 2002;82:637–72.
13. Sohal RS, Weindruch R. Oxidative stress, caloric restriction, and aging. Science. 1996;273:59–63.

14. Madeo F, Carmona-Gutierrez D, Hofer SJ, Kroemer G. Caloric restriction mimetics against age-associated disease: targets, mechanisms, and therapeutic potential. Cell Metab. 2019;29:592–610.
15. Raeini-Sarjaz M, Vanstone CA, Papamandjaris AA, Wykes LJ, Jones PJ. Comparison of the effect of dietary fat restriction with that of energy restriction on human lipid metabolism. Am J Clin Nutr. 2001;73:262–7.
16. Diniz YS, et al. Dietary restriction and fibre supplementation: oxidative stress and metabolic shifting for cardiac health. Can J Physiol Pharmacol. 2003;81:1042–8.
17. Wan R, Camandola S, Mattson MP. Intermittent food deprivation improves cardiovascular and neuroendocrine responses to stress in rats. J Nutr. 2003;133:1921–9.
18. Young JB, Mullen D, Landsberg L. Caloric restriction lowers blood pressure in the spontaneously hypertensive rat. Metabolism. 1978;27:1711–4.
19. Spaulding CC, Walford RL, Effros RB. Calorie restriction inhibits the age-related dysregulation of the cytokines TNF-α and IL-6 in C3B10RF1 mice. Mech Ageing Dev. 1997;93:87–94.
20. Muthukumar A, Zaman K, Lawrence R, Barnes JL, Fernandes G. Food restriction and fish oil suppress atherogenic risk factors in lupus-prone (NZB× NZW) F 1 mice. J Clin Immunol. 2003;23:23–33.
21. Chandrasekar B, Nelson JF, Colston JT, Freeman GL. Calorie restriction attenuates inflammatory responses to myocardial ischemia-reperfusion injury. Am J Physiol Heart Circ Physiol. 2001;280: H2094–102.
22. Ahmet I, Wan R, Mattson MP, Lakatta EG, Talan M. Cardioprotection by intermittent fasting in rats. Circulation. 2005;112:3115–21.
23. Crandall DL, Feirer RP, Griffith DR, Beitz DC. Relative role of caloric restriction and exercise training upon susceptibility to isoproterenol-induced myocardial infarction in male rats. Am J Clin Nutr. 1981;34:841–7.
24. Hatori M, et al. Time-restricted feeding without reducing caloric intake prevents metabolic diseases in mice fed a high-fat diet. Cell Metab. 2012;15: 848–60.
25. Wang CY, Liao JK. A mouse model of diet-induced obesity and insulin resistance. Methods Mol Biol. 2012;821:421–33.
26. Chaix A, Zarrinpar A, Miu P, Panda S. Time-restricted feeding is a preventative and therapeutic intervention against diverse nutritional challenges. Cell Metab. 2014;20:991–1005.
27. Gill S, Le HD, Melkani GC, Panda S. Time-restricted feeding attenuates age-related cardiac decline in Drosophila. Science. 2015;347:1265–9.
28. Lloyd-Jones DM, et al. Defining and setting national goals for cardiovascular health promotion and disease reduction. Circulation. 2010;121:586–613.
29. Yang Q, et al. Trends in cardiovascular health metrics and associations with all-cause and CVD mortality among US adults. JAMA. 2012;307:1273–83.
30. Harvie MN, et al. The effects of intermittent or continuous energy restriction on weight loss and metabolic disease risk markers: a randomized trial in young overweight women. Int J Obes (Lond). 2011;35:714–27.
31. Sundfør TM, Svendsen M, Tonstad S. Effect of intermittent versus continuous energy restriction on weight loss, maintenance and cardiometabolic risk: a randomized 1-year trial. Nutr Metab Cardiovasc Dis. 2018;28:698–706.
32. Quispe R, et al. High-sensitivity C-reactive protein discordance with atherogenic lipid measures and incidence of atherosclerotic cardiovascular disease in primary prevention: the ARIC study. J Am Heart Assoc. 2020;9:e013600.
33. Horne BD, et al. Usefulness of routine periodic fasting to lower risk of coronary artery disease in patients undergoing coronary angiography. Am J Cardiol. 2008;102:814–9.
34. Horne BD, et al. Relation of routine, periodic fasting to risk of diabetes mellitus, and coronary artery disease in patients undergoing coronary angiography. Am J Cardiol. 2012;109:1558–62.
35. Carter S, Clifton PM, Keogh JB. Effect of intermittent compared with continuous energy restricted diet on glycemic control in patients with type 2 diabetes: a randomized noninferiority trial. JAMA Netw Open. 2018;1:e180756.
36. Furmli S, Elmasry R, Ramos M, Fung J. Therapeutic use of intermittent fasting for people with type 2 diabetes as an alternative to insulin. BMJ Case Rep. 2018;2018:bcr2017221854.
37. Corley BT, et al. Intermittent fasting in Type 2 diabetes mellitus and the risk of hypoglycaemia: a randomized controlled trial. Diabet Med. 2018;35:588–94.
38. Horne BD, Grajower MM, Anderson JL. Limited evidence for the health effects and safety of intermittent fasting among patients with type 2 diabetes. JAMA. 2020. https://doi.org/10.1001/jama.2020.3908.
39. Grajower MM, Horne BD. Clinical management of intermittent fasting in patients with diabetes mellitus. Nutrients. 2019;11:873.
40. Trepanowski JF, et al. Effect of alternate-day fasting on weight loss, weight maintenance, and cardioprotection among metabolically healthy obese adults: a randomized clinical trial. JAMA Intern Med. 2017;177:930–8.
41. Varady KA, Bhutani S, Church EC, Klempel MC. Short-term modified alternate-day fasting: a novel dietary strategy for weight loss and cardioprotection in obese adults. Am J Clin Nutr. 2009;90:1138–43.
42. Klempel MC, Kroeger CM, Varady KA. Alternate day fasting (ADF) with a high-fat diet produces similar weight loss and cardio-protection as ADF with a low-fat diet. Metabolism. 2013;62:137–43.
43. Bhutani S, Klempel MC, Kroeger CM, Trepanowski JF, Varady KA. Alternate day fasting and endurance exercise combine to reduce body weight and favorably alter plasma lipids in obese humans. Obesity. 2013;21:1370–9.

44. Eshghinia S, Mohammadzadeh F. The effects of modified alternate-day fasting diet on weight loss and CAD risk factors in overweight and obese women. J Diabetes Metab Disord. 2013;12:4.

45. Cai H, et al. Effects of alternate-day fasting on body weight and dyslipidaemia in patients with non-alcoholic fatty liver disease: a randomised controlled trial. BMC Gastroenterol. 2019;19:219.

46. Stekovic S, et al. Alternate day fasting improves physiological and molecular markers of aging in healthy, non-obese humans. Cell Metab. 2020;31:878–81.

47. Varady KA, et al. Alternate day fasting for weight loss in normal weight and overweight subjects: a randomized controlled trial. Nutr J. 2013;12:146.

48. Heilbronn LK, Smith SR, Martin CK, Anton SD, Ravussin E. Alternate-day fasting in nonobese subjects: effects on body weight, body composition, and energy metabolism. Am J Clin Nutr. 2005;81:69–73.

49. Hoddy KK, et al. Safety of alternate day fasting and effect on disordered eating behaviors. Nutr J. 2015;14:44.

50. Meydani SN, et al. Long-term moderate calorie restriction inhibits inflammation without impairing cell-mediated immunity: a randomized controlled trial in non-obese humans. Aging. 2016;8:1416–31.

51. Schafer AL. Decline in bone mass during weight loss: a cause for concern? J Bone Miner Res. 2016;31:36–9.

52. Villareal DT, et al. Effect of two-year caloric restriction on bone metabolism and bone mineral density in non-obese younger adults: a randomized clinical trial. J Bone Miner Res. 2016;31:40–51.

53. Gill S, Panda S. A smartphone app reveals erratic diurnal eating patterns in humans that can be modulated for health benefits. Cell Metab. 2015;22:789–98.

54. Panda S. Circadian physiology of metabolism. Science. 2016;354:1008–15.

55. Longo VD, Panda S. Fasting, circadian rhythms, and time-restricted feeding in healthy lifespan. Cell Metab. 2016;23:1048–59.

56. Gabel K, et al. Effects of 8-hour time restricted feeding on body weight and metabolic disease risk factors in obese adults: a pilot study. Nutr Healthy Aging. 2018;4:345–53.

57. Cienfuegos S, et al. Effects of 4- and 6-h time-restricted feeding on weight and cardiometabolic health: a randomized controlled trial in adults with obesity. Cell Metab. 2020. https://doi.org/10.1016/j.cmet.2020.06.018.

58. Hutchison AT, et al. Time-restricted feeding improves glucose tolerance in men at risk for type 2 diabetes: a randomized crossover trial. Obesity. 2019;27:724–32.

59. Lowe DA, et al. Effects of time-restricted eating on weight loss and other metabolic parameters in women and men with overweight and obesity: the TREAT randomized clinical trial. JAMA Intern Med. 2020. https://doi.org/10.1001/jamainternmed.2020.4153.

60. Wilkinson MJ, et al. Ten-hour time-restricted eating reduces weight, blood pressure, and atherogenic lipids in patients with metabolic syndrome. Cell Metab. 2020;31:92–104.e5.

61. Sutton EF, et al. Early time-restricted feeding improves insulin sensitivity, blood pressure, and oxidative stress even without weight loss in men with prediabetes. Cell Metab. 2018;27:1212–1221.e3.

62. Morris CJ, et al. The human circadian system has a dominating role in causing the morning/evening difference in diet-induced thermogenesis. Obesity. 2015;23:2053–8.

63. Poggiogalle E, Jamshed H, Peterson CM. Circadian regulation of glucose, lipid, and energy metabolism in humans. Metabolism. 2018;84:11–27.

64. Scheer FAJL, Hilton MF, Mantzoros CS, Shea SA. Adverse metabolic and cardiovascular consequences of circadian misalignment. Proc Natl Acad Sci U S A. 2009;106:4453–8.

65. Garaulet M, et al. Timing of food intake predicts weight loss effectiveness. Int J Obes (Lond). 2013;37:604–11.

66. Jakubowicz D, et al. High-energy breakfast with low-energy dinner decreases overall daily hyperglycaemia in type 2 diabetic patients: a randomised clinical trial. Diabetologia. 2015;58:912–9.

67. Jakubowicz D, Barnea M, Wainstein J, Froy O. High caloric intake at breakfast vs. dinner differentially influences weight loss of overweight and obese women. Obesity. 2013;21:2504–12.

68. Jakubowicz D, Barnea M, Wainstein J, Froy O. Effects of caloric intake timing on insulin resistance and hyperandrogenism in lean women with polycystic ovary syndrome. Clin Sci. 2013;125:423–32.

69. Keim NL, Van Loan MD, Horn WF, Barbieri TF, Mayclin PL. Weight loss is greater with consumption of large morning meals and fat-free mass is preserved with large evening meals in women on a controlled weight reduction regimen. J Nutr. 1997;127:75–82.

70. Ruiz-Lozano T, et al. Timing of food intake is associated with weight loss evolution in severe obese patients after bariatric surgery. Clin Nutr. 2016;35:1308–14.

71. Gabel K, Hoddy KK, Varady KA. Safety of 8-h time restricted feeding in adults with obesity. Appl Physiol Nutr Metab. 2019;44:107–9.

72. Teruya T, Chaleckis R, Takada J, Yanagida M, Kondoh H. Diverse metabolic reactions activated during 58-hr fasting are revealed by non-targeted metabolomic analysis of human blood. Sci Rep. 2019;9:854.

73. Wilhelmi de Toledo F, Grundler F, Bergouignan A, Drinda S, Michalsen A. Safety, health improvement and well-being during a 4 to 21-day fasting period in an observational study including 1422 subjects. PLoS One. 2019;14:e0209353.

74. Li C, et al. Metabolic and psychological response to 7-day fasting in obese patients with and without metabolic syndrome. Forsch Komplementmed. 2013;20:413–20.

75. Li C, et al. Effects of a one-week fasting therapy in patients with type-2 diabetes mellitus and metabolic syndrome – a randomized controlled explorative study. Exp Clin Endocrinol Diabetes. 2017;125:618–24.

76. Thomson TJ, Runcie J, Miller V. Treatment of obesity by total fasting for up to 249 days. Lancet. 1966;2:992–6.
77. Runcie J, Hilditch TE. Energy provision, tissue utilization, and weight loss in prolonged starvation. Br Med J. 1974;2:352–6.
78. Brandhorst S, et al. A periodic diet that mimics fasting promotes multi-system regeneration, enhanced cognitive performance, and healthspan. Cell Metab. 2015;22:86–99.
79. Wei M, et al. Fasting-mimicking diet and markers/risk factors for aging, diabetes, cancer, and cardiovascular disease. Sci Transl Med. 2017;9:eaai8700.
80. Jamshed H, et al. Early time-restricted feeding improves 24-hour glucose levels and affects markers of the circadian clock, aging, and autophagy in humans. Nutrients. 2019;11:1234.

Optimal Dietary Approaches for Those Living with Metabolic Syndrome to Prevent Progression to Diabetes and Reduce the Risk of Cardiovascular Disease

10

Melroy S. D'Souza, Tiffany A. Dong, Devinder S. Dhindsa, Anurag Mehta, and Laurence S. Sperling

Introduction

Cardiovascular disease (CVD) is a preventable condition and the metabolic syndrome (MetS) which consists of various factors that increase the risk for both the development of diabetes mellitus (DM) and CVD. There are ways to prevent and treat the components of the MetS, which require implementation of lifestyle modifications including dietary approaches and exercise.

Various dietary patterns have a favorable impact on the prevention of DM and the progression to CVD. We discuss the Mediterranean dietary pattern (MDP), plant-based dietary pattern (PBD), Dietary Approaches to Stop Hypertension (DASH), and intermittent fasting (IF) and their role to prevent and treat the MetS.

Metabolic Syndrome and Cardiovascular Disease

The MetS is a cluster of gene-behavior-environment interactions that increase one's risk of developing CVD [1, 2]. The main comorbid conditions that comprise the MetS are abdominal obesity, insulin resistance, dyslipidemia, and hypertension [2, 3]. There are nuanced cutoffs used by different health entities, which were summarized by Sperling et al. in a 2015 review [2]. The Cardiometabolic Health Alliance delineated stages of MetS in order to further risk stratify patients and guide management strategies [2].

- Stage A—"at-risk" for MetS based on demographics, body habitus, and family history.
- Stage B—develops ≤ 2 components of MetS and has risk factors for the others.
- Stage C—develops ≥ 3 components of MetS without development of end-organ damage.
- Stage D—MetS components with end-organ damage such as heart disease, renal disease, nonalcoholic fatty liver disease, or diabetes.

Several classifications of MetS, including the one from the World Health Organization, require the presence of impaired fasting glucose along with at least two more additional risk factor

M. S. D'Souza · T. A. Dong
Department of Internal Medicine, Emory University School of Medicine, Atlanta, GA, USA
e-mail: msdsouz@emory.edu;
tiffanydong20@emory.edu

D. S. Dhindsa · A. Mehta · L. S. Sperling (✉)
Emory Clinical Cardiovascular Research Institute, Division of Cardiology, Emory University School of Medicine, Atlanta, GA, USA
e-mail: devinder.singh.dhindsa@emory.edu;
Anurag.mehta@emory.edu; lsperli@emory.edu

© Springer Nature Switzerland AG 2021
M. J. Wilkinson et al. (eds.), *Prevention and Treatment of Cardiovascular Disease*, Contemporary Cardiology, https://doi.org/10.1007/978-3-030-78177-4_10

conditions [4]. This places an emphasis on those at-risk for or who have developed diabetes, as the foundation of MetS. Therefore, the prevention of DM is paramount for the prevention of CVD, especially in individuals who have other risk factors for MetS. Therefore, this chapter will focus on dietary approaches that improve the risk profile of those living with the MetS in the context of preventing the progression to diabetes and the development of CVD.

The presence of one or more risk factors (Fig. 10.1) for MetS exhibits a nonlinear, additive effect on the risk of developing CVD [1]. A meta-analysis by Galassi et al. (2006) demonstrated that individuals with MetS have a higher incidence of CVD (RR 1.53; 95% CI 1.26–1.87) and higher CVD-related mortality (RR 1.74; 95% CI 1.29–2.35) with an increased risk in women (RR 2.10, 95% CI 1.79–2.45) compared to men (RR 1.57; 95% CI 1.41–1.75) with similar profiles [5]. To reduce the incidence of DM, and thus CVD, providers should focus on improving patient's metabolic dysregulation, especially insulin resistance.

The 2018 American Multi-Society Cholesterol Management Guidelines recommend lifestyle modifications as the foundation for preventing of MetS [6]. "Heart-healthy" dietary patterns are an important but not solitary component of lifestyle modification. The Diabetes Prevention Program Research Group demonstrated that a combination of weight loss, regular exercise, and effective dietary pattern together performed better than metformin to reduce the incidence of diabetes in those with elevated fasting glucose [7]. Our discussion emphasizes "dietary approach" instead of the colloquial term "diet" to highlight that the greatest efficacy for prevention is driven by a combination of lifestyle factors.

Dietary Patterns to Treat Metabolic Syndrome

Mediterranean Dietary Pattern

The first indications that the MDP contributed to improved cardiovascular outcomes came from the results of the Seven Countries study [8]. The findings of this seminal epidemiological study defined the relationship between diet and cardiovascular health in Italy and Greece, supporting a beneficial impact of the MDP. Central components of MDP are fresh fruits and vegetables,

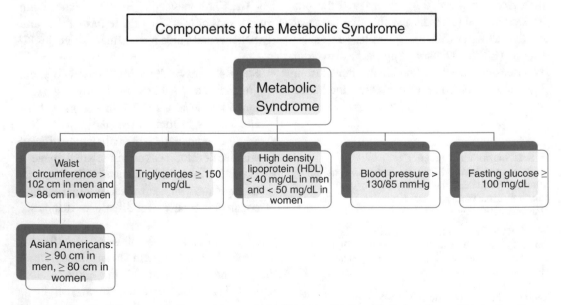

Fig. 10.1 Components of metabolic syndrome, which also represent the risk factors for cardiovascular disease. (Adapted from Ref. [2])

monounsaturated fats in the forms of nuts and olive oil, poultry, fish, and whole grains with minimal consumption of refined grains, sugar, and red meat [9]. In addition to food choices, the Mediterranean approach includes regular physical activity, longer mealtimes, and maintaining a strong social support system [10]. Adherence to this dietary pattern and lifestyle has shown to decrease the incidence of MetS, diabetes, and CVD [11].

Several observational studies have supported the findings for the prevention of MetS with the MDP. The EPIC cohort recruited over half a million participants across various Mediterranean countries. Several analyses were conducted with this cohort and it was found that the MDP was associated with lower blood pressure and body-mass index (BMI) [12]. Similar findings were observed in the Spanish SUN cohort, comprised of 2500 university graduates. The cohort was followed for 6 years and those who had higher adherence to the MDP had a lower incidence of developing MetS [13]. This dose–response relationship was also demonstrated in an analysis of the PREDIMED cohort, where the groups with the highest adherence to the MDP had the lowest odds ratio of developing MetS, OR 0.44; 95% CI 0.27–0.70 [14]. Finally, higher adherence to the MDP was associated with a markedly reduced risk of developing DM in Spanish university graduates [15]. A meta-analysis by Kastorini et al. provided further evidence that the MDP can aid primary prevention of MetS. This analysis included 50 studies and demonstrated that the MDP had a beneficial impact on all components of MetS and was also associated with a lower risk of developing MetS, as a composite outcome [11].

Interventional studies have also demonstrated the benefits of the MDP in participants who had developed or were developing MetS. The Medi-RIVAGE study enrolled participants who had one or more components of MetS and randomized them into the MDP or low-fat diet group [16]. After the 3-month study period, MDP participants saw a significant reduction in BMI, serum triglycerides, serum glucose, serum insulin, and in the homeostatic model assessment for insulin

resistance (HOMA-IR), a marker of insulin resistance [16].

The PREDIMED cohort enrolled over 7000 participants who were at high-risk for CVD but without overt disease and followed them for nearly 5 years [17]. In an analysis of the PREDIMED cohort, participants randomized to the MDP group experienced reductions in blood pressure, fasting serum glucose, serum insulin, HOMA-IR and lipid parameters, while those on a low-fat diet had minimal to no change in these parameters [18]. The MDP has shown to be an effective dietary approach for the prevention and treatment for MetS [10].

In summary, the MDP has demonstrated consistent efficacy for the improvement of MetS components as well as the prevention of diabetes.

Plant-Based Dietary Pattern

A plant-based dietary (PBD) pattern consists of fruits, vegetables, whole grains, nuts, legumes, oils, tea, coffee, and is typically devoid of meat, dairy, and eggs. Studies of PBDs include both vegan and vegetarian approaches; therefore, the reference term PBD will encompass both approaches.

The Seventh-Day Adventist population traditionally adheres to a PBD and the prevalence of diabetes in this population is 55% lower than in the general population [19]. These effects are cumulative over time, as long-term adherence to a vegetarian diet was associated with a 74% reduced risk of developing DM compared to the meat-eating population [19]. A separate study of the Seventh-Day Adventist population found the prevalence of DM decreased from 7.6% in those that chose a nonvegetarian diet to 2.9% in strict vegans [20]. A PBD has also been effective in reducing the risk for diabetes in other populations worldwide such as Taiwanese men, postmenopausal women, and health-care professionals in the USA [21, 22].

A PBD has a positive impact on diabetic individuals. One study followed 20 insulin-dependent males and after adhering to a PBD for 16 days all were able to reduce their dose of exogenous insulin from an average of 26 ± 3 units to 11 ± 3 units (p < 0.001) [23]. Similar results were found by Barnard et al., as 39% of insulin-dependent participants were able to discontinue use of exogenous insulin after adhering to a PBD in addition to exercise [19, 24]. A PBD was also associated with lower postprandial serum glucose and less glycemic variability [25]. A meta-analysis of clinical trials demonstrated that a PBD has an HbA1c lowering effect that equals approximately 50% of the effect seen with metformin [26]. Kahleova et al. randomized diabetic patients to an isocaloric PBD or a low carbohydrate "diabetes diet" outlined by the European Association for the Study of Diabetes. After 24 weeks, 43% of participants in the PBD group were able to reduce the use of diabetes medications compared to only 5% in the control group (p < 0.001) [27]. In summary, plant-based dietary patterns have demonstrated significant efficacy for the prevention and treatment of diabetes.

Several trials have demonstrated that a PBD is superior for weight loss as compared to a more traditional diet. After 6 months of adherence, participants following a vegan and vegetarian diet lost more weight (−7.5 ± 4.5% and −6.3 ± 6.6%, respectively) than those on a pesco-vegetarian (−3.2 ± 3.4%), semi-vegetarian (−3.2 ± 3.8%), and omnivorous diet (−3.1 ± 3.6%) (p < 0.01) [28]. In a trial evaluating a PBD versus a standard New Zealand diet in overweight participants who had ≥1 CVD risk factors , the PBD group saw a significant decrease in BMI compared to controls; reduction at 6 months (4.4 kg × m⁻²; 95% CI 3.7–5.1) and 1 year (4.2 kg × m⁻²; 95% CI 3.4–5) [29]. In a meta-analysis of 12 trials, PBD participants had more weight loss than nonvegetarians did over a median study period of 18 weeks (−2.02 kg; 95% CI −2.80 to −1.23) and vegan diets were associated with more weight loss than vegetarian diets (−2.52 kg; 95% CI: −3.02 to −1.98] versus (−1.48 kg; 95% CI: −3.43 to 0.47) [30]. A plant-based diet, rich in whole grain carbohydrates and fiber, appears to be a favorable dietary pattern for lowering BMI and weight loss maintenance.

Mishra et al. compared the effect of a PBD and a traditional American diet on serum lipids. Of those who completed the 18-week study, those in the PBD group had a greater decrease in total cholesterol and LDL [31]. Meta-analyses have demonstrated that adherence to a PBD is associated with lower total cholesterol, LDL, HDL, and triglycerides [32, 33]. The decrease in HDL seen with PBDs does not adversely affect cardiovascular health [33].

There is an inverse relationship between the intake of fruits, vegetables, whole grains, and blood pressure [34, 35]. The Adventists Health-2 study demonstrated that vegans had the lowest risk of developing hypertension [36]. Chuang et al. confirmed that vegetarians in Taiwan had a much lower risk of developing hypertension [37]. Analysis of observational trials of vegetarian diets demonstrated a reduction in mean systolic and diastolic blood pressure [38]. Participants who consumed a PBD for 4 weeks experienced a decrease in blood pressure and a subsequent reduction in the use of antihypertensive medications [39].

As evidenced by multiple studies, a PBD approach has shown to decrease the incidence of diabetes and other MetS risk factors and is also effective in managing these conditions if they arise.

Dietary Approach to Stop Hypertension

The DASH is a carbohydrate-rich eating plan that emphasizes fruits, vegetables, and low-fat dairy products while reducing saturated fat, total fat, and cholesterol by decreasing consumption of red meat, sweets, and added sugars (Fig. 10.2) [41]. The original study was a feeding trial in which participants were provided with food following DASH recommendations and closely monitored [42]. Results of this and subsequent confirmatory trials demonstrate positive effects of the DASH diet for reducing systolic and diastolic blood pressure and LDL levels [43, 44]. The Prospective Registry Evaluating Outcomes After Myocardial Infarction: Events and Recovery (PREMIER) study implemented DASH via a group-based intervention, teaching participants to purchase

Food Group	Daily servings
Grains	6-8
Meats, poultry, and fish	6 or less
Vegetables	4-5
Fruits	4-5
Low-fat or fat-free dairy products	2-3
Fats and oils	2-3 (avoid saturated or trans fats)
Sodium	Maximum 2,300mg (1500mg associated with further benefit)
	Weekly servings
Nuts, seeds, dry beans, and peas	4-5
Sweets	5 or less

Fig. 10.2 Recommended consumption of various food groups according to the DASH dietary pattern. (Reproduced from National Heart, Lung, and Blood Institute; National Institutes of Health; US Department of Health and Human Services [40])

and prepare DASH foods [45]. Similar to the original DASH feeding trials, improvements in blood pressure levels were observed in PREMIER. In a cohort of young adults with both type I and type II diabetes, higher adherence to the DASH diet was inversely associated with LDL:HDL ratio and HbA1c in multivariable-adjusted models [46]. Youth in the highest adherence tertile had lower low-density LDL:HDL ratio and lower HbA1c levels than those in the lowest tertile after adjustment for potential confounders. These and other studies show that adherence to a DASH pattern could considerably reduce the metabolic risk factors for CVD.

Intermittent Fasting

IF is an approach that is centered around alternating periods of fasting and feeding. There are many iterations of IF, the two most frequently encountered ones are alternate day fasting (ADF) and time-restricted eating (TRE) . A popular form of ADF is a 5:2 strategy where one fasts for 2 days of the week and has ad libitum feeding for the other 5 days, while a popular example of TRE restricts all feeding to an 8-h interval with a 16-h fast.

Wilkinson et al. discussed the impact of a 12-week TRE intervention on participants with MetS [47]. Compared to their baseline, participants had an improvement in BMI (-3%, $p = 0.00011$), waist circumference (-4%, $p = 0.0097$), systolic, and diastolic blood pressure (-4%, $p = 0.041$ and -8%, $p = 0.04$, respectively) , total cholesterol (-7%, $p = 0.030$), and LDL cholesterol (-11%, $p = 0.016$) [47]. The magnitude of these metabolic improvements exceeds the improvement that would be expected from weight loss alone.

While promising overall for MetS, studies reveal mixed results regarding IF on insulin resistance. A group of 8 nonobese males who fasted for 20-h a day for a 2-week period had increased insulin uptake [$6.3 + 0.6$ to $7.3 + 0.3$ mg.kg^{-1}.min^{-1}, ($p = 0.03$)] [48]. In a study of 12 overweight men with prediabetes, following an early TRE regimen for 6 weeks resulted in lower mean insulin levels as compared to the control group [49]. However, two other studies contradict these findings. One study, with 26 obese adults, found no improvement in fasting insulin in either its IF or caloric restriction group after 32 weeks [50]. Trepanowski et al. randomized 100 obese adults to IF, caloric restriction, or ad libitum and found no difference in fasting plasma glucose at either 6 or 12 months [51]. In the aforementioned study by Wilkinson et al. there were promising, yet nonsignificant, improvements in glucose metabolism, decreases in blood glucose (-5%, $p = 0.194$), HbA1c (-2%, $p = 0.058$), and fasting insulin (-21%, $p = 0.064$) [47].

In contrast to diabetes, IF holds more promise for weight loss regardless of BMI category. Premenopausal females lost weight (6.4 kg; 95% CI 4.8–7.9 kg) after 6 months of ADF [52]. Nonobese participants who followed ADF for only 22 days lost 2.5 + 0.5% of initial body weight (p <0.001) and 4 + 1% of their fat mass (p < 0.001) [53]. Nonobese participants who followed an ADF for 10 weeks had reductions in body weight (5.2 + 0.9 kg, p < 0.001) relative to an ad libitum feeding group [54]. However, these findings may be due to reduced caloric consumption rather than the timing of feeding itself.

Some studies of IF have shown a beneficial impact on lipid metabolism. Muslim patrons, who fast from sunrise to sundown for Ramadan, demonstrated lower LDL, triglycerides, and VLDL, which led to a decrease in Framingham risk (13.8–10.8, p < 0.001) [55]. Obese and overweight patients who followed an ADF regimen for 12 weeks reduced serum LDL (10 ± 4%, p < 0.05) and triglycerides (17 ± 5%, p < 0.05) [56]. The positive impact on dyslipidemia may be related to weight loss and/or increasing hepatic production of circadian rhythm factors that help regulate serum lipid levels [57].

IF has also shown benefit in controlling both systolic and diastolic BP. Men with prediabetes who followed TRE for 5 weeks had a reduction of systolic BP (11 + 4 mmHg, p = 0.03) and diastolic BP (10 + 4 mmHg, p = 0.03) [49]. During Ramadan, Muslim patrons had a 3-mmHg reduction in systolic BP (p < 0.05) [55]. These changes may be due to two mechanisms: higher parasympathetic tone and/or lower levels of inflammatory cytokines [58, 59]. Rats undergoing an IF regimen had both lower sympathetic tone and higher parasympathetic tone, as measured by diastolic blood pressure variability and higher frequency heart rate variability [60]. In addition, this higher vagal tone is associated with decreased inflammatory cytokines, including tumor necrosis factor alpha, interleukin-1β, interleukin-6 and interleukin-8 [58].

IF not only lowers cardiovascular risk factors including hypertension, dyslipidemia, and obesity but also appears to reduce inflammatory biomarkers. Caloric restriction is associated with decreased levels of inflammatory cytokines including tumor necrosis factor alpha, interleukin-1β, interleukin-6 and interleukin-8, which are linked to the pathogenesis of atherosclerosis [58]. In an analysis of two studies that enrolled 648 Latter Day Saints patrons, those who underwent a monthly 1-day fast had a lower incidence of coronary heart disease (OR 0.65; CI 0.46–0.94) compared to those who did not fast [59]. A small randomized control trial of nonobese patients showed a significant decrease in CRP (−13 + 17%, p = 0.01) compared to controls [54]. Given the positive results of these observational studies, long-term randomized trials are needed to confirm IF's impact on cardiovascular disease prevention.

Conclusion

The MetS is a complex interaction between genetics, behavior, and environment. The risk factors for MetS carry a cumulative effect for the development of CVD. Dietary approaches can be used for both the prevention and treatment of MetS. In this chapter, we have highlighted the Mediterranean, plant-based, DASH, and IF dietary patterns as effective approaches for managing the MetS. Each approach mitigates the effect of metabolic comorbidities to help avoid the progression of MetSto DM and CVD, along with other components of a healthy lifestyle such as regular exercise. We encourage clinicians and patients to focus on the overlapping themes of these approaches, rather than focusing on the nuances that make them different (Fig. 10.3). Following these general principles will help patients improve their metabolic profile to prevent DM and the development of CVD.

Fig. 10.3 Common principles of all "heart-healthy" dietary practices. Although the consumption of animal products is discouraged by the plant-based diet, the other approaches demonstrate good outcomes with the use of poultry and seafood

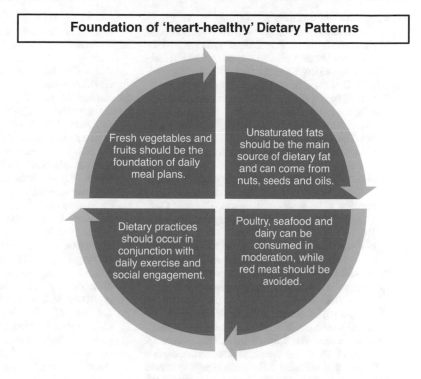

Foundation of 'heart-healthy' Dietary Patterns

Fresh vegetables and fruits should be the foundation of daily meal plans.

Unsaturated fats should be the main source of dietary fat and can come from nuts, seeds and oils.

Dietary practices should occur in conjunction with daily exercise and social engagement.

Poultry, seafood and dairy can be consumed in moderation, while red meat should be avoided.

References

1. Sherling DH, Perumareddi P, Hennekens CH. Metabolic syndrome. J Cardiovasc Pharmacol Ther. 2017;22(4):365–7. https://doi.org/10.1177/1074248416686187.
2. Sperling LS, Mechanick JI, Neeland IJ, Herrick CJ, Despres JP, Ndumele CE, et al. The CardioMetabolic health alliance: working toward a new care model for the metabolic syndrome. J Am Coll Cardiol. 2015;66(9):1050–67. https://doi.org/10.1016/j.jacc.2015.06.1328.
3. Grundy SM, Bryan Brewer H, Cleeman JI, Smith SC, Lenfant C. Definition of metabolic syndrome. Circulation. 2004;109(3):433–8. https://doi.org/10.1161/01.cir.0000111245.75752.c6.
4. Huang PL. A comprehensive definition for metabolic syndrome. Dis Model Mech. 2009;2(5–6):231–7. https://doi.org/10.1242/dmm.001180.
5. Galassi A, Reynolds K, He J. Metabolic syndrome and risk of cardiovascular disease: a meta-analysis. Am J Med. 2006;119(10):812–9. https://doi.org/10.1016/j.amjmed.2006.02.031.
6. Grundy SM, Stone NJ, Bailey AL, Beam C, Birtcher KK, Blumenthal RS, et al. 2018 AHA/ACC/AACVPR/AAPA/ABC/ACPM/ADA/AGS/APhA/ASPC/NLA/PCNA guideline on the management of blood cholesterol: a report of the American College of Cardiology/American Heart Association task force on clinical practice guidelines. Circulation. 2019;139(25) https://doi.org/10.1161/cir.0000000000000625.
7. Knowler WC, Barrett-Connor E, Fowler SE, Hamman RF, Lachin JM, Walker EA, et al. Reduction in the incidence of type 2 diabetes with lifestyle intervention or metformin. N Engl J Med. 2002;346(6):393–403. https://doi.org/10.1056/NEJMoa012512.
8. Keys AAC, Blackburn H, Buzina R, Djordjevi'c BS, et al. Seven countries: a multivariate analysis of death and coronary heart disease. Cambridge, MA: Harvard University Press; 1980.
9. Fung TT, Rexrode KM, Mantzoros CS, Manson JE, Willett WC, Hu FB. Mediterranean diet and incidence of and mortality from coronary heart disease and stroke in women. Circulation. 2009;119(8):1093–100. https://doi.org/10.1161/CIRCULATIONAHA.108.816736.
10. Shen J, Wilmot KA, Ghasemzadeh N, Molloy DL, Burkman G, Mekonnen G, et al. Mediterranean dietary patterns and cardiovascular health. Annu Rev Nutr. 2015;35:425–49. https://doi.org/10.1146/annurev-nutr-011215-025104.

11. Kastorini C-M, Milionis HJ, Esposito K, Giugliano D, Goudevenos JA, Panagiotakos DB. The effect of Mediterranean diet on metabolic syndrome and its components. J Am Coll Cardiol. 2011;57(11):1299–313. https://doi.org/10.1016/j.jacc.2010.09.073.

12. Grosso G, Mistretta A, Frigiola A, Gruttadauria S, Biondi A, Basile F, et al. Mediterranean diet and cardiovascular risk factors: a systematic review. Crit Rev Food Sci Nutr. 2014;54(5):593–610. https://doi.org/10.1080/10408398.2011.596955.

13. Tortosa A, Bes-Rastrollo M, Sanchez-Villegas A, Basterra-Gortari FJ, Nunez-Cordoba JM, Martinez-Gonzalez MA. Mediterranean diet inversely associated with the incidence of metabolic syndrome: the SUN prospective cohort. Diabetes Care. 2007;30(11):2957–9. https://doi.org/10.2337/dc07-1231.

14. Babio N, Bullo M, Basora J, Martinez-Gonzalez MA, Fernandez-Ballart J, Marquez-Sandoval F, et al. Adherence to the Mediterranean diet and risk of metabolic syndrome and its components. Nutr Metab Cardiovasc Dis. 2009;19(8):563–70. https://doi.org/10.1016/j.numecd.2008.10.007.

15. Martinez-Gonzalez MA, de la Fuente-Arrillaga C, Nunez-Cordoba JM, Basterra-Gortari FJ, Beunza JJ, Vazquez Z, et al. Adherence to Mediterranean diet and risk of developing diabetes: prospective cohort study. BMJ. 2008;336(7657):1348–51. https://doi.org/10.1136/bmj.39561.501007.BE.

16. Vincent-Baudry S, et al. The Medi-RIVAGE study: reduction of cardiovascular disease risk factors after a 3-mo intervention with a Mediterranean-type diet or a low-fat diet. Am J Clin Nutr. 2005;82(5):964–71.

17. Estruch R, Ros E, Salas-Salvado J, Covas MI, Corella D, Aros F, et al. Primary prevention of cardiovascular disease with a Mediterranean diet supplemented with extra-virgin olive oil or nuts. N Engl J Med. 2018;378(25):e34. https://doi.org/10.1056/NEJMoa1800389.

18. Estruch R. Effects of a Mediterranean-style diet on cardiovascular risk factors. Ann Intern Med. 2006;145(1):1. https://doi.org/10.7326/0003-4819-145-1-200607040-00004.

19. Barnard ND, Katcher HI, Jenkins DJ, Cohen J, Turner-Mcgrievy G. Vegetarian and vegan diets in type 2 diabetes management. Nutr Rev. 2009;67(5):255–63. https://doi.org/10.1111/j.1753-4887.2009.00198.x.

20. Tonstad S, Butler T, Yan R, Fraser GE. Type of vegetarian diet, body weight, and prevalence of type 2 diabetes. Diabetes Care. 2009;32(5):791–6. https://doi.org/10.2337/dc08-1886.

21. McMacken M, Shah S. A plant-based diet for the prevention and treatment of type 2 diabetes. J Geriatr Cardiol. 2017;14(5):342–54. https://doi.org/10.11909/j.issn.1671-5411.2017.05.009.

22. Satija A, Bhupathiraju SN, Rimm EB, Spiegelman D, Chiuve SE, Borgi L, et al. Plant-based dietary patterns and incidence of type 2 diabetes in US men and women: results from three prospective cohort studies. PLoS Med. 2016;13(6):e1002039. https://doi.org/10.1371/journal.pmed.1002039.

23. Anderson JW, Ward K. High-carbohydrate, high-fiber diets for insulin-treated men with diabetes mellitus. Am J Clin Nutr. 1979;32(11):2312–21. https://doi.org/10.1093/ajcn/32.11.2312.

24. Barnard RJ, Jung T, Inkeles SB. Diet and exercise in the treatment of NIDDM. The need for early emphasis. Diabetes Care. 1994;17(12):1469–72. https://doi.org/10.2337/diacare.17.12.1469.

25. De Natale C, Annuzzi G, Bozzetto L, Mazzarella R, Costabile G, Ciano O, et al. Effects of a plant-based high-carbohydrate/high-fiber diet versus high-monounsaturated fat/low-carbohydrate diet on postprandial lipids in type 2 diabetic patients. Diabetes Care. 2009;32(12):2168–73. https://doi.org/10.2337/dc09-0266.

26. Yokoyama Y, Barnard ND, Levin SM, Watanabe M. Vegetarian diets and glycemic control in diabetes: a systematic review and meta-analysis. Cardiovasc Diagn Ther. 2014;4(5):373–82. https://doi.org/10.3978/j.issn.2223-3652.2014.10.04.

27. Kahleova H, Matoulek M, Malinska H, Oliyarnik O, Kazdova L, Neskudla T, et al. Vegetarian diet improves insulin resistance and oxidative stress markers more than conventional diet in subjects with type 2 diabetes. Diabet Med. 2011;28(5):549–59. https://doi.org/10.1111/j.1464-5491.2010.03209.x.

28. Turner-Mcgrievy GM, Davidson CR, Wingard EE, Wilcox S, Frongillo EA. Comparative effectiveness of plant-based diets for weight loss: a randomized controlled trial of five different diets. Nutrition. 2015;31(2):350–8. https://doi.org/10.1016/j.nut.2014.09.002.

29. Wright N, Wilson L, Smith M, Duncan B, McHugh P. The BROAD study: a randomised controlled trial using a whole food plant-based diet in the community for obesity, ischaemic heart disease or diabetes. Nutr Diabetes. 2017;7(3):e256-e. https://doi.org/10.1038/nutd.2017.3.

30. Huang RY, Huang CC, Hu FB, Chavarro JE. Vegetarian diets and weight reduction: a meta-analysis of randomized controlled trials. J Gen Intern Med. 2016;31(1):109–16. https://doi.org/10.1007/s11606-015-3390-7.

31. Mishra S, Xu J, Agarwal U, Gonzales J, Levin S, Barnard ND. A multicenter randomized controlled trial of a plant-based nutrition program to reduce body weight and cardiovascular risk in the corporate setting: the GEICO study. 2013;67(7):718–24. https://doi.org/10.1038/ejcn.2013.92.

32. Yoko Yokoyama SML, Neal D. Barnard. Association between plant-based diets and plasma lipids: a systematic review and meta-analysis. Nutr Rev. 2017; https://doi.org/10.1093/nutrit/nux030.

33. Ferdowsian HR, Barnard ND. Effects of plant-based diets on plasma. Lipids. 2009;104(7):947–56. https://doi.org/10.1016/j.amjcard.2009.05.032.

34. Steffen LM, Kroenke CH, Yu X, Pereira MA, Slattery ML, Van Horn L, et al. Associations of plant

food, dairy product, and meat intakes with 15-y incidence of elevated blood pressure in young black and white adults: the coronary artery risk development in young adults (CARDIA) study. Am J Clin Nutr. 2005;82(6):1169–77.; quiz 363–4. https://doi.org/10.1093/ajcn/82.6.1169.

35. Chalvon-Demersay T, Azzout-Marniche D, Arfsten J, Egli L, Gaudichon C, Karagounis LG, et al. A systematic review of the effects of plant compared with animal protein sources on features of metabolic syndrome. J Nutr. 2017;147(3):281–92. https://doi.org/10.3945/jn.116.239574.

36. Pettersen BJ, Anousheh R, Fan J, Jaceldo-Siegl K, Fraser GE. Vegetarian diets and blood pressure among white subjects: results from the Adventist Health Study-2 (AHS-2). Public Health Nutr. 2012;15(10):1909–16. https://doi.org/10.1017/s1368980011003454.

37. Chuang SY, Chiu TH, Lee CY, Liu TT, Tsao CK, Hsiung CA, et al. Vegetarian diet reduces the risk of hypertension independent of abdominal obesity and inflammation: a prospective study. J Hypertens. 2016;34(11):2164–71. https://doi.org/10.1097/hjh.0000000000001068.

38. Yokoyama Y, Nishimura K, Barnard ND, Takegami M, Watanabe M, Sekikawa A, et al. Vegetarian diets and blood pressure: a meta-analysis. JAMA Intern Med. 2014;174(4):577–87. https://doi.org/10.1001/jamainternmed.2013.14547.

39. Najjar RS, Moore CE, Montgomery BD. A defined, plant-based diet utilized in an outpatient cardiovascular clinic effectively treats hypercholesterolemia and hypertension and reduces medications. Clin Cardiol. 2018;41(3):307–13. https://doi.org/10.1002/clc.22863.

40. National Heart LaBI. DASH eating plan. https://www.nhlbi.nih.gov/health-topics/dash-eating-plan.

41. Appel LJ, Brands MW, Daniels SR, Karanja N, Elmer PJ, Sacks FM. Dietary approaches to prevent and treat hypertension: a scientific statement from the American Heart Association. Hypertension (Dallas, Tx: 1979). 2006;47(2):296–308. https://doi.org/10.1161/01.hyp.0000202568.01167.b6.

42. Appel LJ, Moore TJ, Obarzanek E, Vollmer WM, Svetkey LP, Sacks FM, et al. A clinical trial of the effects of dietary patterns on blood pressure. N Engl J Med. 1997;336(16):1117–24. https://doi.org/10.1056/nejm199704173361601.

43. Karanja N, Erlinger TP, Pao-Hwa L, Miller ER 3rd, Bray GA. The DASH diet for high blood pressure: from clinical trial to dinner table. Cleve Clin J Med. 2004;71(9):745–53. https://doi.org/10.3949/ccjm.71.9.745.

44. Obarzanek E, Sacks FM, Vollmer WM, Bray GA, Miller ER 3rd, Lin PH, et al. Effects on blood lipids of a blood pressure-lowering diet: the dietary approaches to stop hypertension (DASH) trial. Am J Clin Nutr. 2001;74(1):80–9. https://doi.org/10.1093/ajcn/74.1.80.

45. Funk KL, Elmer PJ, Stevens VJ, Harsha DW, Craddick SR, Lin PH, et al. PREMIER--a trial of lifestyle interventions for blood pressure control: intervention design and rationale. Health Promot Pract. 2008;9(3):271–80. https://doi.org/10.1177/1524839906289035.

46. Liese AD, Bortsov A, Gunther AL, Dabelea D, Reynolds K, Standiford DA, et al. Association of DASH diet with cardiovascular risk factors in youth with diabetes mellitus: the SEARCH for diabetes in youth study. Circulation. 2011;123(13):1410–7. https://doi.org/10.1161/circulationaha.110.955922.

47. Wilkinson MJ, Manoogian ENC, Zadourian A, Lo H, Fakhouri S, Shoghi A, et al. Ten-hour time-restricted eating reduces weight, blood pressure, and atherogenic lipids in patients with metabolic syndrome. Cell Metab. 2020;31(1):92–104. e5. https://doi.org/10.1016/j.cmet.2019.11.004.

48. Halberg N, Henriksen M, Soderhamn N, Stallknecht B, Ploug T, Schjerling P, et al. Effect of intermittent fasting and refeeding on insulin action in healthy men. J Appl Physiol (1985). 2005;99(6):2128–36. https://doi.org/10.1152/japplphysiol.00683.2005.

49. Sutton EF, Beyl R, Early KS, Cefalu WT, Ravussin E, Peterson CM. Early time-restricted feeding improves insulin sensitivity, blood pressure, and oxidative stress even without weight loss in men with prediabetes. Cell Metab. 2018;27(6):1212–21.e3. https://doi.org/10.1016/j.cmet.2018.04.010.

50. Catenacci VA, Pan Z, Ostendorf D, Brannon S, Gozansky WS, Mattson MP, et al. A randomized pilot study comparing zero-calorie alternate-day fasting to daily caloric restriction in adults with obesity. Obesity (Silver Spring). 2016;24(9):1874–83. https://doi.org/10.1002/oby.21581.

51. Trepanowski JF, Kroeger CM, Barnosky A, Klempel MC, Bhutani S, Hoddy KK, et al. Effect of alternate-day fasting on weight loss, weight maintenance, and cardioprotection among metabolically healthy obese adults: a randomized clinical trial. JAMA Intern Med. 2017;177(7):930–8. https://doi.org/10.1001/jamainternmed.2017.0936.

52. Harvie MN, Pegington M, Mattson MP, Frystyk J, Dillon B, Evans G, et al. The effects of intermittent or continuous energy restriction on weight loss and metabolic disease risk markers: a randomized trial in young overweight women. Int J Obes. 2011;35(5):714–27. https://doi.org/10.1038/ijo.2010.171.

53. Heilbronn LK, Smith SR, Martin CK, Anton SD, Ravussin E. Alternate-day fasting in nonobese subjects: effects on body weight, body composition, and energy metabolism. Am J Clin Nutr. 2005;81(1):69–73. https://doi.org/10.1093/ajcn/81.1.69.

54. Varady KA, Bhutani S, Klempel MC, Kroeger CM, Trepanowski JF, Haus JM, et al. Alternate day fasting for weight loss in normal weight and overweight subjects: a randomized controlled trial. Nutr J. 2013;12(1):146. https://doi.org/10.1186/1475-2891-12-146.

55. Nematy M, Alinezhad-Namaghi M, Rashed MM, Mozhdehifard M, Sajjadi SS, Akhlaghi S, et al. Effects of Ramadan fasting on cardiovascular risk factors: a

prospective observational study. Nutr J. 2012;11:69. https://doi.org/10.1186/1475-2891-11-69.

56. Varady KA, Bhutani S, Klempel MC, Kroeger CM. Comparison of effects of diet versus exercise weight loss regimens on LDL and HDL particle size in obese adults. Lipids Health Dis. 2011;10:119. https://doi.org/10.1186/1476-511x-10-119.

57. Froy O, Chapnik N, Miskin R. Effect of intermittent fasting on circadian rhythms in mice depends on feeding time. Mech Ageing Dev. 2009;130(3):154–60. https://doi.org/10.1016/j.mad.2008.10.006.

58. Chandrasekar B, Nelson JF, Colston JT, Freeman GL. Calorie restriction attenuates inflammatory responses to myocardial ischemia-reperfusion injury. Am

J Physiol Heart Circ Physiol. 2001;280(5):H2094–102. https://doi.org/10.1152/ajpheart.2001.280.5.H2094.

59. Horne BD, Muhlestein JB, May HT, Carlquist JF, Lappe DL, Bair TL, et al. Relation of routine, periodic fasting to risk of diabetes mellitus, and coronary artery disease in patients undergoing coronary angiography. Am J Cardiol. 2012;109(11):1558–62. https://doi.org/10.1016/j.amjcard.2012.01.379.

60. Mager DE, Wan R, Brown M, Cheng A, Wareski P, Abernethy DR, et al. Caloric restriction and intermittent fasting alter spectral measures of heart rate and blood pressure variability in rats. FASEB J. 2006;20(6):631–7. https://doi.org/10.1096/fj.05-5263com.

Optimal Diet for Diabetes: Glucose Control, Hemoglobin A1c Reduction, and CV Risk

11

Wahida Karmally and Ira J. Goldberg

Introduction

"With an excess of fat diabetes begins and from an excess of fat diabetics die," Eliot P. Joslin wrote in 1928. This was shortly after the purification of insulin and the emergence of evidence that it could prevent death in patients with type 1 diabetes, many of whom adhered to the Allen high-fat, low-carbohydrate diet. Only after achieving a treatment to prevent death from diabetic keto-acidosis and the starvation-like effects of insulin deficiency did vascular disease emerge as the primary complication of type 1 diabetes. In the late nineteenth century, Osler noted that arteriosclerosis developed "in stout persons who take very little exercise." This observation was likely due to those he observed with co-existing conditions such as diabetes and metabolic syndrome, which are both insulin resistant states. Not until the description of the metabolic syndrome by Reaven in the latter half of the twentieth century [1] was the link between insulin resistance and the development of cardiovascular disease (CVD) defined.

W. Karmally
Columbia University, New York, NY, USA
e-mail: wk2@cumc.columbia.edu

I. J. Goldberg (✉)
Division of Endocrinology, Diabetes and Metabolism,
New York University Grossman School of Medicine,
New York, NY, USA
e-mail: Ira.Goldberg@nyulangone.org

Patients with diabetes often have several CVD risk factors that are affected by diet. Up to 60% of adults with diabetes have hypertension and nearly all have one or more lipid abnormalities [2]. Management of risk factors such as hypertension, dyslipidemia, and hyperglycemia can lead to improved cardiovascular complications in individuals with type 2 diabetes mellitus. A common abnormal lipid problem in individuals with diabetes is an elevation of VLDL triglyceride and cholesterol, a reduction in HDL cholesterol, and an LDL fraction that contains a greater proportion of small, dense LDL particles, and increased postprandial lipemia [3]. Thus, as shown in Fig. 11.1, a special dietary issue for these patients is control of dyslipidemia. Neither simple carbohydrates nor high-saturated fat foods are optimal.

Dietary Composition and Glycemia

Diets rich in simple carbohydrates lead to both greater glycemia and hypertriglyceridemia, the latter referred to as carbohydrate loading. This pattern also increases postprandial lipemia [4]. Complex carbohydrates with fiber and ingestion of carbohydrates in association with other dietary components, most notably unsaturated fats, slow their absorption and subsequent glycemia. For this reason, the glycemic index (GI) of food varies when eaten in combination. More recently, it has become apparent that there is great individual variation in dietary

© Springer Nature Switzerland AG 2021
M. J. Wilkinson et al. (eds.), *Prevention and Treatment of Cardiovascular Disease*, Contemporary
Cardiology, https://doi.org/10.1007/978-3-030-78177-4_11

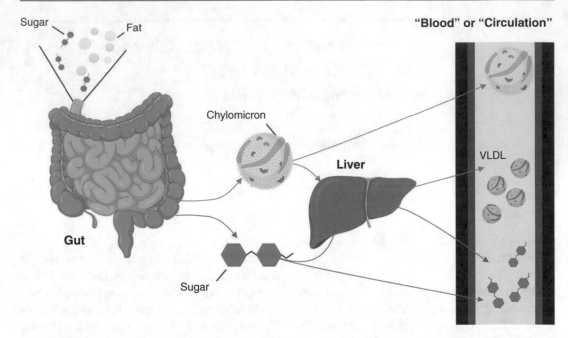

Fig. 11.1 Diabetes and CVD risk. A specific issue for nutritional approach to the patient with diabetes is concomitant control of both circulating glucose and lipids. Fat in the diet enters the lymphatics within chylomicrons. Within the circulation, endothelial cell lipoprotein lipase releases fatty acids for their use by muscles and storage within adipocytes. Sugars, many of which are formed from carbohydrates, enter the portal system and are a substrate for fatty acid synthesis in the liver. These newly formed fatty acids as well as fatty acids returning to the liver from adipose and lipoproteins are secreted within very low density lipoproteins (VLDL). Thus, foods with free sugars or non-complex carbohydrates, which also raise triglyceride levels, should be limited. In addition, high levels of cholesterol and saturated fats should be avoided, as they elevate LDL and also increase postprandial lipemia. For this reason, it is especially important to ascertain food preferences and make healthy substitutions

response with an identical meal. This has been attributed to differences in the microbiome [5], but is likely to also reflect differences in bowel motility, nutrient absorption rates, and the efficiency of enzymatic digestion of starches. With widespread use of continuous glucose monitoring (CGM) devices, patients can determine for themselves their responses to different types of foods, dietary patterns, exercise, and medications. Endocrinologists routinely use CGMs to educate patients with diabetes and pre-diabetes to the relationships of dietary content and exercise to glycemic variability.

Most patients with diabetes note glucose elevations with high-carbohydrate foods such as bread, rice, potatoes, and pasta. For this reason, these foods should be limited. In patients with type 1 diabetes or others on insulin, hyperglycemia due to these foods can be alleviated with injection of rapidly acting insulin. Diabetes educators can often assist the patients to count carbohydrates and develop an insulin sensitivity index to match insulin dosage. In some cases, short-acting insulin secretagogues such as sulfonylureas or inhibitors of intestinal glucose absorption can prevent or dampen hyperglycemia. Other foods with high sugar content also raise glycemia; although patients can often identify sweets such as cakes, cookies, and candy, they sometimes neglect to note the sugars in fruits, juices, and even milk.

Diets and Dyslipidemia

Eating plans that are designed to lower glucose, improve lipid patterns and incorporate regular physical activity are cornerstones in managing lipid disorders and lowering CVD risk in patients with diabetes. All adults with diabetes are candidates for progressively aggressive medical nutrition therapy. The American Diabetes Association (ADA) 2021 Standards of Medical Care in Diabetes recommends intensifying lifestyle therapy and optimizing glycemic control for patients with elevated levels of triglycerides (>150 mg/

dL) and/or low-HDL cholesterol (40 mg/dL in men and >50 mg/dL in women [6]. There is no sufficient evidence to suggest that there is an ideal percentage of calories from carbohydrate, protein, and fat for people with diabetes.

Lifestyle intervention, including weight loss [7], increased physical activity, and medical nutrition therapy, allows some patients to reduce CVD risk factors. Weight loss with hypocaloric diets is as beneficial for improving insulin sensitivity as weight loss achieved with bariatric surgery [8]. Nutrition intervention should be tailored to fit each patient's age, pharmacologic treatment, lipid levels, medical conditions, and metabolic outcomes. Weight loss improves glycemic control and reduces insulin resistance as well as improves lipoproteins (decreases triglycerides and raises HDL cholesterol) [9]. The eating plan based on the individual's caloric needs could provide a total fat intake of 25–35% of calories, with <6% of calories from saturated fatty acids (SFAs). Trans-fatty acids, now less commonly used in commercial food preparation, increase LDL cholesterol (LDL-C) and may decrease HDL cholesterol and should be avoided. Dietary cholesterol intake should be <200 mg/day [10, 11]. The majority of total fat intake should be derived from unsaturated fat sources. Robust evidence indicates that a cardio-protective diet reduces LDL-C by 9–16% in both normo- and hyperlipidemic individuals [12].

Population data support a dietary pattern that promotes the intake of unprocessed foods: fruits and vegetables, plant-based non-tropical oils, lean protein foods, legumes, whole grains, nonfat dairy, and unsalted nuts. Added sugars should be limited to less than 5–10% of daily caloric intake. Vegetables (not including starchy vegetables such as potatoes) and fruits should make up one-half of each meal. Carbohydrate sources should primarily include beans/legumes, whole grains, vegetables of different colors and fruits. An emphasis on monounsaturated fats, such as olive oil, avocados, and nuts, and polyunsaturated fatty acids such as omega-3 fatty acids from chia seeds, flax seeds, fatty fish, and nuts helps reduce risk factors for CVD and **type 2 diabetes.

For individuals with elevated triglycerides (≥150 mg/dL), a calorie-controlled eating plan that avoids extremes in carbohydrate and fat intake and includes physical activity should be recommended. Nutrient-poor calorie sources like alcohol and added sugars should be limited as much as possible. Weight loss of 7–10% of body weight should be encouraged, if indicated. These lifestyle changes lower triglyceride levels. In addition to lifestyle modifications, supplemental eicosapentaenoic acid (EPA) and docosahexaenoic acid (DHA) (2–4 g/day) may be used. These high doses of supplemental EPA and DHA lower triglycerides in individuals with elevated levels (>200 mg/dL) [13]. Multiple studies using a combination of these oils failed to show a CVD benefit. More recently, a trial using EPA in subjects with triglyceride levels >135 mg/dL, many of whom had diabetes, was effective [14]. This surprising result, in conjunction with a previous Japanese EPA study (JELIS) [15] suggests a specific benefit of EPA that might be exclusive of changes in circulating triglycerides.

Eating plans should incorporate fiber-rich foods that contribute at least 25–30 g fiber per day, with special emphasis on soluble fiber sources (7–13 g). Foods rich in soluble fiber include fruits, vegetables, and whole grains, especially high-fiber cereals, oatmeal, and legumes (particularly beans). Eating plans high in total and soluble fiber can further reduce cholesterol by 2–3% and LDL cholesterol up to 7% [16].

Foods enriched with plant sterol and stanol ester may be incorporated into the diet, across two or three times per day, for a total consumption of 2–3 g plant sterol/stanol esters per day. These doses further lower the LDL-C by 7–15% [17]. Doses beyond 3 g have not been shown to provide additional benefit. Plant stanols and plant sterols are also effective in people taking statin drugs, causing further reduction in LDL-C. To prevent weight gain, isocaloric substitutions of nuts and plant stanol/sterol and fiber-containing foods must be made with other foods. The Academy of Nutrition and Dietetics Evidence Analysis Library and ADA nutrition therapy recommendations report limited and mixed evidence regarding the relationship between GI or glycemic load, and CVD.

There is no evidence that adjusting the daily level of protein intake (typically 1–1.5 g/kg body weight/day or 15–20% total calories) will improve health in individuals without diabetic kidney disease, and research is inconclusive regarding the ideal amount of dietary protein to optimize either glycemic management or CVD risk [18].

Finding a Diet That Works

Successful nutrition therapy requires recommendations that maintain the pleasure of eating with a healthful eating pattern. The diet should focus on major strategies: a Mediterranean-style diet [19] or Dietary Approaches to Stop Hypertension eating pattern [20, 21] or other eating patterns based on culture, food preferences, and economic status that focus on the reduction of SFAs and *trans* fatty acids and cholesterol intake; the use of stanols/sterols, omega-3 fatty acids, nuts, and foods containing soluble fiber; and weight loss, if indicated, to achieve a lipid and lipoprotein profile that reduces the risk for vascular disease, achieves glycemic goals, and optimizes micronutrient requirements. Evidence-based nutrition recommendations for diabetes and lipid disorders are provided by the Academy of Nutrition and Dietetics, the American Heart Association/American College of Cardiology (AHA/ACC) (Guidelines [2013]), the American Diabetes Association, and the US Department of Agriculture (USDA) (Dietary Guidelines for Americans 2015). A focus on foods rather than macronutrients can assist patients in understanding the components of a healthy eating pattern. Addressing barriers to following a healthy diet and utilizing an entire healthcare team can empower patients to follow these guidelines. Registered dietitians/nutritionists are especially useful in analyzing individual dietary patterns, making recommendations that require food exchanges, and applying approaches to implement acute and chronic behavioral change.

Nutrition intervention studies lasting ≥1 year, such as Mediterranean-style eating patterns reduced hemoglobin A1C, blood pressure, and body weight and improved serum lipid profile, all of which reduce the risk for developing CVD in participants with both type 1 and type 2 diabetes [19]. Two variants of a Mediterranean diet reduced 24-h ambulatory blood pressure, total cholesterol, and fasting glucose and reduced incidence of major cardiovascular events [22] in participants at high cardiovascular risk (including those with type 2 diabetes). A comparative risk assessment model showed dietary factors were estimated to be associated with a substantial proportion of deaths from heart disease, stroke, and type 2 diabetes [23]. Decreased risk of coronary heart disease and stroke in healthy adults has been strongly and consistently associated with dietary patterns that include the regular consumption of fruits, vegetables, whole grains, nuts, legumes, unsaturated oils, poultry, fish, and low-fat dairy products, and the lower consumption of high-fat dairy products, processed and red meats, and sugar-sweetened foods, and beverages.

Some specific recommendations are needed if the patient also has hypertension. These include paying greater attention to reducing excess body weight through caloric restriction, restricting sodium intake (<2300 mg/day), increasing consumption of fruits and vegetables (8–10 servings per day), and low-fat dairy products (2–3 servings per day), avoiding excessive alcohol consumption (no more than two servings per day in men and no more than one serving per day in women), and increasing activity levels [21, 24].

Ketogenic Diets

Minimizing carbohydrate intake has become a popular approach to weight loss (discussed in other sections, reviewed in Bolla et al.) [25]. Such diets reduce glycemic excursions and, therefore, will reduce hemoglobin A1C levels. When used as an approach to weight loss, these diets can reduce triglyceride levels without raising LDL cholesterol [26] but can lead to marked hyperlipidemia in some patients who need to be monitored. It is likely that substitution of high saturated fats (red meats) and eggs with other forms of fat may alleviate some dietary-driven increases in LDL with these low-carbohydrate diets.

Nutrition Counseling

Nutrition counseling should be tailored to each individual patient to target their specific barriers and increase their motivation to overcome those barriers. An intervention incorporating behavior change strategies is more likely to be effective and meet the patient's individual needs. After identifying the barrier, the next step is to identify how ready the patient is to make a change by identifying their stage of change and ideally moving them forward to the next stage [27]. Patients may be ambivalent about making a change and motivational interviewing can be helpful in resolving uncertainty through listening actively, reflecting, asking open-ended questions, and maintaining a non-judgmental and supportive environment [28].

It is important to allow each patient to identify their own barriers to making changes to further guide them to come up with their own solutions. The patient has a better idea of what is feasible for them and is more likely to follow through with the changes he or she suggests. Additional educational information and solutions can also be provided if patients are empowered to feel like they have autonomy over their eating and lifestyle habits. This can be done by asking the patients what they think about the solution and how helpful it is in overcoming their barrier.

When the patient is ready and has moved into the action phase of the transtheoretical model [29], setting clear and measurable goals is an important next step to the nutrition care process and motivational interviewing. By working together with the patient, realistic, small, achievable goals can be set. Starting with smaller goals

and working up to bigger goals can help the patient gain confidence and feel empowered to meet short- and long-term objectives.

Setting specific and measurable goals is necessary to monitor and evaluate progress. If the patient reports eating fast food four times a week because he/she does not enjoy cooking, examples of small, measurable, short-term goals include the following:

- Replacing fast food items with healthier options
- Providing easy and tasty recipes
- Freezing extra servings to eat on other days

Long-term goals may include the following:

- Eating fast food once a month
- Cooking meals at home four times a week
- Losing weight to achieve healthy body mass index (BMI) between 18.5 and 24.9

Monitoring and Evaluating

After intervention and goal setting, monitoring and evaluating are the next steps to measure progress. This can be done in more than one way by comparing current eating patterns to previous assessments, and taking anthropometric measurements such as height, weight, waist circumference, BMI, and laboratory measurements such as hemoglobin A1C and lipid profile.

Monitoring Apps for Diabetes and Weight Management

Patients can monitor and track their nutrient intake, blood glucose, and weight goals through smartphone apps designed to track food, blood glucose, exercise, weight, and nutrients listed on the Nutrition Facts label. Depending on the app, some also track fitness goals, provide healthy recipes, and customize individual calorie and physical activity plans.

Summary

The approach to patients with diabetes includes similar lifestyle recommendations to those of patients without diabetes because diabetes associates with greater CVD-risk implementation of a heart-healthy dietary pattern is most imperative. Along with reductions in body weight and lipoprotein levels, diets must consider glycemia. The use of CGM technology coupled with a registered dietitian-/nutritionist-prescribed individualized dietary plan should enable better diabetes and CVD-risk reduction for this high-risk population.

References

1. Reaven GM. Role of insulin resistance in human disease (syndrome X): an expanded definition. Annu Rev Med. 1993;44:121–31.
2. Position Statement 8: Cardiovascular disease and risk management. Diabetes Care. 2016;39:S60–S71.
3. Krauss RM. Lipids and lipoproteins in patients with type 2 diabetes. Diabetes Care. 2004;27:1496–504.
4. Chen YD, Coulston AM, Zhou MY, Hollenbeck CB, Reaven GM. Why do low-fat high-carbohydrate diets accentuate postprandial lipemia in patients with NIDDM? Diabetes Care. 1995;18:10–6.
5. Zeevi D, Korem T, Zmora N, Israeli D, Rothschild D, Weinberger A, Ben-Yacov O, Lador D, Avnit-Sagi T, Lotan-Pompan M, Suez J, Mahdi JA, Matot E, Malka G, Kosower N, Rein M, Zilberman-Schapira G, Dohnalová L, Pevsner-Fischer M, Bikovsky R, Halpern Z, Elinav E, Segal E. Personalized nutrition by prediction of glycemic responses. Cell. 2015;163:1079–94.
6. American Diabetes A. Standards of medical care in diabetes-2021 abridged for primary care providers. Clin Diabetes. 2021;39:14–43.
7. Buse JB, Ginsberg HN, Bakris GL, Clark NG, Costa F, Eckel R, Fonseca V, Gerstein HC, Grundy S, Nesto RW, Pignone MP, Plutzky J, Porte D, Redberg R, Stitzel KF, Stone NJ. Primary prevention of cardiovascular diseases in people with diabetes mellitus: a scientific statement from the American Heart Association and the American Diabetes Association. Diabetes Care. 2007;30:162–72.
8. Yoshino M, Kayser BD, Yoshino J, Stein RI, Reeds D, Eagon JC, Eckhouse SR, Watrous JD, Jain M, Knight R, Schechtman K, Patterson BW, Klein S. Effects of diet versus gastric bypass on metabolic function in. Diabetes. 2020;383:721–32.
9. Wing RR, Bolin P, Brancati FL, Bray GA, Clark JM, Coday M, Crow RS, Curtis JM, Egan CM, Espeland MA, Evans M, Foreyt JP, Ghazarian S, Gregg EW, Harrison B, Hazuda HP, Hill JO, Horton ES, Hubbard VS, Jakicic JM, Jeffery RW, Johnson KC, Kahn SE, Kitabchi AE, Knowler WC, Lewis CE, Maschak-Carey BJ, Montez MG, Murillo A, Nathan DM, Patricio J, Peters A, Pi-Sunyer X, Pownall H, Reboussin D, Regensteiner JG, Rickman AD, Ryan DH, Safford M, Wadden TA, Wagenknecht LE, West DS, Williamson DF, Yanovski SZ. Cardiovascular effects of intensive lifestyle intervention in type 2 diabetes. N Engl J Med. 2013;369:145–54.
10. Eckel RH, Jakicic JM, Ard JD, de Jesus JM, Houston Miller N, Hubbard VS, Lee IM, Lichtenstein AH, Loria CM, Millen BE, Nonas CA, Sacks FM, Smith SC Jr, Svetkey LP, Wadden TA, Yanovski SZ, Kendall KA, Morgan LC, Trisolini MG, Velasco G, Wnek J, Anderson JL, Halperin JL, Albert NM, Bozkurt B, Brindis RG, Curtis LH, DeMets D, Hochman JS, Kovacs RJ, Ohman EM, Pressler SJ, Sellke FW, Shen WK, Smith SC Jr, Tomaselli GF. 2013 AHA/ACC guideline on lifestyle management to reduce cardiovascular risk: a report of the American College of Cardiology/American Heart Association task force on practice guidelines. Circulation. 2014;129:S76–99.
11. Jacobson TA, Maki KC, Orringer CE, Jones PH, Kris-Etherton P, Sikand G, La Forge R, Daniels SR, Wilson DP, Morris PB, Wild RA, Grundy SM, Daviglus M, Ferdinand KC, Vijayaraghavan K, Deedwania PC, Aberg JA, Liao KP, McKenney JM, Ross JL, Braun LT, Ito MK, Bays HE, Brown WV, Underberg JA. National lipid association recommendations for patient-centered management of dyslipidemia: part 2. J Clin Lipidol. 2015;9:S1-122.e1.
12. Dietetics AoNa. Disorders of lipid metabolism evidence-based nutrition practice guideline. In: Disorders of Lipid Metabolism. Academy of Nutrition and Dietetics; Chicago, Il: 2011. https://www.andeal.org/topic.cfm?cat=4527.
13. Hartweg J, Perera R, Montori V, Dinneen S, Neil HA, Farmer A. Omega-3 polyunsaturated fatty acids (PUFA) for type 2 diabetes mellitus. Cochrane Database Syst Rev. 2008;1:Cd003205.
14. Bhatt DL, Steg PG, Miller M, Brinton EA, Jacobson TA, Ketchum SB, Doyle RT Jr, Juliano RA, Jiao L, Granowitz C, Tardif JC, Ballantyne CM. Cardiovascular risk reduction with icosapent ethyl for hypertriglyceridemia. N Engl J Med. 2019;380:11–22.
15. Yokoyama M, Origasa H, Matsuzaki M, Matsuzawa Y, Saito Y, Ishikawa Y, Oikawa S, Sasaki J, Hishida H, Itakura H, Kita T, Kitabatake A, Nakaya N, Sakata T, Shimada K, Shirato K. Effects of eicosapentaenoic acid on major coronary events in hypercholesterolaemic patients (JELIS): a randomised open-label, blinded endpoint analysis. Lancet. 2007;369:1090–8.
16. Surampudi P, Enkhmaa B, Anuurad E, Berglund L. Lipid lowering with soluble dietary fiber. Curr Atheroscler Rep. 2016;18:75.
17. Plat J, Baumgartner S, Vanmierlo T, Lütjohann D, Calkins KL, Burrin DG, Guthrie G, Thijs C, Te Velde AA, Vreugdenhil ACE, Sverdlov R, Garssen J, Wout-

ers K, Trautwein EA, Wolfs TG, van Gorp C, Mulder MT, Riksen NP, Groen AK, Mensink RP. Plant-based sterols and stanols in health & disease: "consequences of human development in a plant-based environment?". Prog Lipid Res. 2019;74:87–102.

18. Position Statement 10. Cardiovascular disease and risk management: standards of medical care in diabetes—2020. American Diabetes AssociationDiabetes Care J. 2020;43(Supple 1):S111–S134.

19. Estruch R, Ros E, Salas-Salvadó J, Covas MI, Corella D, Arós F, Gómez-Gracia E, Ruiz-Gutiérrez V, Fiol M, Lapetra J, Lamuela-Raventos RM, Serra-Majem L, Pintó X, Basora J, Muñoz MA, Sorlí JV, Martínez JA, Fitó M, Gea A, Hernán MA, Martínez-González MA. Primary prevention of cardiovascular disease with a Mediterranean diet supplemented with extra-virgin olive oil or nuts. N Engl J Med. 2018;378:e34.

20. Azadbakht L, Fard NR, Karimi M, Baghaei MH, Surkan PJ, Rahimi M, Esmaillzadeh A, Willett WC. Effects of the dietary approaches to stop hypertension (DASH) eating plan on cardiovascular risks among type 2 diabetic patients: a randomized crossover clinical trial. Diabetes Care. 2011;34:55–7.

21. Liese AD, Bortsov A, Günther AL, Dabelea D, Reynolds K, Standiford DA, Liu L, Williams DE, Mayer-Davis EJ, D'Agostino RB Jr, Bell R, Marcovina S. Association of DASH diet with cardiovascular risk factors in youth with diabetes mellitus: the SEARCH for diabetes in youth study. Circulation. 2011;123:1410–7.

22. Lasa A, Miranda J, Bulló M, Casas R, Salas-Salvadó J, Larretxi I, Estruch R, Ruiz-Gutiérrez V, Portillo MP. Comparative effect of two Mediterranean diets versus a low-fat diet on glycaemic control in individuals with type 2 diabetes. Eur J Clin Nutr. 2014;68:767–72.

23. Micha R, Peñalvo JL, Cudhea F, Imamura F, Rehm CD, Mozaffarian D. Association between dietary factors and mortality from heart disease, stroke, and type 2 diabetes in the United States. JAMA. 2017;317: 912–24.

24. Sacks FM, Svetkey LP, Vollmer WM, Appel LJ, Bray GA, Harsha D, Obarzanek E, Conlin PR, Miller ER 3rd, Simons-Morton DG, Karanja N, Lin PH. Effects on blood pressure of reduced dietary sodium and the dietary approaches to stop hypertension (DASH) diet. DASH-sodium collaborative research group. N Engl J Med. 2001;344:3–10.

25. Bolla AM, Caretto A, Laurenzi A, Scavini M, Piemonti L. Low-carb and ketogenic diets in type 1 and type 2 diabetes. Nutrients. 2019;11:962.

26. Kirkpatrick CF, Bolick JP, Kris-Etherton PM, Sikand G, Aspry KE, Soffer DE, Willard KE, Maki KC. Review of current evidence and clinical recommendations on the effects of low-carbohydrate and very-low-carbohydrate (including ketogenic) diets for the management of body weight and other cardiometabolic risk factors: a scientific statement from the National Lipid Association Nutrition and lifestyle task force. J Clin Lipidol. 2019;13:689–711.

27. Di Noia J, Prochaska JO. Dietary stages of change and decisional balance: a meta-analytic review. Am J Health Behav. 2010;34:618–32.

28. Armstrong MJ, Mottershead TA, Ronksley PE, Sigal RJ, Campbell TS, Hemmelgarn BR. Motivational interviewing to improve weight loss in overweight and/or obese patients: a systematic review and meta-analysis of randomized controlled trials. Obes Rev. 2011;12:709–23.

29. Resnicow K, McMaster F. Motivational interviewing: moving from why to how with autonomy support. Int J Behav Nutr Phys Act. 2012;9:19.

Dietary and Lifestyle Cardiometabolic Risk Reduction Strategies in Pro-inflammatory Diseases

12

Ashira Blazer, Kinjan Parikh, David I. Fudman, and Michael S. Garshick

Introduction

Appropriate regulation of both innate and adaptive immunity is a critical component of host defense, wound healing, and physiologic regulation (among many other functions) [1]. Immune system activation with concomitant upregulated chemotactic cytokines, termed systemic inflammation for the purpose of this chapter, are a response to changes in physiologic and patho-

A. Blazer
Division of Rheumatology, Department of Medicine, New York University Langone Health, New York, NY, USA
e-mail: Ashira.blazer@nyulangone.org

K. Parikh
Leon H. Charney Division of Cardiology, Department of Medicine, New York University Langone Health, New York, NY, USA
e-mail: Kinjan.parikh@nyulangone.org

D. I. Fudman
Division of Digestive and Liver Diseases, Department of Medicine, University of Texas Southwestern Medical Center, Dallas, TX, USA
e-mail: David.Fudman@UTSouthwestern.edu

M. S. Garshick (✉)
Leon H. Charney Division of Cardiology, Department of Medicine, New York University Langone Health, New York, NY, USA

Center for the Prevention of Cardiovascular Disease, New York University Langone Health, New York, NY, USA
e-mail: Michael.garshick@nyulangone.org

physiologic conditions (e.g., viral/bacterial infections). When this response is maladaptive or directed against the host, as is the case with autoimmune and autoinflammatory conditions, an inappropriate pro-inflammatory state develops. This dysregulated immune response characterizes such conditions as psoriasis, inflammatory arthritis, inflammatory bowel disease (IBD), systemic lupus erythematosus (SLE), and human immunodeficiency virus (HIV).

The concept that pro-inflammatory conditions relate to vascular disease dates back over 60 years, when physicians recognized the systemic cardiovascular disease (CVD) complications of many autoimmune conditions [2]. Relatively more recently, innate and adaptive immune activation came to also be considered a core component of CVD development [3]. It is now well recognized and supported by large epidemiologic and clinical-translational literature that atherosclerotic cardiovascular (CV) events are a complication of pro-inflammatory conditions. Professional societies including the American Heart Association (AHA) and American College of Cardiology (ACC) now consider pro-inflammatory diseases as CV risk enhancers and place emphasis on the need to provide appropriate CV risk reduction therapies to these patients outside of other risk factors [4]. Recognizing this inherent increased CV risk, the aim of this chapter is to discuss dietary and lifestyle interventions in these patient populations in an attempt to improve CV-related outcomes.

© Springer Nature Switzerland AG 2021
M. J. Wilkinson et al. (eds.), *Prevention and Treatment of Cardiovascular Disease*, Contemporary Cardiology, https://doi.org/10.1007/978-3-030-78177-4_12

Inflammation, Atherosclerosis, and Clinical CVD

The development and progression of atherosclerosis is a lifelong process and involves a complex interplay between the endothelium, circulating lipids, platelets, and one's innate and adaptive immunity [5]. On a pathologic level, progression of atherosclerosis includes endothelial dysfunction, lipid accumulation with intimal fatty streak formation, translocation of leukocytes and foam cell formation, and lesion progression including smooth muscle cell migration and synthesis of extracellular matrix proteinases [5]. At each stage, immune system activation is a key regulator of this process.

The impact of systemic inflammation on atherosclerosis development is seen early as endothelial pro-inflammatory activation occurs via cytokine stimulation. Upregulated vascular adhesion and chemotactic molecules attract immune cells including monocyte and T lymphocytes. Intimal monocytes mature into macrophages that phagocytose modified lipid particles. Foam cells are formed with enhanced local singling driving smooth muscle cell proliferation [6]. Modified lipoproteins and activated platelets adhering to damaged endothelium send their own pro-inflammatory signals (e.g., S100A8/A9), thus further enhancing the inflammatory milieu in atherosclerosis [6]. In summary, an atherosclerotic plaque is a heterogeneous composite of not just monocyte-derived lipid laden macrophages, but also B and T lymphocytes, mast cells, and neutrophils. [6]

A variety of pro-inflammatory cytokines including chemokines and those from the interleukin (IL), tumor necrosis factor (TNF), interferon (IFN), and colony-stimulating factor (CSF) families are each implicated in atherosclerosis and are shown to correlate with clinical CVD (Fig. 12.1). [7] Key inflammatory cytokines promoting this atherosclerotic march include NLRP3 inflammasome-activated IL-1β and IL-18 with downstream IL-6 production [8]. The clinical importance of this pathway has since been confirmed in clinical trials in which inhibiting IL-1β in patients with a history of myocardial infarction

and elevated high-sensitivity C-reactive protein (hs-CRP) reduced recurrent cardiac events [9]. Other pro-atherosclerotic and pro-inflammatory cytokines include TNFα and IFNγ [10]. Based on this evolving understanding of pathophysiology, it is not surprising that pro-inflammatory conditions in which the primary disturbances are those of either innate or adaptive immunity also potentiate atherosclerosis and elevate CV risk.

Rheumatoid Arthritis

Rheumatoid arthritis (RA) is the most common autoimmune inflammatory arthritis affecting up to 1% of the US population [11]. The incidence of RA is twice as high in women as men with the highest incidence occurring in middle-aged to older individuals [11]. The pathogenesis of RA is multifactorial owing to a combination of genetic and environmental causes. Post-translational protein citrullination by peptidylarginine deiminase is a major contributor to self-antigen production and immune stimulation. [12] The resultant citrullinated peptides cause innate immune activation; a first step in systemic and synovial inflammation [12]. An adaptive immune response is elicited in lymphoid tissues with T-cell and B-cell activation, thus producing antibodies including anti-citrullinated peptide (CCP) antibodies and rheumatoid factor [12]. The synovium is the primary target of a systemic immune response in RA. Innate immune cells and macrophage-like synoviocytes produce cytokines and chemokines that attract a host of leukocytes, most notably memory CD4+ T cells. Interestingly, these T cells form ectopic germinal centers with mature B cells in the synovium causing the production of auto-antibodies in the joint tissue [12]. Cytokine signatures in RA are characterized by pro-atherosclerotic mediators including IL-1, IL-6, and TNFα [12].

In comparison to individuals without RA, CV mortality and ischemic heart disease in patients with RA are up to 50% and 59% higher, respectively [13]. Chronic systemic and vascular inflammation is felt to play a dominant role in enhancing CV risk [13]. Vascular arterial FDG-

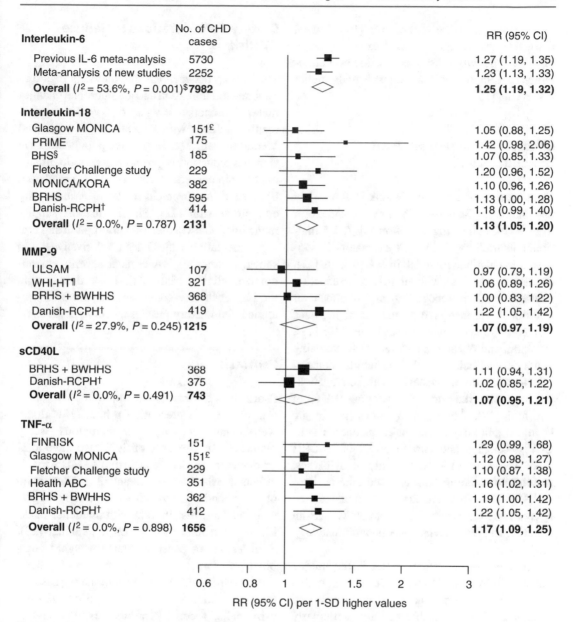

Fig. 12.1 Meta-analysis assessing the association between pro-inflammatory cytokines and risk of non-fatal myocardial infarction or coronary heart disease death. Box with line indicates relative risk with 95% confidence interval. Diamond indicates composite relative risk with 95% confidence interval. (Adapted from Kaptoge et al. [7])

PET studies show that disease activity, presence of rheumatoid nodules, and higher anti-CCP antibody titers are associated with ascending aortic inflammation [14]. ESR and hs-CRP in RA also track with enhanced CV risk [15]. While specific mechanisms to explain vascular inflammation in RA remain under investigation, upregulated IL-6 and TNFα, a dominant role of T lymphocytes and macrophages, along with the contribution of endothelial dysfunction, platelet activation and hypercoagulability promote atherosclerosis [13]. Patients with RA are also often prescribed glucocorticoids and NSAIDs, which can independently elevate risk further [12]. Tofacitinib, a JAK inhibitor approved for the treatment of rheumatoid arthritis (and ulcerative colitis), may further elevate the risk of thrombosis [16]. Finally, a well-described lipid paradox exists, whereby higher RA activity is associated with lower circulating LDL-cholesterol and unexpectedly higher CV events [15].

Lifestyle Management in RA to Reduce CV Risk

Identification of elevated CV risk in RA is key and major medical societies now consider RA to be a risk enhancing condition [4]. A 1.5 multiplier to traditional CV risk estimators is suggested to calculate total risk in RA patients [17]. Similar to a patient without RA, risk reduction strategies include recognition and treatment of traditional risk factors, especially as higher rates of metabolic syndrome (upwards of 30%) [18], smoking, and obesity are present [18]. Smoking is not only associated with RA, but also contributes to disease pathogenesis, with active smoking increasing the odds of developing RA up to two-fold [19]. Among many other pathologic changes, smoking is shown to potentiate anti-CCP antibodies and elevate levels of hs-CRP, IL-6, TNFα, and the IL-1 family of cytokines, thereby potentiating both RA and atherosclerosis [19]. Therefore, smoking cessation must be aggressively emphasized, for both the CV health benefits and to alleviate RA symptomatology [19].

Another consideration in RA is the unique physical activity and mobility restriction which may make a recommended 30 minutes a day 5 days a week of aerobic activity particularly challenging. It is not yet clear if exercise regimens in the RA population lead to a decrease in biomarkers of inflammation [20]. However, clinical trials in the RA population show that aerobic activity is feasible and safe with 70% of RA patients able to tolerate prescribed exercise programs. The beneficial CV health impact of exercise is similar among patients with and without RA and such activity should be encouraged [21].

Dietary Considerations to Reduce CV Risk

The overlap between RA and diet with regard to systemic inflammation and gut microbial changes makes diet another key part of CV risk management of patients with RA. Studies of vegan and Mediterranean diets in the RA population have shown a reduction in pro-atherosclerotic inflammatory biomarkers, decreased BMI, circulating lipids, and improvement in RA disease severity and progression [22]. Finally, fish-oil supplementation, both via dietary consumption and oral supplementation with Omega-3 derivatives, was shown to improve RA clinical severity in randomized clinical trials [22]. These data portray the impact dietary counseling can have on systemic inflammatory profiles and CV risk in RA.

Psoriasis

Psoriasis is a chronic, pro-inflammatory condition of the skin presenting primarily as thick, well-demarcated, and erythematous scaly plaques [23]. Upwards of 20% also have joint involvement (psoriatic arthritis) [23]. Psoriasis affects 2–3% of all Americans [23]. There is no obvious gender predilection and studies suggest a bimodal age distribution with incidence peaking between 30–39 and 50–69 years of age [23]. Skin lesions of psoriasis start through a combination of environmental stimuli and genetic predisposition driving an inflammatory cascade (termed initiation phase) composed of dendritic cells, T cells, keratinocytes, and neutrophils. Cytokines produced during this process include type I and II interferons, TNFα, IL-6, and IL-1β. Activation of myeloid dendritic cells produces IL-12/23 leading to further T-cell differentiation with the production of IL-17 family of cytokines. Inflammatory mediators and cross-talk between the innate and adaptive immune systems drive keratinocyte activation and proliferation. A pro-inflammatory feedback loop is generated with Th17 production of

IL17A [23]. Breaking of the positive feedback loop is a mainstay of anti-inflammatory therapies in psoriasis.

Meta-analyses support an approximate 50% increased risk of CVD in patients with psoriasis, and CV-risk stratification guidelines now consider psoriasis a risk enhancing condition [24]. Psoriasis disease severity directly associates with not just pro-atherosclerotic biomarkers such as IL-6 and hs-CRP, but also endothelial and vascular inflammation [25]. Inflammasome signaling, IL-6 [26], and a synergistic component of IFNγ, TNFα, and the IL17 family contribute to vascular arterial inflammation in psoraisis [25, 27]. Direct immunologic mechanisms linking psoriasis with early atherosclerosis are heterogeneous and still under investigation. Lymphoid abnormalities (including upregulated TH1 and TH17 cells) associate with many pro-inflammatory pro-atherosclerotic processes in psoriasis [28]. However, recent work has shifted to the contribution of myeloid cells including neutrophils, classical monocytes, and platelet activation to further explain mechanisms that drive atherosclerosis in psoriasis [29].

Lifestyle Management in Psoriasis to Reduce Cardiometabolic Disease

Comorbidities in psoriasis are frequently underdiagnosed and undertreated [30]. The odds of having a coexisting CV risk factor (obesity, smoking, hypertension, and hyperlipidemia) with psoriasis varies depending on the population studied but can range between 1.03–1.31 for mild and 1.31–2.23 for severe psoriasis [30]. For example, obesity doubles the risk of developing psoriasis [31] and enhances vascular inflammation [32]. The odds of metabolic syndrome is up to two-fold higher and hyperlipidemia upwards of four-fold higher than controls [33]. Smoking itself can increase the risk of psoriasis by over 70% (in some studies up to two-fold) and worsens the severity of psoriasis [34]. Therefore, management of CV risk in psoriasis requires aggressive

lifestyle modification to reduce and treat known CV risk factors.

In obese psoriasis patients, a hypocaloric diet and those patient who undergo bariatric surgery for weight loss (specifically those with initial BMI > 40 kg/m^2) have a 50% reduced risk of psoriasis disease progression in addition to other CV benefits [35]. In a Cochrane review of over 1000 obese patients with psoriasis or psoriatic arthritis, structured exercise along with dietary programs to achieve weight loss improved quality of life and provided up to a 75% improvement in the severity of psoriasis skin lesions [36]. These data suggest obesity assessment and treatment is a critical part of psoriasis management. Finally, while smoking cessation should strongly be encouraged and probably improves psoriasis severity [37], clinical trials evaluating this are limited [36].

Specific Dietary Consideration in Psoriasis to Reduce Cardiometabolic Disease

Dietary free fatty acids (such as in fried foods) in psoriasis are shown to amplify the pro-inflammatory phenotype and skin inflammation in psoriasis including enhanced inflammasome production of IL-1β and IL-18 [31]. As such, specific diets have been evaluated in overweight-obese psoriasis including the Ornish and South Beach to induce weight loss, but it is not clear if these specifically improve psoriasis severity [38]. Gluten-free diets are shown to improve psoriasis severity only in those with known celiac disease [38]. Recognizing the impact weight and diet can have on psoriasis severity and CV risk, the National Psoriasis Foundation recently published dietary recommendations [38]. Overall, a generalized hypocaloric diet is recommended in psoriasis. However, a Mediterranean diet should be considered due to its known CV benefits and high in omega-3 fatty acid content, as well as association with reduced psoriasis skin severity and systemic inflammatory markers such as hs-CRP [38].

Systemic Lupus Erythematosus

SLE is a heterogeneous clinical autoimmune disorder characterized by systemic immune activation and multi-organ system tissue injury [39]. In a recent US population-based registry, prevalent SLE was found to be 62.2 per 100,000 person years with nine-fold higher rates in women compared to men [40]. SLE disproportionately affects racial and ethnic minorities with three- and two-fold higher rates in non-Hispanic Black and Hispanic women, respectively [40]. SLE pathogenesis is driven both by dysfunctional clearance of apoptotic debris, and the production of auto-reactive antibodies [41]. Apoptotic-derived nucleic acids stimulate pattern recognition receptors, most notably toll-like receptors (TLRs), which are an integral part of the innate and adaptive immune response to viral pathogens [41]. TLR ligation produces type I IFNs, strongly associated with SLE, which promote B-cell differentiation and loss of adaptive immune tolerance [41]. Persistent auto-reactive B cells produce the somatically mutated IgG anti-nuclear antibodies pathognomonic of SLE [41].

Importantly SLE carries a significant risk of morbidity and mortality with late deaths most often due to CV [42]. In a recent nested case–control study using the National Inpatient Sample, SLE patients exhibited higher prevalent atherosclerotic CVD compared to age- and sex-matched controls at an adjusted odds ratio of 1.46 [43]. Notably, the CVD prevalence disparity was most pronounced at younger ages with SLE patients developing atherosclerosis in their 20s [43]. SLE patients have increased carotid artery intima-media thickness with plaque detected in 21% of patients under 35, and nearly 100% of those over 65 years of age [44]. Clinically, SLE can produce CVD by several mechanisms including accelerated atherosclerosis, arteritis, thrombosis, and vasospasm among others [45]. As a primary target of inflammatory cytokines, the endothelial barrier function is compromised in SLE [39]. Pro-inflammatory soluble mediators, such as TNF-α and IL-1, cause the endothelium to express adhesion molecules and chemokines [46].

Macrophages, foam cells, platelet activation, and reactive oxygen species all drive endothelial dysfunction and accelerated atherosclerotic plaque production in SLE [39].

Lifestyle Management in SLE to Reduce Cardiometabolic Disease

Risk assessment, the first step in reduction, is notoriously difficult in SLE due to disease heterogeneity [47]. Though SLE patients tend to have high prevalence of traditional CV risk factors, this phenomenon does not fully account for excess atherosclerotic disease [48]. SLE activity, medication use, particularly prednisone, and prevalence of anti-phospholipid antibodies are all contributory [45]. CV risk scores developed in general populations such as Framingham (FRS) and the American College of Cardiology/American Heart Association (ACC/AHA) pooled cohort equation consistently under-estimate risk in SLE patients [49].

The approach to CV risk reduction in SLE should be aimed at healthful behavior change in addition to pharmacological interventions. Counseling on diet and exercise is of crucial importance [50]. SLE patients often experience fatigue, musculoskeletal pain, and/or require prednisone, all of which may reduce the opportunity for exercise and promote obesity [51]. Sleeplessness and fatigue are widely reported in SLE and are major barriers to maintaining healthy lifestyle choices that prevent CVD [51]. SLE patients experiencing high levels of fatigue, are shown to sleep less, exercise less, and smoke more [51]. Strategies to improve fatigue and, therefore, quality of life include recommending greater than 7 h of sleep per night, and a regular exercise regimen [51]. Aerobic exercise at least three times per week has been shown to improve exercise tolerance, fatigue scores, and maximum oxygen consumption [19]. Exercise also improves brachial artery flow-mediated dilation over 16 weeks, a proxy for vascular health [52]. Finally, smoking cessation should be a cornerstone of CV risk management in SLE [44]. Smoking has been associated both with worsened

SLE disease activity and CVD events in multiple, high-quality observational studies [53].

Dietary Consideration in SLE to Reduce Cardiometabolic Disease

A balanced heart-healthy diet should be aimed at maintaining a BMI less than 25 kg/m^2 with both low-calorie and low-glycemic-index diets shown to promote healthy body weight in SLE [50]. Upwards of 60% of SLE patients have a co-existing diagnosis of dyslipidemia characterized by elevated total cholesterol, triglycerides, and LDL-C, along with decreased HDL-C [54]. Dyslipidemia and particularly elevated triglycerides have been independently associated with CV events in SLE, and therefore, should be managed aggressively through diet, pharmacologic interventions, and minimizing glucocorticoid dosing [55]. Omega-3 fatty acid supplementation may also be beneficial to improving endothelial function as measured by FMD in SLE patients [50]. Supporting this, in an observational study of 114 patients with SLE, higher adipose tissue EPA and DHA levels associated with a lower incidence of carotid intimal medial thickness in SLE [56]. Conversely, diets high in carbohydrates associate with SLE-characteristic dyslipidemia [56]. SLE patients should be monitored for adequate vitamin D levels, and supplementation should be provided if required, as low vitamin D levels in SLE track with elevated CV risk factors including hypertension, hyperlipidemia, elevated CRP, higher SLE disease activity, and CV events [57].

Inflammatory Bowel Disease

Inflammatory bowel disease, including Crohn's disease and ulcerative colitis (UC), is a chronic inflammatory disease of the gastrointestinal (GI) tract. The incidence of IBD is rising worldwide, with overall prevalence expected to soon reach 1% [58]. Its pathophysiology involves an interaction between environmental, genetic, and host–microbial commensal flora that initiates a localized autoimmune reaction including epithe-

lial damage within the GI tract [59]. The resulting inflammatory cascade occurs across multiple cell lines such as those of myeloid lineage and CD4$^+$ Th1-derived T lymphocytes. Upregulated cytokines in this process include TNF, IL-1β, IFNs, IL-12/23 along with disturbances in the TH17 and IL-17 pathways, which are critical for maintaining gut epithelial homeostasis [59]. The importance of these cytokines in the pathogenesis of IBD is further emphasized by the efficacy of treatment with anti-TNF and IL-12/23 biologics and the potential worsening of disease in those given IL-17 inhibitors [60].

With regard to vascular complications, venous thromboembolism (VTE) may be the most common and is reported to be between 1.7-fold and 5.5-fold higher than in those without IBD [61]. Atherosclerotic and arterial thromboembolic CV complications are also elevated, with rates approximately 20% higher than patients without IBD [62]. The relative impact of IBD on CV risk may be higher in women (RR 1.35; 95% CI [1.21–1.51]) with IBD as compared to males (RR 1.19; 95% CI [1.03–1.38]) [63]. As opposed to other pro-inflammatory conditions, it is not yet clear if traditional CVD risk factors in IBD including obesity, metabolic syndrome, and hypertension exhibit a higher prevalence [64]. In fact, circulating lipids may actually be lower when compared to matched non-IBD patients [65]. Therefore, hypothesized mechanisms to relate IBD to CVD focus less on the impact of traditional CV risk factors and more on how cytokines such as IL-6, TNFα, and low-grade endotoxemia driven by disturbances in intestinal barrier homeostasis impart elevated CV risk [66].

Lifestyle Management to Reduce Cardiometabolic Disease in IBD

While minimal data exist on how lifestyle and dietary management can improve CV risk specifically in the IBD population, recommendations to reduce inflammatory activity in IBD often overlap with standard CVD prevention techniques. Similar to other pro-inflammatory conditions, smoking is shown to promote inflammation in Crohn's disease and patients with Crohn's who smoke have worse outcomes, further highlighting the importance of smoking cessation in this population [67]. Physical activity is also associated with a lower incidence of Crohn's disease and in some studies was shown to decrease disease flares [68].

Dietary Considerations to Reduce Cardiometabolic Disease in IBD

Although the etiology of IBD is clearly multifactorial, epidemiologic data point to a definite role of environmental factors in triggering the inflammation underlying the disease, and a growing body of evidence supports diet and its effect on the microbiome playing at least part of that environmental role. A "Western diet," high in saturated fat and animal intake and low in plants is linked to not just enhanced CVD but also felt to be associated with the development of IBD [69]. In addition, some evidence suggests that high fiber intake – and foods rich in Omega-3 and Omega-6, which are important in CV prevention – are associated with a lower risk of development of IBD, most notably Crohn's disease, and maybe beneficial in those diagnosed with Crohn's [70].

While its evidence base is quite limited, the most well-known diet promoted to reduce intestinal inflammation is the specific carbohydrate diet, a restrictive diet that eliminates poorly absorbed carbohydrates under the theory that these lead to intestinal damage via promotion of a pro-inflammatory gut microbiome. Other proposed diets or dietary modifications to reduce inflammation in IBD (and presumably reduce CV risk) include a semi-vegetarian diet, the Mediterranean diet, red meat reduction, and increasing fruit and vegetable intake (importantly, in those with Crohn's this last dietary modification includes only those patients who do not have intestinal strictures) [71]. Finally, a unique consideration in IBD patients, as compared to other populations with pro-inflammatory conditions, is the risk for protein-calorie malnutrition [72]. Protein-calorie malnutrition in IBD is associated with a 3.5-fold in-hospital mortality likely reflecting a substan-

tial burden of disease in this population [73]. In summary, nutritional status and nutrient intake play an important role in IBD management which may also have implications for CV outcomes.

Human Immunodeficiency Virus

HIV infection can be divided into three phases: the viral transmission phase, the acute phase, and then chronic phase, which eventually progresses into acquired immunodeficiency syndrome (AIDS). The advent of effective antiretroviral therapy (ART) has transformed HIV from almost uniformly fatal, into a chronic illness where the causes of morbidity and mortality are often no longer AIDS-related complications but rather CVD [74]. In a simplified manner, HIV infection is characterized by a destruction and dysregulation of $CD4^+$ T cells and activation of cytotoxic $CD8^+$ T cells. While many immune system abnormalities normalize after initiation of ART, others do not. Specifically in chronic, treated HIV, destruction of $CD4^+$ Th17 T cells, essential in gut epithelial homeostasis, lead to chronic microbial translocation and endotoxemia driving monocyte activation and pro-inflammatory cytokines such as IL-6, IL-1β, TNFα, MCP1 as well as platelet activation [75]. Increased B-cell activation is also present often leading to a higher percentage of B-cell malignancies. [76] Finally, a strong type I IFN signature is also felt to play a role in the chronic inflammation of HIV [77].

Not surprisingly, and in part because of these immune abnormalities, CVD plays a significant role in enhanced morbidity and mortality of HIV with a 1.5–2-fold increased rate of CV events compared to those not infected with HIV [74]. Dyslipidemia, particularly hypertriglyceridemia, is common in HIV and correlated with the degree of viremia [74]. Hypertension, metabolic syndrome, diabetes, smoking, and heavy alcohol use are also more prevalent, especially in developed nations. Although multifactorial, the pro-inflammatory disease state which defines chronic HIV is felt to play a role in potentiating CV risk [74]. For example, in the Strategies for Management of Antiretroviral Therapy (SMART) study to test CD4 guided vs continuous ART, higher CRP and IL-6 levels were associated with an eight-fold increase in risk of all-cause mortality [78]. Both endothelial damage and vascular inflammation (in FDG-PET studies) are increased in HIV and associated with monocyte activation [79], thus enhancing atherosclerosis development. Based on these observations, CV guidelines now recommend treating HIV as a CV risk enhancing condition [80].

Lifestyle Management in HIV to Reduce Cardiometabolic Disease

The conventional lifestyle and unhealthy dietary patterns that drive CVD development in the non-HIV population have also been studied in the HIV population [74]. In developed nations, up to 40% of those with HIV are active smokers, highlighting the importance of smoking cessation [74]. Those HIV patients with low-physical activity, also exhibit depression, reduced adherence to ART, and higher viral load [74]. In survey studies of HIV individuals, specific barriers to a healthy lifestyle include the higher cost of obtaining nutritious foods, an environment not conducive toward healthy eating, and lack of a social support system [81]. For example, having a strong patient–provider relationship improves ART adherence and healthy behavior patterns [81]. Finally, dietary and lifestyle interventions can work and are beneficial in HIV [82]. Regular exercise (e.g., 1-h, 3× week gym class combined with nutritional counseling) is shown to decrease fat mass, waist circumference, and glucose while raising CD4+ T cells, muscle mass, and improving quality of life [82]. These data suggest that in HIV individuals, similar to the general population, adherence to healthy diet and exercise regimens can improve patient CV outcomes.

Dietary Consideration in HIV to Reduce Cardiometabolic Disease

The appropriate macro- and micro-nutrient intake of the HIV individual potentially impact-

ing overall CV health is an active area of investigation. While we have discussed many of the increased risks in the developed world, the developing world often faces different problems. The resting energy expenditure of HIV is approximately 10% higher than in healthy individuals [83], exacerbating problems of malnutrition due to food insecurity and poverty in HIV health and management. In these countries, supplementation with multivitamins including vitamin D, and increasing protein intake can increase CD4 count, potentially reduce hs-CRP [84], and subsequently reduce HIV progression and mortality [83]. These data have led to position statements from the American Dietetic Association highlighting the importance of food security, nutrition education, and nutrition supplementation when appropriate in the individual living with HIV [85].

In chronic HIV infection, especially in developed nations for those on ART, obesity, metabolic syndrome, hyperlipidemia, and hypertriglyceridemia are of significant concern and have dietary implications. Studies evaluating nutrient intervention in HIV show a beneficial impact on overall health. In a randomized trial of a reduced-fat diet in HIV individuals initiated on ART, those who underwent dietary intervention reduced triglycerides by 25%. At the end of the study, 21% in the treated and 68% in the untreated groups met the criteria for dyslipidemia [86]. Given its CV risk reduction benefits, the Mediterranean diet has also been studied in HIV. Adherence to a Mediterranean lifestyle in HIV is associated with less insulin resistance, higher HDL-C, and a trend toward lower triglycerides [87]. Omega-3 supplementation, especially in those with hypertriglyceridemia, is shown to be effective, and in light of the negative impact of elevated triglycerides in CVD progression, can be considered in those with have an inadequate response to dietary interventions [88]. In summary, a dietary approach to reduce CV risk in chronic HIV has to be customized to baseline nutritional status, feasibility, and individual metabolic abnormalities. Interventions designed to improve cardiometabolic profiles in HIV are shown to be successful and should be considered in those with HIV.

Conclusion

In summary, atherosclerosis development is a complex interplay between the endothelium, vasculature, lipids, platelets, innate, and adaptive immunity. The systemic inflammation derived from autoimmune and autoinflammatory conditions creates a predisposition to atherosclerosis development, thus leading to elevated rates of adverse CV events. A general approach to managing CV risk in these patients is to ensure appropriate screening of traditional CV risk factors (hypertension, obesity, smoking, dyslipidemia, and diabetes). Once recognized, lifestyle modification including smoking cessation, exercise, and dietary regimens (including omega-3 and vitamin D supplementation) can have an impact not just on CV risk, but also on autoimmune disease severity and control.

References

1. Chaplin DD. Overview of the immune response. J Allergy Clin Immunol. 2010;125:S3–23.
2. Garshick MS. Editorial commentary: psoriasis, inflammation and cardiometabolic disease. Will we ever get to the heart of the matter? Trends Cardiovasc Med. 2020;30:479–480.
3. Hansson GK. Immune and inflammatory mechanisms in the development of atherosclerosis. Br Heart J. 1993;69:S38–41.
4. Arnett DK, Blumenthal RS, Albert MA et al. ACC/AHA Guideline on the Primary Prevention of Cardiovascular Disease: Executive Summary: A Report of the American College of Cardiology/American Heart Association Task Force on Clinical Practice Guidelines. J Am Coll Cardiol 2019;74:1376–1414.
5. Libby P, Ridker PM, Hansson GK. Progress and challenges in translating the biology of atherosclerosis. Nature. 2011;473:317–25.
6. Libby P. Inflammation in atherosclerosis. Arterioscler Thromb Vasc Biol. 2012;32:2045–51.
7. Kaptoge S, Seshasai SR, Gao P, Freitag DF, Butterworth AS, Borglykke A, Di Angelantonio E, Gudnason V, Rumley A, Lowe GD, Jorgensen T, Danesh J. Inflammatory cytokines and risk of coronary heart disease: new prospective study and updated meta-analysis. Eur Heart J. 2014;35:578–89. https://doi.org/10.1093/eurheartj/eht367.
8. Back M, Yurdagul A Jr, Tabas I, Oorni K, Kovanen PT. Inflammation and its resolution in atherosclerosis: mediators and therapeutic opportunities. Nat Rev Cardiol. 2019;16:389–406.
9. Ridker PM, Everett BM, Thuren T, et al. Antiinflammatory therapy with canakinumab for atherosclerotic disease. N Engl J Med. 2017;377:1119–31.
10. Tousoulis D, Oikonomou E, Economou EK, Crea F, Kaski JC. Inflammatory cytokines in atherosclerosis: current therapeutic approaches. Eur Heart J. 2016;37:1723–32.
11. Crowson CS, Matteson EL, Myasoedova E, Michet CJ, Ernste FC, Warrington KJ, Davis JM 3rd, Hunder GG, Therneau TM, Gabriel SE. The lifetime risk of adult-onset rheumatoid arthritis and other inflammatory autoimmune rheumatic diseases. Arthritis Rheum. 2011;63:633–9.
12. Smolen JS, Aletaha D, Barton A, Burmester GR, Emery P, Firestein GS, Kavanaugh A, McInnes IB, Solomon DH, Strand V, Yamamoto K. Rheumatoid arthritis. Nat Rev Dis Primers. 2018;4:18001.
13. Avina-Zubieta JA, Choi HK, Sadatsafavi M, Etminan M, Esdaile JM, Lacaille D. Risk of cardiovascular mortality in patients with rheumatoid arthritis: a meta-analysis of observational studies. Arthritis Rheum. 2008;59:1690–7.
14. Geraldino-Pardilla L, Zartoshti A, Ozbek AB, Giles JT, Weinberg R, Kinkhabwala M, Bokhari S, Bathon JM. Arterial inflammation detected with (18) F-fluorodeoxyglucose-positron emission tomography in rheumatoid arthritis. Arthritis Rheumatol. 2018;70:30–9.
15. Amezaga Urruela M, Suarez-Almazor ME. Lipid paradox in rheumatoid arthritis: changes with rheumatoid arthritis therapies. Curr Rheumatol Rep. 2012;14:428–37.
16. Scott IC, Hider SL, Scott DL. Thromboembolism with Janus Kinase (JAK) inhibitors for rheumatoid arthritis: how real is the risk? Drug Saf. 2018;41:645–53.
17. Agca R, Heslinga SC, Rollefstad S, et al. EULAR recommendations for cardiovascular disease risk management in patients with rheumatoid arthritis and other forms of inflammatory joint disorders: 2015/2016 update. Ann Rheum Dis. 2017;76:17–28.
18. Kerekes G, Nurmohamed MT, Gonzalez-Gay MA, Seres I, Paragh G, Kardos Z, Barath Z, Tamasi L, Soltesz P, Szekanecz Z. Rheumatoid arthritis and metabolic syndrome. Nat Rev Rheumatol. 2014;10:691–6.
19. Chang K, Yang SM, Kim SH, Han KH, Park SJ, Shin JI. Smoking and rheumatoid arthritis. Int J Mol Sci. 2014;15:22279–95.
20. Burghardt RD, Kazim MA, Ruther W, Niemeier A, Strahl A. The impact of physical activity on serum levels of inflammatory markers in rheumatoid arthritis: a systematic literature review. Rheumatol Int. 2019;39:793–804.
21. Rausch Osthoff AK, Niedermann K, Braun J, et al. 2018 EULAR recommendations for physical activity in people with inflammatory arthritis and osteoarthritis. Ann Rheum Dis. 2018;77:1251–60.
22. Khanna S, Jaiswal KS, Gupta B. Managing rheumatoid arthritis with dietary interventions. Front Nutr. 2017;4:52.

23. Greb JE, Goldminz AM, Elder JT, Lebwohl MG, Gladman DD, Wu JJ, Mehta NN, Finlay AY, Gottlieb AB. Psoriasis. Nat Rev Dis Primers. 2016;2:16082.
24. Miller IM, Ellervik C, Yazdanyar S, Jemec GB. Meta-analysis of psoriasis, cardiovascular disease, and associated risk factors. J Am Acad Dermatol. 2013;69:1014–24.
25. Garshick MS, Barrett T, Wechter T, Azarchi S, Scher J, Neimann A, Katz S, Fuentes-Duculan J, Cannizzaro MV, Jelic S, Fisher EA, Krueger JG, Berger JS. Inflammasome signaling and impaired vascular health in psoriasis. Arterioscler Thromb Vasc Biol. 2019;39(4):787–98.
26. Wang Y, Golden JB, Fritz Y, Zhang X, Diaconu D, Camhi MI, Gao H, Dawes SM, Xing X, Ganesh SK, Gudjonsson JE, Simon DI, McCormick TS, Ward NL. Interleukin 6 regulates psoriasiform inflammation-associated thrombosis. JCI Insight. 2016;1:e89384.
27. Mehta NN, Teague HL, Swindell WR, et al. IFN-gamma and TNF-alpha synergism may provide a link between psoriasis and inflammatory atherogenesis. Sci Rep. 2017;7:13831.
28. Armstrong AW, Voyles SV, Armstrong EJ, Fuller EN, Rutledge JC. A tale of two plaques: convergent mechanisms of T-cell-mediated inflammation in psoriasis and atherosclerosis. Exp Dermatol. 2011;20:544–9.
29. Teague HL, Aksentijevich M, Stansky E, et al. Cells of myeloid origin partly mediate the association between psoriasis severity and coronary plaque. J Invest Dermatol. 2020;140:912–915 e1.
30. Neimann AL, Shin DB, Wang X, Margolis DJ, Troxel AB, Gelfand JM. Prevalence of cardiovascular risk factors in patients with psoriasis. J Am Acad Dermatol. 2006;55:829–35.
31. Kunz M, Simon JC, Saalbach A. Psoriasis: obesity and fatty acids. Front Immunol. 2019;10:1807.
32. Rivers JP, Powell-Wiley TM, Dey AK, et al. Visceral adiposity in psoriasis is associated with vascular inflammation by (18)F-fluorodeoxyglucose positron-emission tomography/computed tomography beyond cardiometabolic disease risk factors in an observational cohort study. JACC Cardiovasc Imaging. 2018;11:349–57.
33. Elmets CA, Leonardi CL, Davis DMR, et al. Joint AAD-NPF guidelines of care for the management and treatment of psoriasis with awareness and attention to comorbidities. J Am Acad Dermatol. 2019;80(4):1073–113.
34. Naldi L. Psoriasis and smoking: links and risks. Psoriasis (Auckl). 2016;6:65–71.
35. Alotaibi HA. Effects of weight loss on psoriasis: a review of clinical trials. Cureus. 2018;10:e3491.
36. Ko SH, Chi CC, Yeh ML, Wang SH, Tsai YS, Hsu MY. Lifestyle changes for treating psoriasis. Cochrane Database Syst Rev. 2019;7:CD011972.
37. Li W, Han J, Choi HK, Qureshi AA. Smoking and risk of incident psoriasis among women and men in the United States: a combined analysis. Am J Epidemiol. 2012;175:402–13.
38. Ford AR, Siegel M, Bagel J, et al. Dietary recommendations for adults with psoriasis or psoriatic arthritis from the medical board of the national psoriasis foundation: a systematic review. JAMA Dermatol. 2018;154:934–50.
39. Kahlenberg JM, Kaplan MJ. The interplay of inflammation and cardiovascular disease in systemic lupus erythematosus. Arthritis Res Ther. 2011;13:203.
40. Izmirly PM, Wan I, Sahl S, et al. The incidence and prevalence of systemic lupus erythematosus in New York county (Manhattan), New York: the Manhattan lupus surveillance program. Arthritis Rheumatol. 2017;69:2006–17.
41. Tsokos GC, Lo MS, Costa Reis P, Sullivan KE. New insights into the immunopathogenesis of systemic lupus erythematosus. Nat Rev Rheumatol. 2016;12:716–30.
42. Danila MI, Pons-Estel GJ, Zhang J, Vila LM, Reveille JD, Alarcon GS. Renal damage is the most important predictor of mortality within the damage index: data from LUMINA LXIV, a multiethnic US cohort. Rheumatology (Oxford). 2009;48:542–5.
43. Katz G, Smilowitz NR, Blazer A, Clancy R, Buyon JP, Berger JS. Systemic lupus erythematosus and increased prevalence of atherosclerotic cardiovascular disease in hospitalized patients. Mayo Clin Proc. 2019;94:1436–43.
44. Tselios K, Sheane BJ, Gladman DD, Urowitz MB. Optimal monitoring for coronary heart disease risk in patients with systemic lupus erythematosus: a systematic review. J Rheumatol. 2016;43:54–65.
45. Petri MA, Barr E, Magder LS. Development of a systemic lupus erythematosus cardiovascular risk equation. Lupus Sci Med. 2019;6:e000346.
46. Ramji DP, Davies TS. Cytokines in atherosclerosis: key players in all stages of disease and promising therapeutic targets. Cytokine Growth Factor Rev. 2015;26:673–85.
47. Boulos D, Koelmeyer RL, Morand EF, Hoi AY. Cardiovascular risk profiles in a lupus cohort: what do different calculators tell us? Lupus Sci Med. 2017;4:e000212.
48. Masson W, Rossi E, Mora-Crespo LM, Cornejo-Pena G, Pessio C, Gago M, Alvarado RN, Scolnik M. Cardiovascular risk stratification and appropriate use of statins in patients with systemic lupus erythematosus according to different strategies. Clin Rheumatol. 2020;39:455–62.
49. Sivakumaran J, Harvey P, Omar A, Urowitz MB, Gladman DD, Anderson N, Su J, Touma Z. 291 assessment of the QRISK2, QRISK3, SLE cardiovascular risk equation, modified Framingham and Framingham risk calculators as predictors of cardiovascular disease events in systemic lupus erythematosus. Lupus Sci Med. 2019;6:A211–2.
50. Andrades C, Fuego C, Manrique-Arija S, Fernandez-Nebro A. Management of cardiovascular risk in systemic lupus erythematosus: a systematic review. Lupus. 2017;26:1407–19.

51. Rodriguez Huerta MD, Trujillo-Martin MM, Rua-Figueroa I, Cuellar-Pompa L, Quiros-Lopez R, Serrano-Aguilar P, Spanish SLE CPG Development Group. Healthy lifestyle habits for patients with systemic lupus erythematosus: a systemic review. Semin Arthritis Rheum. 2016;45:463–70.

52. Barnes JN, Nualnim N, Dhindsa M, Renzi CP, Tanaka H. Macro- and microvascular function in habitually exercising systemic lupus erythematosus patients. Scand J Rheumatol. 2014;43:209–16.

53. Bruce IN, O'Keeffe AG, Farewell V, et al. Factors associated with damage accrual in patients with systemic lupus erythematosus: results from the systemic lupus international collaborating clinics (SLICC) inception cohort. Ann Rheum Dis. 2015;74:1706–13.

54. Tselios K, Koumaras C, Gladman DD, Urowitz MB. Dyslipidemia in systemic lupus erythematosus: just another comorbidity? Semin Arthritis Rheum. 2016;45:604–10.

55. Ballocca F, D'Ascenzo F, Moretti C, Omede P, Cerrato E, Barbero U, Abbate A, Bertero MT, Zoccai GB, Gaita F. Predictors of cardiovascular events in patients with systemic lupus erythematosus (SLE): a systematic review and meta-analysis. Eur J Prev Cardiol. 2015;22:1435–41.

56. Elkan AC, Anania C, Gustafsson T, Jogestrand T, Hafstrom I, Frostegard J. Diet and fatty acid pattern among patients with SLE: associations with disease activity, blood lipids and atherosclerosis. Lupus. 2012;21:1405–11.

57. Lertratanakul A, Wu P, Dyer A, et al. 25-hydroxyvitamin D and cardiovascular disease in patients with systemic lupus erythematosus: data from a large international inception cohort. Arthritis Care Res (Hoboken). 2014;66:1167–76.

58. Ng SC, Shi HY, Hamidi N, Underwood FE, Tang W, Benchimol EI, Panaccione R, Ghosh S, Wu JCY, Chan FKL, Sung JJY, Kaplan GG. Worldwide incidence and prevalence of inflammatory bowel disease in the 21st century: a systematic review of population-based studies. Lancet. 2018;390:2769–78.

59. Guan Q. A comprehensive review and update on the pathogenesis of inflammatory bowel disease. J Immunol Res. 2019;2019:7247238.

60. Rawla P, Sunkara T, Raj JP. Role of biologics and biosimilars in inflammatory bowel disease: current trends and future perspectives. J Inflamm Res. 2018;11:215–26.

61. Bunu DM, Timofte CE, Ciocoiu M, Floria M, Tarniceriu CC, Barboi OB, Tanase DM. Cardiovascular manifestations of inflammatory bowel disease: pathogenesis, diagnosis, and preventive strategies. Gastroenterol Res Pract. 2019;2019:3012509.

62. Zezos P, Kouklakis G, Saibil F. Inflammatory bowel disease and thromboembolism. World J Gastroenterol. 2014;20:13863–78.

63. Feng W, Chen G, Cai D, Zhao S, Cheng J, Shen H. Inflammatory bowel disease and risk of ischemic heart disease: an updated meta-analysis of cohort studies. J Am Heart Assoc. 2017;6:e005892.

64. Singh S, Dulai PS, Zarrinpar A, Ramamoorthy S, Sandborn WJ. Obesity in IBD: epidemiology, pathogenesis, disease course and treatment outcomes. Nat Rev Gastroenterol Hepatol. 2017;14:110–21.

65. Aarestrup J, Jess T, Kobylecki CJ, Nordestgaard BG, Allin KH. Cardiovascular risk profile among patients with inflammatory bowel disease: a population-based study of more than 100 000 individuals. J Crohns Colitis. 2019;13:319–23.

66. Schicho R, Marsche G, Storr M. Cardiovascular complications in inflammatory bowel disease. Curr Drug Targets. 2015;16:181–8.

67. Nos P, Domenech E. Management of Crohn's disease in smokers: is an alternative approach necessary? World J Gastroenterol. 2011;17:3567–74.

68. Jones PD, Kappelman MD, Martin CF, Chen W, Sandler RS, Long MD. Exercise decreases risk of future active disease in patients with inflammatory bowel disease in remission. Inflamm Bowel Dis. 2015;21:1063–71.

69. Rizzello F, Spisni E, Giovanardi E, Imbesi V, Salice M, Alvisi P, Valerii MC, Gionchetti P. Implications of the westernized diet in the onset and progression of IBD. Nutrients. 2019;11:1033.

70. Amre DK, D'Souza S, Morgan K, et al. Imbalances in dietary consumption of fatty acids, vegetables, and fruits are associated with risk for Crohn's disease in children. Am J Gastroenterol. 2007;102: 2016–25.

71. Levine A, Rhodes JM, Lindsay JO, et al. Dietary guidance from the international organization for the study of inflammatory bowel diseases. Clin Gastroenterol Hepatol. 2020;18:1381–92.

72. Rocha R, Santana GO, Almeida N, Lyra AC. Analysis of fat and muscle mass in patients with inflammatory bowel disease during remission and active phase. Br J Nutr. 2009;101:676–9.

73. Nguyen GC, Munsell M, Harris ML. Nationwide prevalence and prognostic significance of clinically diagnosable protein-calorie malnutrition in hospitalized inflammatory bowel disease patients. Inflamm Bowel Dis. 2008;14:1105–11.

74. Feinstein MJ, Hsue PY, Benjamin LA, Bloomfield GS, Currier JS, Freiberg MS, Grinspoon SK, Levin J, Longenecker CT, Post WS. Characteristics, prevention, and management of cardiovascular disease in people living with HIV: a scientific statement from the American Heart Association. Circulation. 2019;140:e98–e124.

75. Somsouk M, Estes JD, Deleage C, Dunham RM, Albright R, Inadomi JM, Martin JN, Deeks SG, McCune JM, Hunt PW. Gut epithelial barrier and systemic inflammation during chronic HIV infection. AIDS. 2015;29:43–51.

76. Moir S, Fauci AS. B cells in HIV infection and disease. Nat Rev Immunol. 2009;9:235–45.

77. Teigler JE, Leyre L, Chomont N, et al. Distinct biomarker signatures in HIV acute infection associate

with viral dynamics and reservoir size. JCI Insight. 2018;3:e98420.

78. Kuller LH, Tracy R, Belloso W, De Wit S, Drummond F, Lane HC, Ledergerber B, Lundgren J, Neuhaus J, Nixon D, Paton NI, Neaton JD, Group ISS. Inflammatory and coagulation biomarkers and mortality in patients with HIV infection. PLoS Med. 2008;5:e203.

79. Nou E, Lo J, Grinspoon SK. Inflammation, immune activation, and cardiovascular disease in HIV. AIDS. 2016;30:1495–509.

80. Arnett DK, Blumenthal RS, Albert MA, et al. 2019 ACC/AHA guideline on the primary prevention of cardiovascular disease: executive summary. Circulation. 2019;140(11):e563–95.

81. Capili B, Anastasi JK, Chang M, Ogedegbe O. Barriers and facilitators to engagement in lifestyle interventions among individuals with HIV. J Assoc Nurses AIDS Care. 2014;25:450–7.

82. d'Ettorre G, Ceccarelli G, Giustini N, Mastroianni CM, Silvestri G, Vullo V. Taming HIV-related inflammation with physical activity: a matter of timing. AIDS Res Hum Retrovir. 2014;30:936–44.

83. Botros D, Somarriba G, Neri D, Miller TL. Interventions to address chronic disease and HIV: strategies to promote exercise and nutrition among HIV-infected individuals. Curr HIV/AIDS Rep. 2012;9:351–63.

84. Poudel-Tandukar K, Chandyo RK. Dietary B vitamins and serum C-reactive protein in persons with human immunodeficiency virus infection: the positive living with HIV (POLH) study. Food Nutr Bull. 2016;37:517–28.

85. Fields-Gardner C, Campa A, American Dietetics Association. Position of the American Dietetic Association: nutrition intervention and human immunodeficiency virus infection. J Am Diet Assoc. 2010;110:1105–19.

86. Lazzaretti RK, Kuhmmer R, Sprinz E, Polanczyk CA, Ribeiro JP. Dietary intervention prevents dyslipidemia associated with highly active antiretroviral therapy in human immunodeficiency virus type 1-infected individuals: a randomized trial. J Am Coll Cardiol. 2012;59:979–88.

87. Tsiodras S, Poulia KA, Yannakoulia M, Chimienti SN, Wadhwa S, Karchmer AW, Mantzoros CS. Adherence to Mediterranean diet is favorably associated with metabolic parameters in HIV-positive patients with the highly active antiretroviral therapy-induced metabolic syndrome and lipodystrophy. Metabolism. 2009;58:854–9.

88. Oliveira JM, Rondo PH. Omega-3 fatty acids and hypertriglyceridemia in HIV-infected subjects on antiretroviral therapy: systematic review and meta-analysis. HIV Clin Trials. 2011;12:268–74.

Parag Anilkumar Chevli and Michael D. Shapiro

Introduction

Low-Density Lipoprotein and Atherosclerosis

Atherosclerosis is a complex process that involves many factors, but the cholesterol rich apolipoprotein B (apoB)-containing lipoproteins have emerged as the chief initiating and driving factor. Cholesterol and triglycerides, water-insoluble lipids, require protein-containing complexes called lipoproteins for solubilization in the aqueous plasma and for transport to tissue. ApoB is the major structural protein (apolipoprotein) found on atherogenic lipoproteins and serves as the scaffold for lipidation and as a ligand for receptor binding. The five major atherogenic lipoproteins include chylomicron remnants, very-low-density lipoprotein, intermediate-density lipoprotein, low-density lipoprotein (LDL), and lipoprotein(a). Although LDL is the principle atherogenic lipoprotein, largely due to its relatively high plasma concentrations relative to other lipoproteins, other apoB-containing lipoproteins (up to about 70 nm in diameter) also play a role in the

initiation and progression of atherosclerosis [1]. LDL particles penetrate the arterial endothelial cell lining, especially in the presence of endothelial dysfunction, and enter the subendothelial space where they interact with positively charged intimal proteoglycans to become retained in the arterial wall [2]. The subendothelial retention of apoB-containing lipoprotein particles leads to a complex interplay between metabolic and inflammatory processes that leads to the initiation of an atheroma. Early atherogenesis can be impacted by many factors including hyperlipidemia, lipoprotein influx, lipoprotein modification, turbulent blood flow, and alterations in the endothelium, smooth muscle cells, and matrix. According to the response-to-retention hypothesis of early atherogenesis, lipoprotein retention is an absolute prerequisite for lesion development and appears to be sufficient in the majority of circumstances to provoke otherwise normal cellular and matrix elements to participate in a stream of events leading to atherosclerosis [3].

Importance of Lowering LDL Cholesterol for Primary Prevention of Cardiovascular Disease

Data from numerous observational studies suggest that, even in the absence of other risk factors, severe hypercholesterolemia (e.g., LDL-cholesterol [LDL-C] $\geq$ 190 mg/dL) is associated with signifi-

P. A. Chevli · M. D. Shapiro (✉)
Center for Prevention of Cardiovascular Disease, Section on Cardiovascular Medicine, Wake Forest University Baptist Medical Center, Medical Center Boulevard, Winston Salem, NC, USA
e-mail: pchevli@wakehealth.edu;
mdshapir@wakehealth.edu

© Springer Nature Switzerland AG 2021
M. J. Wilkinson et al. (eds.), *Prevention and Treatment of Cardiovascular Disease*, Contemporary Cardiology, https://doi.org/10.1007/978-3-030-78177-4_13

cantly increased risk for atherosclerotic cardiovascular disease (ASCVD) [4]. One of the earlier trials evaluating the efficacy of decreasing cholesterol in reducing the risk of coronary heart disease (CHD) was the LRC-CCPT (Lipid Research Clinics Coronary Primary Prevention Trial), including 3806 asymptomatic middle-aged men. The study revealed that treatment with bile acid sequestrant cholestyramine was associated with a 20% reduction in LDL-C with an associated 19% reduction in the incidence of CHD [5]. In the Air Force/ Texas Coronary Atherosclerosis Prevention Study (AFCAPS/TexCAPS), treatment with lovastatin reduced LDL-C by 25% compared to placebo and reduced the incidence of first acute major coronary events after 5.2 years [6]. The (HOPE)-3 (Heart Outcomes Prevention Evaluation) trial studied the effect of statins in 12,705 intermediate-risk, ethnically diverse participants without cardiovascular disease [7]. Rosuvastatin reduced LDL-C level by 27% compared to the placebo at 5 years. Treatment with rosuvastatin resulted in a 24% reduction in the primary composite outcome of death from CVD, non-fatal myocardial infarction, or nonfatal stroke. The JUPITER (Justification for the Use of Statins in Prevention: an Intervention Trial Evaluating Rosuvastatin) trial, included 17,802 men and women free of cardiovascular disease at baseline with LDL-C levels <130 mg/dL and high-sensitivity C-reactive protein levels ≥2.0 mg/L and randomized them to rosuvastatin 20 mg daily vs. placebo. Rosuvastatin reduced LDL-C levels by 50% and significantly reduced the incidence of a first major cardiovascular event by 44% [8]. It is clear from the evidence that there is a significant benefit associated with LDL-C lowering in the primary prevention of ASCVD (Table 13.1).

Importance of Lowering LDL Cholesterol for Secondary Prevention of Cardiovascular Disease

Many large clinical trials assessed the impact of LDL-C lowering in patients with known CVD. In the 4S (Scandinavian Simvastatin Survival Study), 4444 patients with known CHD were randomly

assigned to simvastatin (10–40 mg daily) or placebo [9]. At the end of 5.4 years, simvastatin reduced LDL-C level by 35%. Treatment with simvastatin resulted in a 42% reduction in coronary mortality and a 35% reduction in major coronary events. More recently, non-statin therapies were evaluated in patients with ASCVD in the IMPROVE-IT (Improved Reduction of Outcomes: Vytorin Efficacy International Trial). This study enrolled 18,144 patients with a recent acute coronary syndrome (within 10 days of enrollment) and randomly assigned participants to receive simvastatin 40 mg plus ezetimibe 10 mg or simvastatin 40 mg daily plus placebo. The median time–weighted average LDL-C level during the study was 53.7 mg/dL in the simvastatin/ezetimibe group as compared with 69.5 mg/dL in the simvastatin monotherapy group [10]. At the conclusion of the study, there was a 6.5% proportional reduction in major cardiovascular events (cardiovascular death, non-fatal MI, unstable angina requiring hospitalization, coronary revascularization ≥30 days after randomization, or non-fatal stroke) with combination therapy compared to simvastatin/placebo. The study concluded that reducing LDL-C to levels below previous targets provided additional benefit (e.g., even lower LDL-C is even better). The discovery of proprotein convertase subtilisin/kexin type 9 (PCSK9) and the recent development and approval of the PCSK9 inhibitors have transformed our understanding of lipoprotein metabolism and our ability to manage patients with hypercholesterolemia and/or ASCVD. The FOURIER (Further Cardiovascular Outcomes Research with PCSK9 Inhibition in Subjects with Elevated Risk) trial assessed the efficacy of evolocumab when added to statin therapy in patients with clinically evident ASCVD [11]. In total, 27,564 participants with ASCVD and LDL-C levels of 70 mg/dL or higher who were on optimized statin therapy were randomly assigned to receive evolocumab (either 140 mg every 2 weeks or 420 mg monthly) or placebo. After a median follow-up of 2.2 years, treatment with evolocumab, as compared with placebo, led to a reduction in LDL-C from a median baseline value of 92–30 mg/dL corresponding to 59% reduction. There was a significant 15% reduction

Table 13.1 Primary prevention trials of lipid-lowering drugs

Trial	Study design	Sample size	Participants	Drug dosage	Follow-up time	Mean baseline LDL-C (mg/dL) and change with intervention	Primary outcome
AFCAPS/ TexCAPS [6]	RCT	6605	Participants without clinical evidence of ASCVD	Lovastatin (20–40 mg daily) or placebo	5.2 years	150, ↓ 25%	Incidence of first acute major coronary events ↓ 37%
ASCOT-LLA [89]	RCT	10,305	Hypertensive patients	Atorvastatin 10 mg daily or placebo	3.3 years	131, ↓ 30%	Non-fatal MI and fatal CHD ↓ 36%
HOPE-3 (7)	RCT	12,705	Intermediate-risk participants without CVD	Rosuvastatin 10 mg daily or placebo	5.6 years	128, ↓ 27%	Primary composite outcome of death from CVD, non-fatal MI, or non-fatal stroke ↓ 24%
JUPITER [8]	RCT	17,802	Participants free of CVD at baseline with LDL-C levels <130 mg/dL and high-sensitivity CRP levels ≥2.0 mg/L	Rosuvastatin 20 mg daily or placebo	1.9 years	108, ↓ 50%	First major cardiovascular event ↓ 44%
LRC-CPPT [5]	RCT	3806	Asymptomatic middle-aged men with primary hypercholesterolemia	Bile acid sequestrant cholestyramine resin or placebo	7.4 years	205, ↓ 20%	Definite CHD death ↓ 19% Non-fatal MI ↓ 24%
WOSCOPS [90]	RCT	2560	Participants with LDL-C ≥ 190 mg/dL and without evidence of vascular disease	Pravastatin 40 mg daily or placebo	4.9 years	206, ↓ 20%	CHD ↓ 27% MACE ↓ 25%

AFCAPS/TexCAPS Air Force/Texas Coronary Atherosclerosis Prevention Study, *ASCOT-LLA* Anglo Scandinavian Cardiac Outcomes Trial-Lipid Lowering Arm, *ASCVD* atherosclerotic cardiovascular disease, *CHD* coronary heart disease, *CRP* C-reactive protein, *CVD* cardiovascular disease, *HOPE-3* Heart Outcomes Prevention Evaluation Study 3, *JUPITER* Justification for the Use of Statins in Primary Prevention: An Intervention Trial Evaluating Rosuvastatin trial, *LDL-C* low-density lipoprotein cholesterol, *LRC-CPPT* Lipid Research Clinics Coronary Primary Prevention Trial, *MACE* major adverse cardiovascular event, *MI* myocardial infarction, *RCT* randomized controlled trial, *WOSCOPS* West of Scotland Coronary Prevention Study

in the risk of the primary composite endpoint of cardiovascular death, myocardial infarction, stroke, hospitalization for unstable angina, or coronary revascularization with evolocumab treatment above and beyond background optimal medical therapy. Several meta-analyses have also suggested similar cardiovascular benefits with an intensive lowering of LDL-C in patients with ASCVD [12–14]. In conclusion, the totality of the evidence indicates that reducing plasma LDL-C level is an integral component of secondary prevention of ASCVD (Table 13.2).

Table 13.2 Secondary prevention trials of lipid-lowering drugs

Trial	Study design	Sample size	Participants	Drug dosage	Follow-up time	Mean baseline LDL-C (mg/dL) and change with intervention	Primary outcome
4S [9]	RCT	4444	Patients with CHD	Simvastatin (10–40 mg daily) or placebo	5.4 years	188, ↓ 25%	Coronary mortality ↓ 42% Major coronary events ↓ 35%
CARE [91]	RCT	4159	Patients with MI	Pravastatin 40 mg daily or placebo	5 years	139, ↓ 32%	Fatal CHD or confirmed MI ↓ 24%
FOURIER [11]	RCT	27,564	Patients with ASCVD	Evolocumab (either 140 mg every 2 weeks or 420 mg monthly) or placebo	2.2 years	92, ↓ 59%	Primary composite outcome of cardiovascular death, MI, stroke, hospitalization for UA, or coronary revascularization ↓ 15%
IMPROVE-IT [10]	RCT	18,144	Patients who were hospitalized for an ACS within the preceding 10 days	Simvastatin (40 mg) and ezetimibe (10 mg) or simvastatin (40 mg) and placebo	6 years	94, ↓ 24%	Primary composite outcome of death from CVD, a major coronary event, or non-fatal stroke ↓ 6.5%
PROSPER [92]	RCT	5804	Patients with history of, or risk factors for, vascular disease	Pravastatin 40 mg daily or placebo	3.2 years	147, ↓ 34%	Primary composite outcome of death from CHD, non-fatal MI, and fatal or non-fatal stroke ↓ 15%
ODYSSEY [93]	RCT	18,924	Patients with ACS within the preceding 1–12 months	Alirocumab or 75 mg every 2 weeks or placebo	2.8 years	92, ↓ 55%	Primary composite endpoint of death from CHD, non-fatal MI, fatal or non-fatal ischemic stroke, or UA requiring hospitalization

4S Scandinavian Simvastatin Survival Study, *ACS* acute coronary syndrome, *ASCVD* atherosclerotic cardiovascular disease, *CARE* Cholesterol and Recurrent Events, *CHD* coronary heart disease, *CVD* cardiovascular disease, *FOURIER* Further Cardiovascular Outcomes Research with PCSK9 Inhibition in Subjects with Elevated Risk, *IMPROVE-IT* Improved Reduction of Outcomes: Vytorin Efficacy International Trial, *LDL-C* low-density lipoprotein cholesterol, *MI* myocardial infarction, *PROSPER* PROspective Study of Pravastatin in the Elderly at Risk, *RCT* randomized controlled trial, *UA* unstable angina

Impact of Diet on LDL-C

Dietary Fat and LDL

The relationship between macronutrient intake in the diet and plasma LDL-C concentrations is well known. Historically, there was an emphasis on the reduction of total dietary fat intake. In aggregate, clinical studies have failed to reveal a favorable impact on CVD by taking this approach [15]. However, it is now understood that the specific type of fat is far more critical in influencing plasma lipids and CVD outcomes [16].

Dietary Cholesterol

The main sources of dietary cholesterol are egg yolks. The other major sources include dairy products, shrimp, beef, pork, and poultry. A systematic review and meta-analysis of randomized controlled trials exploring the quantitative effect of egg consumption on serum lipid concentrations demonstrated that compared with non-egg-consumers, consumption of eggs increased LDL-C by 5.5 mg/dL [17]. However, the consumption of eggs also increased HDL-C, and there was no effect on the LDL-C: HDL-C ratio. A meta-analysis of 13 randomized controlled trials investigating the impact of dietary cholesterol interventions on serum LDL-C showed a significant increase in LDL-C when comparing intervention with control doses of dietary cholesterol [18]. The "National Lipid Association Recommendations for Patient-Centered Management of Dyslipidemia" recommend limiting cholesterol intake to <200 mg/day to maintain a cardioprotective eating pattern [19]. It is important to note that intestinal absorption of cholesterol is variable with both hyper- and hypo-absorbers. Some individuals show little or no increases in LDL-C in response to a higher intake of dietary cholesterol, while others show responses well above the average [19, 20]. Dietary Guidelines for Americans (2015–2020) do not limit the consumption of dietary cholesterol to 300 mg per day in contrast to the 2010 Dietary Guidelines [21]. However, the guideline suggests that limiting dietary cholesterol is an integral part of building a healthy eating pattern. It is particularly important that individuals with inherited hypercholesterolemia (e.g., familial hypercholesterolemia) continue to limit dietary cholesterol intake.

Saturated Fatty Acids

High concentrations of saturated fatty acids are found in red meat, dairy products, and plant-derived products such as palm kernel oil and coconut oil. Saturated fats increase LDL-C through different mechanisms (Fig. 13.1). However, issues related to saturated fats and their impacts on LDL-C are considerably more nuanced. The LDL-C raising effect of saturated fatty acids progressively increases as the chain length of saturated fat diminishes. Specifically, lauric acid (C12:0) is more potent than myristic acid (C14:0) and palmitic acid (C16:0) in increasing LDL-C. On the other hand, lauric acid has also been shown to increase high-density lipoprotein (HDL)-cholesterol (HDL-C), though the clinical significance of this effect is unclear [22]. The DELTA (Dietary Effects on Lipoproteins and Thrombogenic Activity) study compared the average American diet containing 15% of total calories from saturated fat to a low saturated fat diet containing 6.1% of total calories from saturated fat. The lower saturated fat diet was associated with an 11% reduction in LDL-C as compared to the typical American diet [23]. However, the evidence suggests that the effect of saturated fatty acids on LDL-C is modified by the food source within which they are consumed [24]. A randomized controlled trial of 49 participants demonstrated that cheese consumption was associated with lower LDL-C when compared with butter intake of equal fat content [25]. A meta-analysis of 36 randomized control trials of red meat consumption in comparison with other diets exhibited no significant difference in plasma LDL-C concentration [26]. Similarly, evidence has suggested that a higher intake of processed meat is associated with a neutral or increased risk of CVD, while

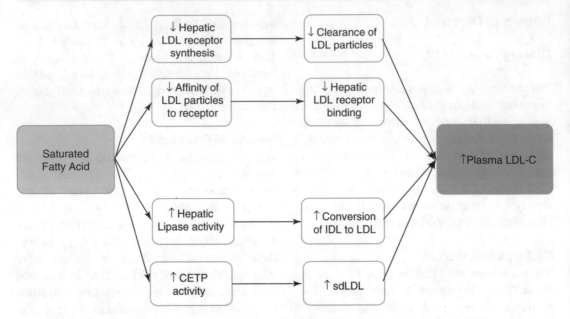

Fig. 13.1 Impact of saturated fatty acids on plasma LDL-C. CETP cholesteryl ester transfer protein, IDL intermediate-density lipoprotein, LDL-C low-density lipoprotein cholesterol, sdLDL small dense low-density lipoprotein

dairy products have a neutral or beneficial effect on CVD [16]. Evidence, as provided in these examples, has called into question the recommendation to keep total saturated fat consumption below 10% of total calories. In fact, many experts suggest evaluating the quality of dietary nutrients, components, and patterns rather than a rigid reliance on absolute proportions of macronutrients [27].

Polyunsaturated Fatty Acids

Omega-3 (ω-3) and Omega-6 (ω-6) fatty acids are polyunsaturated fatty acids (PUFAs) as they contain more than one *cis* double bond in the long-carbon fatty acid chain. Unlike saturated and monounsaturated fats, humans cannot synthesize PUFA because they lack desaturase enzymes necessary to insert a *cis* double bond at the n-3 and n-6 positions of a fatty acid. Hence, PUFA are considered essential fatty acids. Dietary ω-3 PUFA include eicosapentaenoic acid (EPA), docosahexaenoic acid (DHA), and α-linolenic acid (ALA). Oily fish such as herring, salmon, sardines, oysters, and tuna are the richest dietary sources of EPA and DHA. Flaxseed, chia seed, and walnuts are the primary dietary

sources of ALA. Most studies investigating the effect of ω-3 PUFA on plasma lipids are notable for the consistent triglyceride-lowering properties of EPA and DHA, particularly at high doses (4 grams per day). On the other hand, ω-3 PUFA have shown either no effect or a slight increase in LDL-C [28]. A 2018 Cochrane systematic review of 79 RCTs revealed no beneficial effect of EPA, DHA, or ALA on LDL-C [29]. However, most studies demonstrated an increase in mean LDL particle size without an increase in LDL particle number [29]. This shift toward large LDL particles may confer cardiovascular benefit, as small dense LDL (sdLDL) particles have relatively greater atherogenic potential [30]. Mechanisms by which sdLDL may facilitate atherogenesis are illustrated in Fig. 13.2.

The main dietary ω-6 PUFA are linoleic acid (LA) and arachidonic acid (AA). LA is found in vegetable oils such as safflower oil, sunflower oil, and corn oil, as well as nuts and seeds. AA is present in small amounts in eggs, meat, and poultry. A meta-analysis of 27 RCTs suggested a beneficial effect of LA on LDL-C [31]. A Cochrane systematic review of 19 RCTs, including 6461 participants, demonstrated that replacing dietary

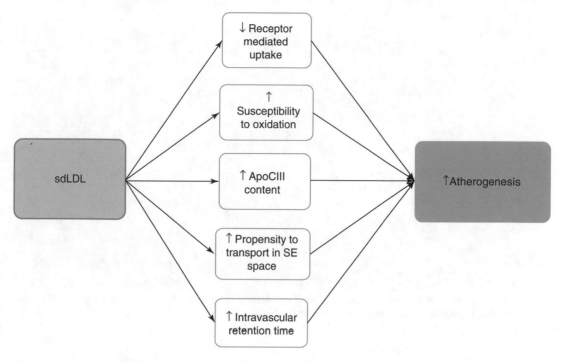

Fig. 13.2 Putative mechanisms for enhanced atherogenicity of small, dense LDL. ApoCIII apolipoprotein CIII, sdLDL small dense low-density lipoprotein, SE subendothelial space

saturated fatty acids with ω-6 PUFA lowered total blood cholesterol. Still, there was no evidence of LDL-C reducing benefits [32].

Monounsaturated Fatty Acids

In contrast to PUFA, monounsaturated fatty acid (MUFA) contains only one *cis* double bond. The primary source of MUFA includes dairy products, red meat, and plant-based oil, including olive oil. MUFA is also found in avocados, peanut butter, and other nuts and seeds. An RCT of 58 participants tested the effect of replacing saturated fat with MUFA or PUFA [33]. At the end of the study period, the serum LDL-C level decreased by 18% in those on the MUFA diet and by 13% in those on the PUFA diet. The study concluded that a diet rich in MUFA was as efficacious as a diet rich in PUFA in lowering LDL-C. In the OmniHeart (Optimal Macronutrient Intake Trial to Prevent Heart Disease) study, replacing saturated fat with MUFA led to a significant decrease in LDL-C [34]. A similar reduction in LDL-C was observed in a meta-

analysis of 27 trials investigating the replacement of saturated fat with MUFA [31].

Trans Fatty Acids

There are two main sources of *trans* fatty acids (TFA). Naturally occurring TFA can be found in small amounts from meat and dairy products. However, the major dietary source is synthetic TFA found in processed foods. The partial hydrogenation of unsaturated fat found in vegetable oil leads to the formation of TFA. This process is used by the food industry to increase the shelf-life of processed foods and to enhance flavor. A meta-analysis of 32 clinical trials demonstrated that a high intake of industrial TFA lead to increases in serum LDL-C [35]. Another meta-analysis of 12 randomized controlled trials on isocaloric replacement of saturated fat or *cis* unsaturated fats with TFA revealed that the consumption of TFA increases LDL-C as compared with the consumption of an equal number of calories from saturated or *cis* unsaturated fats [36]. Given their harmful effects on atherogenic lipid levels, sys-

Table 13.3 Dietary fats and LDL-C

	Cholesterol	SFA	ω-3 PUFA	ω-6 PUFA	MUFA	TFA
Sources	Egg yolks, chicken, beef, pork, shrimp, cheese, butter	Red meat, cheese, butter, whole milk, palm kernel oil, coconut oil	Oily fish such as herring, salmon, sardines, oysters, and tuna; flaxseed, chia seed, walnut	Vegetable oils such as safflower oil, sunflower oil, and corn oil; flaxseed, pumpkin seeds, walnuts	Vegetable oils such as olive oil, canola oil, peanut oil, sunflower, and safflower oils; avocados, peanut butter	Processed food, dairy products, beef, lamb
Effect on LDL-C	↑ LDL-C	↑ LDL-C	No effect on LDL-C	No effect on LDL-C	↓ LDL-C	↑ LDL-C
Recommendation	Limit cholesterol intake to reduce ASCVD risk	Limit SFA intake to less than 7% of total daily calories intake to reduce ASCVD risk	Replace SFA with PUFA to reduce ASCVD risk	Replace SFA with PUFA to reduce ASCVD risk	Replace SFA with MUFA to reduce ASCVD risk	Avoid TFA to reduce ASCVD risk

ASCVD atherosclerotic cardiovascular disease, *LDL-C* low-density lipoprotein cholesterol, *MUFA* monounsaturated fatty acids, *PUFA* polyunsaturated fatty acids, *SFA* saturated fatty acids

temic inflammation, and ASCVD, the 2019 ACC/AHA Guideline on the Primary Prevention of Cardiovascular Disease recommended minimizing the consumption of TFA [37].

In summary, dietary cholesterol is associated with increased LDL-C. The effect of saturated fat on LDL-C is modulated by the food source. EPA and DHA may not reduce LDL-C but could confer CVD protection through increasing LDL size and triglyceride lowering. Replacement of saturated fat with MUFA seems to have a beneficial effect on LDL-C. The consumption of TFA has been consistently shown to increase LDL-C (Table 13.3).

Dietary Sugars and LDL

The major source of added sugar among US adults aged 20 and overcomes from sugar-sweetened beverages such as fruit-flavored drinks, sodas, and sports drinks [38]. Low-calorie sweetened beverages and 100% fruit juices are frequently considered as a healthier alternative to sugar-sweetened beverages. A cross-sectional analysis from the National Health and Nutrition Examination Survey (NHANES) demonstrated that intake of added sugar was positively associated with higher LDL-C [39]. A prospective cohort of the Coronary Artery Risk Development in Young Adults (CARDIA) Study demonstrated that higher consumption of sugar-sweetened beverages was associated with increased risk of high LDL-C at 20 years [40]. A longitudinal study from the FOS (Framingham Offspring Study) and GEN3 (Generation Three) cohorts examined the association of sugar-sweetened beverages, low-calorie sweetened beverages, and fruit juice consumption with changes in the lipid profile [41]. The study demonstrated that the regular consumption of sugar-sweetened beverages was associated with decreased HDL-C and increased triglycerides. Moreover, recent low-calorie sweetened beverage consumption was associated with increased LDL-C. Sugar-sweetened beverages are sweetened primarily with fructose, sucrose, or high-fructose corn syrup (HFCS) [42]. A meta-analysis of 19 controlled feeding trials indicated that there was a dose–response relationship between fructose consumption and LDL-C [43]. Fructose intake >100 g/day significantly increased LDL-C by 11.6 mg/dL. A

2-week parallel-arm trial, including a total of 187 participants, demonstrated that consumption of beverages containing 10%, 17.5%, or 25% of energy requirements from HFCS produced significant linear dose-response increase fasting LDL cholesterol [44]. Hence, the 2019 ACC/AHA Guideline and the Dietary Guidelines for Americans (2015–2020) recommend minimizing or entirely eliminating sugar-sweetened beverage consumption [21, 37].

Dietary Fibers and LDL

Dietary fibers represent the indigestible part of plant foods. Dietary fibers are classified based on their solubility in water as soluble fibers or insoluble fibers. They are mainly found in vegetables, fruits, oats, nuts, barley, and legumes. Dietary fibers are also available as supplements that contain psyllium, methylcellulose, and wheat dextrin. A meta-analysis of 67 randomized controlled trials evaluating the effect of soluble fibers on plasma lipids found that soluble fiber consumption of 1 g/day was associated with approximately a 2 mg/dL reduction of LDL-C [45]. A randomized control trial of 68 patients evaluated the LDL-C lowering effect of psyllium added to simvastatin [46]. The study found that the addition of 15 g of daily psyllium fiber to 10 mg simvastatin/day achieved a similar 36% LDL-C reduction to that achieved with 20 mg simvastatin/day. A more recent meta-analysis of 28 randomized controlled trials evaluating the effects of psyllium on LDL-C found that the supplementation of 10.2 g/day of psyllium reduced the LDL-C by an average of 12.9 mg/dL. The National Lipid Association (NLA) and the 2016 ACC Expert Consensus Decision Pathway (ECDP), recommend the incorporation of soluble dietary fiber as a dietary adjunct for lowering LDL-C in patients with dyslipidemia [19, 47].

Phytosterols and LDL

Plant sterols and plant stanols are commonly referred to as phytosterols (plant-based ste-

rols) that are similar in structure to cholesterol. Phytosterols are found in foods of plant origin, including vegetable oils, nuts, whole grains, seeds, and legumes. There are also dietary supplements fortified with phytosterols available commercially. Numerous studies have demonstrated the beneficial effects of the consumption of foods enriched with free or esterified forms of phytosterols on LDL-C [48, 49]. A meta-analysis of 124 studies examining the LDL-C lowering effect of phytosterols demonstrated that the consumption of 0.6–3.3 g/day of phytosterols was associated with a 6–12% reduction in LDL-C in a dose-response fashion [50]. In one meta-analysis including 15 trials, phytosterols consumption of 1.8–6 g/day in patients treated with statins was associated with 11.7 mg/dL lower LDL-C compared with a statin alone [51]. The NLA and the 2016 ACC ECDP, recommend considering the use of phytosterols as a part of lifestyle modification to reduce LDL-C for primary and secondary prevention of ASCVD [19, 47].

Dietary Patterns and LDL

The 2019 ACC/AHA Guideline on the Primary Prevention of Cardiovascular Disease placed a significant emphasis on the benefits of a healthy diet [37]. In the following section, we will review some of the dietary patterns associated with improvements in the lipid profile, including LDL-C.

DASH Diet
The DASH (Dietary Approaches to Stop Hypertension) trial was an outpatient controlled feeding study including 459 participants who were randomized to either a control dietary pattern, similar to an average American diet or two experimental diets: FV (fruits, vegetable) diet or the DASH diet [52]. The FV dietary pattern contained more fruit, vegetables, and whole grains and fewer sweets but had macronutrient content similar to that of the control diet. The DASH diet was a combination of dietary patterns, and compared with the control and FV diet, it was higher

in protein and calcium and lower in saturated fat, total fat, and cholesterol. At the end of 8 weeks, the DASH diet, compared with the control diet, led to a significantly lower mean LDL-C level (−10.7 mg/dL), which represented a 9% net reduction [53]. The DASH-Sodium trial was a multicenter, randomized feeding trial, where participants were randomly assigned to a typical American control diet or the DASH diet, each prepared with three levels of sodium [54]. The study revealed that compared with the control diet, the DASH diet significantly lowered LDL-C. Further improvement in LDL-C was found when part of the carbohydrate content in the DASH diet was replaced with either unsaturated fat or protein in the OmniHeart trial [34]. The OmniHeart was a randomized, three-period crossover design comparing the effect of three healthful diets on serum lipids and blood pressure. The three diets included a carbohydrate-rich diet, similar to the DASH diet, a protein-rich diet, and a diet rich in unsaturated fat. The study demonstrated that the DASH diet decreased mean LDL-C by an absolute 11.6 mg/dL from baseline. Compared with the DASH diet, the protein-rich diet, but not the diet rich in unsaturated fat, significantly lowered LDL-C levels.

Mediterranean Diet

The Mediterranean dietary pattern represents the dietary habits of populations bordering the Mediterranean Sea. While there is considerable regional variation in the Mediterranean diet, perhaps more appropriately referred to as the Mediterranean pattern, there are some general similarities found in this dietary pattern. This diet is enriched in fruits, vegetables, complex carbohydrates, including whole grains, nuts, and seeds [55, 56]. Olive oil is a principal source of fat in this diet. Also, the typical Mediterranean diet is low in animal fat and simple sugars. The Med-RIVAGE (Mediterranean Diet, Cardiovascular Risks, and Gene Polymorphisms) study, including 212 participants with moderate CVD risk, demonstrated a beneficial effect on LDL-C with the Mediterranean-type diet [57]. The Indo-Mediterranean Diet Heart Study random-

ized 1000 patients with angina pectoris, myocardial infarction, or surrogate risk factors for CVD to receive either a diet rich in whole grains, fruits, vegetables, walnuts, and almonds or the Step 1 NCEP (National Cholesterol Education Program) diet. At the end of 2 years, both groups demonstrated a significant reduction in LDL-C. However, the effect was greater in the Mediterranean diet group [58]. A recent meta-analysis including 30 randomized control trials, including 12,461 participants comparing the Mediterranean dietary intervention versus usual care or another dietary intervention (e.g., low-fat, the traditional diet of that country, national recommendations/disease-specific guidance, and vegetarian), demonstrated that the Mediterranean diet produced small beneficial or no effect on LDL-C levels [59]. The PREDIMED (Prevención con Dieta Mediterránea) study is the largest randomized control study to evaluate the health effects of the Mediterranean diet on 7447 subjects at high risk for cardiovascular disease [60]. The participants were assigned to one of three diets: a Mediterranean diet supplemented with extra-virgin olive oil, a Mediterranean diet supplemented with mixed nuts, or a control diet (low-fat diet). The original trial, which was published in 2013, demonstrated a beneficial effect of the Mediterranean diet supplemented with extra-virgin olive oil or nuts on major cardiovascular events. However, it was retracted after identifying protocol deviations, including enrollment of household members without randomization, assignment to a study group without randomization of some participants at 1 of 11 study sites, and apparent inconsistent use of randomization tables at another site. After the omission of 1588 participants whose study-group assignments were known or suspected to have departed from the protocol, the results did not change [61]. A random subsample of 210 individuals from the PREDIMED study revealed that the Mediterranean diet supplemented with extra-virgin olive oil led to a statistically significant absolute 10.5 mg/dL decrease of LDL-C level. Moreover, measures of LDL oxidation and LDL particle size were improved in participants randomized to the Mediterranean diet supplemented with extra-virgin olive oil compared to the low-fat diet [62]. The Mediterranean diet supplemented with nuts exhibited similar trends but did not reach statistical significance.

Plant-Based Vegetarian Diet

There are many variations to the vegetarian diet, including the pescovegetarian diet (seafood with or without eggs and dairy), lactovegetarian diet (dairy), lacto-ovo-vegetarian diet (eggs and dairy), and vegan diet (no animal products). A plant-based vegetarian diet incorporates vegetables and fruits as well as whole grains, beans, legumes, nuts, and seeds. The Oxford Vegetarian Study was an observational study of 11,040 participants residing in the United Kingdom and revealed that vegans exhibited lower LDL-C compared to meat-eaters [63]. One of the earliest trials to examine the impact of lifestyle changes on the progression of coronary atherosclerosis was the Lifestyle Heart Trial, which was a randomized controlled trial conducted from 1986 to 1992, including 48 patients with moderate to severe coronary heart disease [64]. The participants in the experimental group were prescribed an intensive lifestyle program that included adhering to a vegetarian diet in addition to other lifestyle modifications (smoking cessation, exercise, and stress management). After 1 year, LDL-C levels decreased by 40% in the experimental group compared to a 1.2% decrease in LDL-C in the control group. In a crossover experiment, Cooper et al. examined the effects of a lactovegetarian diet in 15 healthy, nonsmoking physicians and medical students [65]. The participants were randomly assigned to a low-saturated fat vegetarian diet or a "typical American diet." Compared to the omnivorous diet, participants consuming the vegetarian diet experienced a 14.7% decrease in LDL-C. In the GEICO (Government Employees Insurance Company) study, 291 participants with a body mass index (BMI) $\geq 25\,kg/m2$ and/or a previous diagnosis of Type 2 diabetes were randomized to either a low-fat vegan diet or a group without any dietary changes [66]. After 18 weeks, LDL-C was reduced by 8.1 mg/dL for the participants consuming a low-fat vegan diet compared with

only 0.9 mg/dL reduction in LDL-C in the control group. Another randomized control trial investigated the impact of a low-fat vegan diet on cardiovascular risk factors in 99 individuals with Type 2 diabetes [67]. The participants were randomized to a low-fat, low-glycemic index vegan diet or to the American Diabetes Association (ADA) diet. After 22 weeks, the participants consuming a vegan diet experienced a 21.2% reduction in LDL-C compared to a 10.7% reduction in those consuming the ADA diet. It is important to note that the benefits of the vegetarian diet could be due to specific components of the diet with lipid-lowering properties. The "portfolio" diet is a vegan diet with emphasis on plant sterols, soy foods, viscous fibers, and almonds. In a randomized control trial of 25 individuals with hyperlipidemia, participants were randomized to either a portfolio diet or a lacto-ovo-vegetarian diet [68]. At the end of the trial, LDL-C was reduced by 12.1% in the participants assigned to a lacto-ovo-vegetarian diet while the portfolio diet led to a 35% reduction in LDL-C. Another study examining the impact of the portfolio diet enrolled 45 hyperlipidemic individuals to determine whether the portfolio diet leads to cholesterol reduction similar to statins [69]. The participants were randomly assigned to either a low-fat diet, a low-fat diet plus lovastatin, or a vegetarian portfolio diet. Interestingly, the portfolio diet group and the low-fat diet plus statin group demonstrated significant and comparable reductions in LDL-C. A 2017 meta-analysis, including 49 studies (30 observational studies and 19 clinical trials), demonstrated that compared to the omnivorous diet, the plant-based vegetarian diet lowered LDL-C by 15–30% [70]. The CARDIVEG (Cardiovascular Prevention With Vegetarian Diet) was the first randomized control trial assessing the effects of a lacto-ovo-vegetarian diet compared to a Mediterranean diet on CVD risk factors [71]. After 3 months of dietary intervention, compared with the Mediterranean diet, the vegetarian diet led to a significant reduction in LDL-C. The plant-based vegetarian diets may reduce serum LDL-C through multiple mechanisms [72]. The plant-based vegetarian diet, including fruits, vegetables, whole grains, legumes, nuts, and various soy products, contain a number of phytochemicals including plant sterols and/or stanols, phytoestrogen, and flavonoids [73]. The beneficial effect of plant sterols/stanols and flavonoids is likely related to inhibition of cholesterol absorption in the small intestine [74]. The phytoestrogen content of soy facilitates plasma LDL-C reduction through an increase in the excretion of bile acids with concomitant increased LDL receptor expression on hepatocytes [75]. Phytoestrogens can also inhibit the oxidation of LDL [76].

Ketogenic Diet

The ketogenic diet is a high-fat, low-carbohydrate diet that has generated a lot of interest and has led to a great deal of debate, especially regarding its safety and long-term effects on cardiovascular health [77]. There are many versions of a ketogenic diet with a different ratio of macronutrients. In general, the typical ketogenic diet consists of 70–80% calories from fat, 10–20% calories from protein, and 5–10% from carbohydrate. The ketogenic diet causes the body to break down fat into ketones, which becomes the primary source of energy. The hypothesized favorable mechanisms of ketosis include appetite suppressant action of the ketone bodies, increased lipolysis, and greater metabolic efficiency in consuming fats [78]. A randomized control trial of 30 normal-weight, healthy individuals, assessed the impact of the ketogenic diet on LDL-C. The participants were assigned to either a ketogenic diet or a habitual diet for 3 weeks. There was a 44% increase in LDL-C among the participants allocated to the ketogenic diet at the end of 3 weeks, while LDL-C remained unchanged in the control group [79]. Similarly, several meta-analyses also demonstrated deleterious effects on plasma LDL-C associated with the ketogenic diet [80–82].

Intermittent Fasting

Intermittent fasting (IF) includes different eating patterns such as time-restricted feeding, alternate-day fasting, and 5:2 intermittent fasting (fasting 2 days each week) [83]. The exact underlying mechanism of the potentially ben-

eficial effects of IF is not entirely understood but may involve bolstering cellular stress resistance and metabolic switching [84]. In a single-arm, paired-sample trial, 19 participants with metabolic syndrome underwent 10 h of time-restricted feeding for 12 weeks [85]. At the end of 12 weeks, participants observed a significant reduction in LDL-C (-12 ± 19 mg/dL [-11%], $p = 0.016$), and this effect was independent of weight loss. Another study examined the effect of alternate-day fasting on CVD risk factors in obese individuals. The study enrolled 16 individuals who completed the 10-week trial consisting of three phases: (1) a 2-week control phase, (2) a 4-week weight loss/alternate-day fasting controlled food intake phase, and (3) a 4-week weight loss/alternate-day fasting self-selected food intake phase. At the study conclusion, there was a 25% reduction in LDL-C. Several other studies have also demonstrated the LDL-C lowering effect of IF [86–88].

Conclusion

LDL is in the causal pathway of ASCVD, and, as such, it is the primary target of therapy in all major international guidelines. Lifestyle modifications, including the adoption of a healthy dietary pattern, remain paramount in the prevention and management of ASCVD. The focus has shifted from restricting the total fat intake to a focus on the quality of specific types of fat as a means to reduce LDL-C and mitigate the risk of ASCVD. In general, the effect of dietary fat on LDL-C is complex. Moreover, humans consume food that contains different types and ratios of macronutrients like fats rather than eating in isolation. In recognition of the complexity of the impact of isolated nutrients on LDL-C, it is crucial to focus on a healthy dietary pattern. The totality of the evidence suggests that any dietary pattern that incorporates more vegetables, fruits, whole grains, and nuts optimizes LDL-C lowering and is associated with improved cardiovascular outcomes (Table 13.4).

Table 13.4 Dietary patterns and LDL-C

	Study design	Sample size	Control/ baseline diet	Intervention diet	Change in LDL-C with intervention diet
DASH diet					
DASH [53]	RCT	459	Typical American diet	The fruits and vegetable diet or the DASH diet	↓ 9% from baseline with the DASH diet
OmniHeart [34]	RCT	164	Typical American diet	The carbohydrate (DASH) diet, the protein diet or the unsaturated fat diet	↓ 10% from baseline with the DASH diet
Mediterranean diet					
Med-RIVAGE [57]	RCT	212	Western-type diet	Mediterranean diet or a low-fat American Heart Association-type diet	↓ 11% from baseline with a Mediterranean diet
PREDIMED [61, 62]	RCT	210	Low-fat diet	Mediterranean diet supplemented with extra-virgin olive oil or a Mediterranean diet supplemented with mixed nuts	↓ 8% from baseline with a Mediterranean diet supplemented with extra-virgin olive oil
Plant-based vegetarian diet					
LIFESTYLE Heart [64]	RCT	48	Regular diet	Low-fat vegetarian diet	↓ 40% from baseline with a low-fat vegetarian diet
CARDIVEG [71]	RCT	118	Mediterranean diet	Lacto-ovo-vegetarian diet	↓ 5.5% from baseline with a Lacto-ovo-vegetarian diet

CARDIVEG Cardiovascular Prevention With Vegetarian Diet, *DASH* Dietary Approaches to Stop Hypertension, *Med-RIVAGE* Mediterranean Diet, Cardiovascular Risks, and Gene Polymorphisms, *PREDIMED* Prevención con Dieta Mediterránea, *RCT* randomized controlled trial

Conflicts of Interest Michael D. Shapiro: reports scientific advisory activities with Amgen, Esperion, and Regeneron as well as consultant activities with Novartis. Parag Anilkumar Chevli: declares no conflicts of interest.

References

1. Boren J, Williams KJ. The central role of arterial retention of cholesterol-rich apolipoprotein-B-containing lipoproteins in the pathogenesis of atherosclerosis: a triumph of simplicity. Curr Opin Lipidol. 2016;27(5):473–83.
2. Tabas I, Williams KJ, Boren J. Subendothelial lipoprotein retention as the initiating process in atherosclerosis - update and therapeutic implications. Circulation. 2007;116(16):1832–44.
3. Williams KJ, Tabas I. The response-to-retention hypothesis of early atherogenesis. Arterioscler Thromb Vasc Biol. 1995;15(5):551–61.
4. Perak AM, Ning H, de Ferranti SD, Gooding HC, Wilkins JT, Lloyd-Jones DM. Long-term risk of atherosclerotic cardiovascular disease in US adults with the familial hypercholesterolemia phenotype. Circulation. 2016;134(1):9–19.
5. The Lipid Research Clinics Coronary Primary Prevention Trial results. I. Reduction in incidence of coronary heart disease. JAMA. 1984;251(3):351–64.
6. Downs JR, Clearfield M, Weis S, Whitney E, Shapiro DR, Beere PA, et al. Primary prevention of acute coronary events with lovastatin in men and women with average cholesterol levels: results of AFCAPS/TexCAPS. Air Force/Texas Coronary Atherosclerosis Prevention Study. JAMA. 1998;279(20):1615–22.
7. Yusuf S, Bosch J, Dagenais G, Zhu J, Xavier D, Liu L, et al. Cholesterol lowering in intermediate-risk persons without cardiovascular disease. N Engl J Med. 2016;374(21):2021–31.
8. Ridker PM, Danielson E, Fonseca FA, Genest J, Gotto AM Jr, Kastelein JJ, et al. Rosuvastatin to prevent vascular events in men and women with elevated C-reactive protein. N Engl J Med. 2008;359(21):2195–207.
9. Pedersen TR, Kjekshus J, Berg K, Haghfelt T, Faergeman O, Thorgeirsson G, et al. Randomized trial of cholesterol-lowering in 4444 patients with coronary-heart-disease – the Scandinavian Simvastatin Survival Study (4s). Lancet. 1994;344(8934):1383–9.
10. Cannon CP, Blazing MA, Giugliano RP, McCagg A, White JA, Theroux P, et al. Ezetimibe added to statin therapy after acute coronary syndromes. N Engl J Med. 2015;372(25):2387–97.
11. Sabatine MS, Giugliano RP, Keech AC, Honarpour N, Wiviott SD, Murphy SA, et al. Evolocumab and clinical outcomes in patients with cardiovascular disease. N Engl J Med. 2017;376(18):1713–22.
12. LaRosa JC, Grundy SM, Waters DD, Shear C, Barter P, Fruchart J, et al. Intensive lipid lowering with

atorvastatin in patients with stable coronary disease. N Engl J Med. 2005;352(14):1425–35.

13. Baigent C, Blackwell L, Emberson J, Holland LE, Reith C, Bhala N, et al. Efficacy and safety of more intensive lowering of LDL cholesterol: a meta-analysis of data from 170 000 participants in 26 randomised trials. Lancet. 2010;376(9753):1670–81.

14. Mills EJ, O'Regan C, Eyawo O, Wu P, Mills F, Berwanger O, et al. Intensive statin therapy compared with moderate dosing for prevention of cardiovascular events: a meta-analysis of > 40 000 patients. Eur Heart J. 2011;32(11):1409–U138.

15. Harcombe Z, Baker JS, DiNicolantonio JJ, Grace F, Davies B. Evidence from randomised controlled trials does not support current dietary fat guidelines: a systematic review and meta-analysis. Open Heart. 2016;3(2):e000409.

16. Siri-Tarino PW, Chiu S, Bergeron N, Krauss RM. Saturated fats versus polyunsaturated fats versus carbohydrates for cardiovascular disease prevention and treatment. Annu Rev Nutr. 2015;35:517–43.

17. Rouhani MH, Rashidi-Pourfard N, Salehi-Abargouei A, Karimi M, Haghighatdoost F. Effects of egg consumption on blood lipids: a systematic review and meta-analysis of randomized clinical trials. J Am Coll Nutr. 2018;37(2):99–110.

18. Berger S, Raman G, Vishwanathan R, Jacques PF, Johnson EJ. Dietary cholesterol and cardiovascular disease: a systematic review and meta-analysis. Am J Clin Nutr. 2015;102(2):276–94.

19. Jacobson TA, Maki KC, Orringer CE, Jones PH, Kris-Etherton P, Sikand G, et al. National Lipid Association recommendations for patient-centered management of dyslipidemia: part 2. J Clin Lipidol. 2015;9(6): S1–S122.

20. Griffin JD, Lichtenstein AH. Dietary cholesterol and plasma lipoprotein profiles: randomized-controlled trials. Curr Nutr Rep. 2013;2(4):274–82.

21. US Department of Health and Human Services; US Department of Agriculture. 2015–2020 Dietary Guidelines for Americans. 8th ed. Washington, DC: US Dept of Health and Human Services; December 2015. http://www.health.gov/DietaryGuidelines. Accessed Aug 2020.

22. Mensink RP, Zock PL, Kester ADM, Katan MB. Effects of dietary fatty acids and carbohydrates on the ratio of serum total to HDL cholesterol and on serum lipids and apolipoproteins: a meta-analysis of 60 controlled trials. Am J Clin Nutr. 2003;77(5): 146–55.

23. Ginsberg HN, Kris-Etherton P, Dennis B, Elmer PJ, Ershow A, Lefevre M, et al. Effects of reducing dietary saturated fatty acids on plasma lipids and lipoproteins in healthy subjects: the DELTA Study, protocol 1. Arterioscler Thromb Vasc Biol. 1998;18(3):441–9.

24. Astrup A, Dyerberg J, Elwood P, Hermansen K, Hu FB, Jakobsen MU, et al. The role of reducing intakes of saturated fat in the prevention of cardiovascular disease: where does the evidence stand in 2010? Am J Clin Nutr. 2011;93(4):684–8.

25. Hjerpsted J, Leedo E, Tholstrup T. Cheese intake in large amounts lowers LDL-cholesterol concentrations compared with butter intake of equal fat content. Am J Clin Nutr. 2011;94(6):1479–84.

26. Guasch-Ferre M, Satija A, Blondin SA, Janiszewski M, Emlen E, O'Connor LE, et al. Meta-analysis of randomized controlled trials of red meat consumption in comparison with various comparison diets on cardiovascular risk factors. Circulation. 2019;139(15):1828–45.

27. Freeland-Graves JH, Nitzke S, Academy of Nutrition and Dietetics. Position of the academy of nutrition and dietetics: total diet approach to healthy eating. J Acad Nutr Diet. 2013;113(2):307–17.

28. Oscarsson J, Hurt-Camejo E. Omega-3 fatty acids eicosapentaenoic acid and docosahexaenoic acid and their mechanisms of action on apolipoprotein Bcontaining lipoproteins in humans: a review. Lipids Health Dis. 2017;16(1):149.

29. Abdelhamid AS, Brown TJ, Brainard JS, Biswas P, Thorpe GC, Moore HJ, et al. Omega-3 fatty acids for the primary and secondary prevention of cardiovascular disease. Cochrane Database Syst Rev. 2018;7:CD003177.

30. Berneis KK, Krauss RM. Metabolic origins and clinical significance of LDL heterogeneity. J Lipid Res. 2002;43(9):1363–79.

31. Mensink RP, Katan MB. Effect of dietary fatty acids on serum lipids and lipoproteins. A meta-analysis of 27 trials. Arterioscler Thromb. 1992;12(8):911–9.

32. Hooper L, Al-Khudairy L, Abdelhamid AS, Rees K, Brainard JS, Brown TJ, et al. Omega-6 fats for the primary and secondary prevention of cardiovascular disease. Cochrane Database Syst Rev. 2018;7: CD011094.

33. Mensink RP, Katan MB. Effect of a diet enriched with monounsaturated or polyunsaturated fatty acids on levels of low-density and high-density lipoprotein cholesterol in healthy women and men. N Engl J Med. 1989;321(7):436–41.

34. Appel LJ, Sacks FM, Carey VJ, Obarzanek E, Swain JF, Miller ER, et al. Effects of protein, monounsaturated fat, and carbohydrate intake on blood pressure and serum lipids – results of the OmniHeart randomized trial. JAMA. 2005;294(19):2455–64.

35. Liska DJ, Cook CM, Wang DD, Gaine PC, Baer DJ. Trans fatty acids and cholesterol levels: an evidence map of the available science. Food Chem Toxicol. 2016;98:269–81.

36. Mozaffarian D, Katan MB, Ascherio A, Stampfer MJ, Willett WC. Medical progress – trans fatty acids and cardiovascular disease. N Engl J Med. 2006;354(15):1601–13.

37. Arnett DK, Blumenthal RS, Albert MA, Buroker AB, Goldberger ZD, Hahn EJ, et al. 2019 ACC/AHA guideline on the primary prevention of cardiovascular disease: executive summary: a report of the American College of Cardiology/American Heart Association task force on clinical practice guidelines. Circulation. 2019;140(11):E563–E95.

38. Rosinger A, Herrick K, Gahche J, Park S. Sugar-sweetened beverage consumption among U.S. youth, 2011–2014. NCHS Data Brief. 2017(271):1–8.

39. Welsh JA, Sharma A, Cunningham SA, Vos MB. Consumption of added sugars and indicators of cardiovascular disease risk among US adolescents. Circulation. 2011;123(3):249–57.

40. Duffey KJ, Gordon-Larsen P, Steffen LM, Jacobs DR, Popkin BM. Drinking caloric beverages increases the risk of adverse cardiometabolic outcomes in the Coronary Artery Risk Development in Young Adults (CARDIA) Study. Am J Clin Nutr. 2010;92(4):954–9.

41. Haslam DE, Peloso GM, Herman MA, Dupuis J, Lichtenstein AH, Smith CE, et al. Beverage consumption and longitudinal changes in lipoprotein concentrations and incident dyslipidemia in US adults: the Framingham Heart Study. J Am Heart Assoc. 2020;9(5):e014083.

42. Ventura EE, Davis JN, Goran MI. Sugar content of popular sweetened beverages based on objective laboratory analysis: focus on fructose content. Obesity (Silver Spring). 2011;19(4):868–74.

43. Zhang YH, An T, Zhang RC, Zhou Q, Huang Y, Zhang J. Very high fructose intake increases serum LDL-cholesterol and total cholesterol: a meta-analysis of controlled feeding trials. J Nutr. 2013;143(9):1391–8.

44. Stanhope KL, Medici V, Bremer AA, Lee V, Lam HD, Nunez MV, et al. A dose-response study of consuming high-fructose corn syrup-sweetened beverages on lipid/lipoprotein risk factors for cardiovascular disease in young adults. Am J Clin Nutr. 2015;101(6): 1144–54.

45. Brown L, Rosner B, Willett WW, Sacks FM. Cholesterol-lowering effects of dietary fiber: a meta-analysis. Am J Clin Nutr. 1999;69(1):30–42.

46. Moreyra AE, Wilson AC, Koraym A. Effect of combining psyllium fiber with simvastatin in lowering cholesterol. Arch Intern Med. 2005;165(10):1161–6.

47. Lloyd-Jones DM, Morris PB, Ballantyne CM, Birtcher KK, Daly DD Jr, DePalma SM, et al. 2017 focused update of the 2016 ACC expert consensus decision pathway on the role of non-statin therapies for LDL-cholesterol lowering in the management of atherosclerotic cardiovascular disease risk: a report of the American College of Cardiology Task Force on Expert Consensus Decision Pathways. J Am Coll Cardiol. 2017;70(14):1785–822.

48. Miettinen TA, Puska P, Gylling H, Vanhanen H, Vartiainen E. Reduction of serum cholesterol with sitostanol-ester margarine in a mildly hypercholesterolemic population. N Engl J Med. 1995;333(20):1308–12.

49. Katan MB, Grundy SM, Jones P, Law M, Miettinen T, Paoletti R, et al. Efficacy and safety of plant stanols and sterols in the management of blood cholesterol levels. Mayo Clin Proc. 2003;78(8):965–78.

50. Ras RT, Geleijnse JM, Trautwein EA. LDL-cholesterol-lowering effect of plant sterols and stanols across different dose ranges: a meta-analysis of randomised controlled studies. Br J Nutr. 2014;112(2): 214–9.

51. Han S, Jiao J, Xu J, Zimmermann D, Actis-Goretta L, Guan L, et al. Effects of plant stanol or sterol-enriched diets on lipid profiles in patients treated with statins: systematic review and meta-analysis. Sci Rep. 2016;6:31337.

52. Appel LJ, Moore TJ, Obarzanek E, Vollmer WM, Svetkey LP, Sacks FM, et al. A clinical trial of the effects of dietary patterns on blood pressure. DASH Collaborative Research Group. N Engl J Med. 1997;336(16):1117–24.

53. Obarzanek E, Sacks FM, Vollmer WM, Bray GA, Miller ER 3rd, Lin PH, et al. Effects on blood lipids of a blood pressure-lowering diet: the Dietary Approaches to Stop Hypertension (DASH) trial. Am J Clin Nutr. 2001;74(1):80–9.

54. Harsha DW, Sacks FM, Obarzanek E, Svetkey LP, Lin PH, Bray GA, et al. Effect of dietary sodium intake on blood lipids – results from the DASH-Sodium trial. Hypertension. 2004;43(2):393–8.

55. Willett WC, Sacks F, Trichopoulou A, Drescher G, Ferroluzzi A, Helsing E, et al. Mediterranean diet pyramid – a cultural model for healthy eating. Am J Clin Nutr. 1995;61(6):1402s–6s.

56. Shen J, Wilmot KA, Ghasemzadeh N, Molloy DL, Burkman G, Mekonnen G, et al. Mediterranean dietary patterns and cardiovascular health. Annu Rev Nutr. 2015;35:425–49.

57. Vincent-Baudry S, Defoort C, Gerber M, Bernard MC, Verger P, Helal O, et al. The Medi-RIVAGE study: reduction of cardiovascular disease risk factors after a 3-mo intervention with a Mediterranean-type diet or a low fat diet. Am J Clin Nutr. 2005;82(5):964–71.

58. Singh RB, Dubnov G, Niaz MA, Ghosh S, Singh R, Rastogi SS, et al. Effect of an indo-Mediterranean diet on progression of coronary artery disease in high risk patients (Indo-Mediterranean Diet Heart Study): a randomised single-blind trial. Lancet. 2002;360(9344):1455–61.

59. Rees K, Takeda A, Martin N, Ellis L, Wijesekara D, Vepa A, et al. Mediterranean-style diet for the primary and secondary prevention of cardiovascular disease. Cochrane Database Syst Rev. 2019;3:CD009825.

60. Estruch R, Ros E, Salas-Salvado J, Covas MI, Corella D, Aros F, et al. Primary prevention of cardiovascular disease with a Mediterranean diet. N Engl J Med. 2013;368(14):1279–90.

61. Estruch R, Ros E, Salas-Salvado J, Covas MI, Corella D, Aros F, et al. Primary prevention of cardiovascular disease with a Mediterranean diet supplemented with extra-virgin olive oil or nuts. N Engl J Med. 2018;378(25):e34.

62. Hernáez Á, Castañer O, Goday A, Ros E, Pintó X, Estruch R, et al. The Mediterranean Diet decreases LDL atherogenicity in high cardiovascular risk individuals: a randomized controlled trial. 2017;61(9):1601015.

63. Thorogood M, Carter R, Benfield L, McPherson K, Mann JI. Plasma lipids and lipoprotein cholesterol concentrations in people with different diets in Britain. Br Med J (Clin Res Ed). 1987;295(6594):351–3.

64. Ornish D, Scherwitz LW, Billings JH, Brown SE, Gould KL, Merritt TA, et al. Intensive lifestyle changes for reversal of coronary heart disease. JAMA. 1998;280(23):2001–7.

65. Cooper RS, Goldberg RB, Trevisan M, Tsong Y, Liu K, Stamler J, et al. The selective lipid-lowering effect of vegetarianism on low-density lipoproteins in a crossover experiment. Atherosclerosis. 1982;44(3):293–305.

66. Mishra S, Xu J, Agarwal U, Gonzales J, Levin S, Barnard ND. A multicenter randomized controlled trial of a plant-based nutrition program to reduce body weight and cardiovascular risk in the corporate setting: the GEICO study. Eur J Clin Nutr. 2013;67(7):718–24.

67. Barnard ND, Cohen J, Jenkins DJA, Turner-McGrievy G, Gloede L, Jaster B, et al. A low-fat vegan diet improves glycemic control and cardiovascular risk factors in a randomized clinical trial in individuals with type 2 diabetes. Diabetes Care. 2006;29(8):1777–83.

68. Jenkins DJA, Kendall CWC, Marchie A, Faulkner D, Vidgen E, Lapsley KG, et al. The effect of combining plant sterols, soy protein, viscous fibers, and almonds in treating hypercholesterolemia. Metab-Clin Exp. 2003;52(11):1478–83.

69. Jenkins DJA, Kendall CWC, Marchie A, Faulkner DA, Wong JMW, de Souza R, et al. Effects of a dietary portfolio of cholesterol-lowering foods vs lovastatin on serum lipids and C-reactive protein. JAMA. 2003;290(4):502–10.

70. Yokoyama Y, Levin SM, Barnard ND. Association between plant-based diets and plasma lipids: a systematic review and meta-analysis. Nutr Rev. 2017;75(9):683–98.

71. Sofi F, Dinu M, Pagliai G, Cesari F, Gori AM, Sereni A, et al. Low-calorie vegetarian versus Mediterranean diets for reducing body weight and improving cardiovascular risk profile CARDIVEG study (cardiovascular prevention with vegetarian diet). Circulation. 2018;137(11):1103–13.

72. Ferdowsian HR, Barnard ND. Effects of plant-based diets on plasma lipids. Am J Cardiol. 2009;104(7):947–56.

73. deLorgeril M, Salen P, Martin JL, Mamelle N, Monjaud I, Touboul P, et al. Effect of a Mediterranean type of diet on the rate of cardiovascular complications in patients with coronary artery disease – insights into the cardioprotective effect of certain nutriments. J Am Coll Cardiol. 1996;28(5):1103–8.

74. Tilvis RS, Miettinen TA. Serum plant sterols and their relation to cholesterol absorption. Am J Clin Nutr. 1986;43(1):92–7.

75. Erdman JW, Comm AN. Soy protein and cardiovascular disease – a statement for healthcare professionals from the Nutrition Committee of the AHA. Circulation. 2000;102(20):2555–9.

76. Damasceno NRT, Apolinario E, Flauzino FD, Fernandes I, Abdalla DSP. Soy isoflavones reduce electronegative low-density lipoprotein (LDL-) and anti-LDL- autoantibodies in experimental atherosclerosis. Eur J Nutr. 2007;46(3):125–32.

77. O'Neill B, Raggi P. The ketogenic diet: pros and cons. Atherosclerosis. 2020;292:119–26.

78. Paoli A. Ketogenic diet for obesity: friend or foe? Int J Environ Res Public Health. 2014;11(2):2092–107.

79. Retterstol K, Svendsen M, Narverud I, Holven KB. Effect of low carbohydrate high fat diet on LDL cholesterol and gene expression in normal-weight, young adults: a randomized controlled study. Atherosclerosis. 2018;279:52–61.

80. Bueno NB, de Melo ISV, de Oliveira SL, Ataide TD. Very-low-carbohydrate ketogenic diet v. low-fat diet for long-term weight loss: a meta-analysis of randomised controlled trials. Br J Nutr. 2013;110(7):1178–87.

81. Dong T, Guo M, Zhang P, Sun G, Chen B. The effects of low-carbohydrate diets on cardiovascular risk factors: a meta-analysis. PLoS One. 2020;15(1):e0225348.

82. Mansoor N, Vinknes KJ, Veierod MB, Retterstol K. Effects of low-carbohydrate diets v. low-fat diets on body weight and cardiovascular risk factors: a meta-analysis of randomised controlled trials. Br J Nutr. 2016;115(3):466–79.

83. Anton SD, Moehl K, Donahoo WT, Marosi K, Lee SA, Mainous AG 3rd, et al. Flipping the Metabolic Switch: Understanding and Applying the Health Benefits of Fasting. Obesity (Silver Spring). 2018;26(2):254–68.

84. de Cabo R, Mattson MP. Effects of intermittent fasting on health, aging, and disease. N Engl J Med. 2019;381(26):2541–51.

85. Wilkinson MJ, Manoogian ENC, Zadourian A, Lo H, Fakhouri S, Shoghi A, et al. Ten-hour time-restricted eating reduces weight, blood pressure, and atherogenic lipids in patients with metabolic syndrome. Cell Metab. 2020;31(1):92–104. e5

86. Most J, Gilmore LA, Smith SR, Han H, Ravussin E, Redman LM. Significant improvement in cardiometabolic health in healthy nonobese individuals during caloric restriction-induced weight loss and weight loss maintenance. Am J Physiol Endocrinol Metab. 2018;314(4):E396–405.

87. Lefevre M, Redman LM, Heilbronn LK, Smith JV, Martin CK, Rood JC, et al. Caloric restriction alone and with exercise improves CVD risk in healthy nonobese individuals. Atherosclerosis. 2009;203(1):206–13.

88. Kroeger CM, Klempel MC, Bhutani S, Trepanowski JF, Tangney CC, Varady KA. Improvement in coronary heart disease risk factors during an intermittent fasting/calorie restriction regimen: relationship to adipokine modulations. Nutr Metab (Lond). 2012;9(1):98.

89. Sever PS, Dahlof B, Poulter NR, Wedel H, Beevers G, Caulfield M, et al. Prevention of coronary and stroke events with atorvastatin in hypertensive patients who have average or lower-than-average cholesterol concentrations, in the Anglo-Scandinavian Cardiac Outcomes Trial-Lipid Lowering Arm (ASCOT-LLA):

a multicentre randomised controlled trial. Lancet. 2003;361(9364):1149–58.

90. Vallejo-Vaz AJ, Robertson M, Catapano AL, Watts GF, Kastelein JJ, Packard CJ, et al. Low-density lipoprotein cholesterol lowering for the primary prevention of cardiovascular disease among men with primary elevations of low-density lipoprotein cholesterol levels of 190 mg/dL or above analyses from the WOSCOPS (West of Scotland Coronary Prevention Study) 5-year randomized trial and 20-year observational follow-up. Circulation. 2017;136(20):1878–+.

91. Sacks FM, Pfeffer MA, Moye LA, Rouleau JL, Rutherford JD, Cole TG, et al. The effect of pravastatin on coronary events after myocardial infarction in patients with average cholesterol levels. N Engl J Med. 1996;335(14):1001–9.

92. Shepherd J, Blauw GJ, Murphy MB, Bollen ELEM, Buckley BM, Cobbe SM, et al. Pravastatin in elderly individuals at risk of vascular disease (PROSPER): a randomised controlled trial. Lancet. 2002;360(9346):1623–30.

93. Schwartz GG, Steg PG, Szarek M, Bhatt DL, Bittner VA, Diaz R, et al. Alirocumab and cardiovascular outcomes after acute coronary syndrome. N Engl J Med. 2018;379(22):2097–107.

Lifestyle Approaches to Lowering Triglycerides

14

Stephen J. Hankinson, Michael Miller, and Andrew M. Freeman

Introduction

Approximately one-quarter of American adults age 20 and over have hypertriglyceridemia (HTG), defined as fasting blood triglyceride (TG) levels >150 mg/dL [1]. In the USA, the percentage of adults with TGs above 150, 200, 500, and 1000 mg/dL are 33, 18, 1.7, and 0.4%, respectively [2]. The prevalence of HTG is substantially higher in patients who are overweight and obese [3]. Other factors that contribute to elevated TG levels include physical inactivity, excessive alcohol intake, poor dietary choices including ultra-processed foods, hypothyroidism, and Type 2 diabetes mellitus (T2DM) [4]. Epidemiological studies suggest that high TGs are associated with an elevated risk of atherosclerotic cardiovascular disease (ASCVD) [5, 6]. Genetic studies using Mendelian randomization demonstrate that high TGs are causally related to ASCVD [7–9]. Other genetic studies suggest individuals with mutations of apolipoprotein C-III (APOC3)

and angiopoietin-like 4 (ANGPTL4), an inhibitor of lipoprotein lipase (LPL), have lower TGs and reduced risk of ASCVD [10–12]. While TGs do not accumulate in atherosclerotic plaques, they promote a pro-inflammatory milieu due to enrichment of apolipoprotein B (ApoB) and apolipoprotein C3 (ApoC3) containing particles, that contribute to the development and acceleration of atherosclerosis [13, 14]. Conversely, Mendelian randomization studies have found that genetic variants associated with reduced TG (e.g., LPL) or with low-density lipoprotein cholesterol (LDL-C) were associated with a similarly lower risk of ASCVD per unit difference in ApoB, suggesting that all ApoB-containing lipoproteins have similar effects on the risk of ASCVD [15].

Overview of Management

Mild-Moderate Hypertriglyceridemia

The 2018 American Heart Association (AHA)/ American College of Cardiology (ACC) Guidelines recommend that patients age 40–75 years old and ASCVD risk ≥7.5% with persistently elevated TGs should consider statin therapy to lower atherogenic lipoproteins. The guidelines also recommend in adults with moderate HTG (175–499 mg/dL) clinicians should address diet, exercise, secondary factors, and medications that increase TG levels [16]. Lifestyle modification through a

S. J. Hankinson · M. Miller (✉)
Division of Cardiology, Department of Medicine, University of Maryland School of Medicine, Baltimore, MD, USA
e-mail: shankinson@som.umaryland.edu; mmiller@som.umaryland.edu

A. M. Freeman
Division of Cardiology, Department of Medicine, National Jewish Health, Denver, CO, USA
e-mail: andrew@docandrew.com

© Springer Nature Switzerland AG 2021
M. J. Wilkinson et al. (eds.), *Prevention and Treatment of Cardiovascular Disease*, Contemporary Cardiology, https://doi.org/10.1007/978-3-030-78177-4_14

hypocaloric, low-fat diet, and aerobic exercise are particularly important for patients with mild-moderate HTG who are overweight or obese [4].

Severe Hypertriglyceridemia

The 2018 AHA/ACC Guidelines recommend that adults with severe HTG (≥500 mg/mL) have secondary causes of HTG ruled out and/or treated. With persistently elevated TGs, recommendations include weight loss via caloric restriction, avoidance of refined carbohydrates and alcohol, dietary fat reduction, consumption of omega-3 polyunsaturated fatty acids (PUFAs), and/or fibrate therapy to prevent pancreatitis [16].

Lifestyle Modifications

HTG in adults is commonly encountered in association with visceral adiposity, physical inactivity and a diet enriched in simple/refined carbohydrates [17]. Treatment of HTG has two distinct objectives: prevention of pancreatitis in patients with severe HTG (≥500 mg/dL) and reduction of global ASCVD risk [18] in those with more moderate HTG (200–500 mg/dL). Weight loss, dietary changes, and moderate-to-high aerobic exercise may offer pronounced reductions in TG, approximating 50% or greater when used in combination [19, 20]. Furthermore, regular physical exercise has been demonstrated to reduce TGs irrespective of weight loss or diet [21, 22].

Weight Loss

Weight loss is the most effective non-pharmacologic method to lower TG levels [23]. Aiming for 200–300 kcal/day via energy expenditure in association with reduced caloric intake that approximates 300–500 kcal/day may result in

significant TG reduction [19]; in overweight and obese patients, a 5–10% reduction in body weight lowers TG 20–30% [24] and ameliorates other ASCVD risk factors [25]. The AHA recommends weight loss of up to 5% of body weight for moderate HTG (150–199 mg/dL) and weight loss of 5–10% of body weight for high (200–499 mg/dL) or very high (>500 mg/dL) HTG [20].

Exercise

Moderate-to-heavy aerobic exercise is associated with improvement of the lipid profile by reducing TG levels and increasing high-density lipoprotein cholesterol (HDL-C) concentrations [19]. Aerobic exercise lowers TGs via upregulation of LPL activity and increased utilization of TGs by skeletal muscle [26]. Baseline TG levels, exercise intensity, caloric expenditure, and duration of activity predict the extent of TG lowering [20]. Guidelines recommend that patients with dyslipidemia participate in regular physical exercise of moderate intensity for ≥30 min/day [19].

Dietary Management

Dietary modification with specific foods and supplements should be part of the initial therapy for patients with HTG [27, 28]. Dietary strategies to reduce TG levels include overall fat reduction, elimination of trans fatty acids (TFAs), increased consumption of omega-3 PUFAs, substitution of saturated fatty acids (SFAs) derived from animal and plant sources (e.g., tropical oils) with monounsaturated fatty acids (MUFAs) and PUFAs, and replacement of refined starchy foods and simple sugars with fiber-rich foods like fruits, vegetables, and whole grains [19]. An example of helpful lifestyle tips for lowering triglycerides has been provided by the National Lipid Association (Fig. 14.1). In patients with very severe HTG

Lifestyle Changes to Reduce Triglycerides
Advice from the National Lipid Association Clinician's Lifestyle Modification Toolbox

What are triglycerides?

Triglycerides (TGs) are one form of fatin your blood. High levels of TGs can increase your risk of heart disease, stroke, and pancreatitis. Eating healthy and being physically active can help lower yourTG level.

Blood levels of TGs (mg/dL) are:

Normal: less than 150   **Borderline:**150-199   **High:**200-499   *Very High:*more than 500

Helpful Tips to Lower Your Triglycerides

Limit Starchy Foods – Some can Increase TGs
like white b reads , cereals, corn, crackers, pasta, potatoes, and white rice.When choosing star chy foods, keep portions small. **Rather than white,choose 100% whole grain** breads, cereals, crackers, pasta, and brown rice. Oats and dried beans and peas are also great choices.

Avoid Alcohol or Consume Small Amounts – It can Increase TGs
Alcohol can increase your TGs, especially binge drinking with a high-fat meal. Alcohol also has extra calories that may cause you to be over weight. Extra body fat can increase your TGs.

Limit Foods High in Sugar–They can Increase TGs
Try to limit foods high in both natural and added sugar (see box below). The National Lipid Association supports the American Heart Association (AHA) guideline to **limit** *added* sugar to no more than 6 teaspoons for women and 9 teaspoons for men each day .

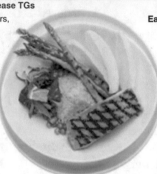

Include *Healthy* Fat at Meals
Eat foods with healthy fats. Choose small amounts of vegetable oil (canola, corn, olive, safflower, or soybean). Within your total daily calories, choose unsalted nuts, seeds, nutbutters, or avocado at meals and snacks. **Eat fewer foods with unhealthy fats** like fatty meats, and high - fat dairy foods and desserts.

Aim for a Healthy Weight
If you are overweight, eat smaller portions of high calorie foods and larger portions of vegetables and other low-calorie foods. Even a small amount of weight loss (5-10% of your current weight) may lower your TGs.

Make Exercise Part of Your Day
Get at least 30 minutes of moderate-intensity exercise   most days, or **at least 150 minutes** of exercise each week.To better lower your TGs and for weight loss, **work toward 200 to 300 minutes** of moderate-intensity exercise each week.

How Much Sugar are You Eating and Drinking?	
Drinks and Foods with Added Sugars	
Sugar-sweetened soda,**12 oz.**	10–11 teaspoons
Cranberry juice cocktail,**12 oz.**	10 teaspoons
Lemonade,**12 oz.**	10 teaspoons
Coffee Frappuccino,**12 oz.**	9 teaspoons
Regular sports drink,**12 oz.**	5 teaspoons
Yogurt, regular,**6 oz.**	7 teaspoons
Pudding,**½ cup**	5 teaspoons
Ice Cream, regular,**½ cup**	4.5 teaspoons
Drinks and Foods with Natural Sugars	
100% grape juice,**12 oz.**	13 teaspoons
100% orange juice,**12 oz.**	9 teaspoons
Grapes,**1 cup**	5.5 teaspoons
Orange,**1 medium**	3 teaspoons

Tips to Achieve Your AHA D aily Added Sugar Goal and Lower Your Triglycerides
• Limit high -sugar foods like candy, cakes cookies, cheesecake, Ice cream , pastries, pies , pudding, and some yogurts   .
• Avoid sugary drinks like regular soda, fruit-flavored drinks, lemonade, coffee drinks, sports drinks, and energy drinks.

Watch for Foods High in Natural Sugars
• Fruit and 100% fruit juices are high in natural sugars, but also many nutrients.Fruit can be part of a healthy eating pattern   .
• Choose whole fruits at meals and for snacks.
• Limit fruit juice (even 100% fruit juice); a serving = ½ cup (4 oz.).

*If your TGs are over 500 mg/dL, you will need to follow a special nutrition plan. Please consult your healthcare provider for additional treatment. This will often includea referral to a registered dietitian nutritionist (RDN).
A RDN can help you make a heart-healthy meal plan that works best for your lifestyle, and support you in your journey to change your nutrition habits.

This information is provided as part of the *Clinician's Lifestyle Modification Toolbox* **courtesy of the National Lipid Association.**

Fig. 14.1 Helpful tips for lowering triglycerides from the National Lipid Association. (Reproduced from the NLA as open access https://www.lipid.org/sites/default/files/lifestyle_changes_to_reduce_triglycerides.final_edits.7.17.16_0.pdf)

whereby fasting levels exceed 1000 mg/dL (e.g., familial chylomicronemia syndrome), dietary recommendations include very low fat intake (e.g., <15 g/day), avoidance of alcohol and restriction of refined carbohydrates to lower the potential risk of pancreatitis [16, 19]. Medium chain triglyceride oil may be used as a caloric source as these fatty acids are directly taken up via the portal circulation rather than being processed into chylomicrons [29].

Fructose

Consumption of significant amounts of dietary fructose (particularly without fiber, i.e., juices) contributes to HTG [30]. Fructose has been shown to have a dose-dependent increase in TGs [31] through stimulating de novo lipogenesis in the liver and reducing LPL activity [32, 33]. In contrast to glucose metabolism, which is regulated by phosphofructokinase, fructose metabolism is relatively unregulated [34]. A cross-sectional study of US adults demonstrated that the lowest TG levels were observed in low-sugar diets and the highest TG levels were observed in high-sugar diets [35]. The importance of limiting simple carbohydrates was demonstrated in a meta-analysis of trials that demonstrated that replacement of carbohydrates with any class of fatty acids decreased fasting serum TG levels [36].

Trans Fatty Acids

TFAs originate from industrial partial hydrogenation of unsaturated fatty acids and occur naturally in ruminant meat and dairy products [37, 38]. TFAs are associated with both increased ASCVD and all-cause mortality [39]. Risk is reduced most effectively when TFAs and SFAs are replaced with *cis* unsaturated fatty acids [36]. Moreover, a diet that replaced TFAs with *cis*-PUFAs was shown to lower TGs [40].

Alcohol

Moderate alcohol consumption (≤10 g/day; the equivalent of ~1–12-ounce bottle of beer, 4 ounces of table wine, or 1 ounce of spirits) for men and women is acceptable if TGs are not elevated [19]. Moderate alcohol use has a weak association between increased TGs [41, 42]; however, higher consumption of alcohol is associated with increased levels of TGs [43]. Alcohol-induced HTG may occur with a high-fat meal due to inhibition of LPL-mediated hydrolysis of chylomicrons [44]. Therefore, alcohol consumption should generally be avoided in patients with severe HTG due to the potential increased risk of precipitating pancreatitis [45].

Mediterranean Diet

The Mediterranean diet is characterized by high intake of virgin olive oil, fruits, vegetables, whole grains, nuts, and legumes, moderate intake of fish and shellfish, low intake of meat, dairy and meat products, and consumption of moderate amounts of wine during meals [46]. Meta-analyses have suggested that the Mediterranean diet lowers ASCVD risk [46–48]. The Prevención con Dieta Mediterránea (PREDIMED) trial found that a Mediterranean diet, supplemented with either extra virgin olive oil or nuts, had a significantly lower combined endpoint of major adverse cardiovascular events such as myocardial infarction (MI), stroke, or cardiovascular death when compared with a reduced-fat diet; however, improved outcomes were largely driven by a reduction in stroke with no significant improvement in mortality or non-fatal MI compared to controls [49]. A systematic review and meta-analysis of 30 randomized controlled trials (RCTs) concluded that uncertainty still remains with regard to the effects of the Mediterranean diet on clinical endpoints and ASVCD risk factors [50]. The systematic review and meta-analysis concluded that there was moderate-quality evidence for a small reduction of TGs when subscribing to the Mediterranean diet compared to other diets tested in primary ASCVD prevention [50]. In overweight and obese adults, the PREDIMED-Plus RCT demonstrated that an energy-restricted Mediterranean diet with physical activity promotion and behavioral support significantly decreased TG levels in comparison to an unrestricted Mediterranean diet after 12 months [51]. Furthermore, a meta-analysis demonstrated that a Mediterranean diet improved TG levels in patients with T2DM [52]. These findings suggest that the Mediterranean diet may also be a useful adjuvant with lifestyle modification to lower TG levels in overweight, obese, and T2DM patients.

Dietary Approaches to Stop Hypertension Diet

The Dietary Approaches to Stop Hypertension (DASH) diet is typically high in fruits, vegetables, and fiber and low in dairy, animal protein, and SFAs [53]. The most relevant difference between the Mediterranean diet and the DASH diet is the emphasis of the former on virgin olive oil [19]. The DASH diet has not been demonstrated to lower TG levels [54–56], which may in part, reflect the relatively high carbohydrate content of the diet [54]. In contrast, the Optimal Macronutrient Intake (OmniHeart) Trial, in which the carbohydrate content of the DASH diet was reduced and partially replaced with either protein or unsaturated fat, demonstrated lower TGs in both treatment arms [57]. These results suggest that substitution of carbs with moderate intake of (predominately) unsaturated fatty acids and plant-based proteins yields a TG-lowering effect approximating 10% [20].

Low-Carbohydrate Diet

In absolute terms, low-carbohydrate diets include "non-ketogenic low-carbohydrate diets" containing 50–150 g of carbohydrates and "ketogenic low-carbohydrate diets" containing a maximum of 50 g of carbohydrates [58]. In overweight and obese adults, a meta-analysis of RCTs compared the effects of balanced diets with low-carbohydrate diets found little or no difference in either weight loss or changes in cardiovascular risk factors (including TG levels) after 2 years of follow-up [59]. A meta-analysis of RCTs found overweight patients on low-carbohydrate diets, when compared to overweight patients on low-fat diets, exhibited greater reduction in body weight and TG levels and a greater increase in HDL-C and LDL-C levels [60]. Furthermore, a meta-analysis of very-low-carbohydrate ketogenic diets, when compared to low-fat diets, found significantly greater reductions in body weight and TG levels and greater increases in HDL-C and LDL-C levels [61]. Of note is that ketogenic diets may increase levels of LDL-C and the total number of apoB containing lipoproteins [62, 63], both of which contribute to the initiation and acceleration of atherogenesis [64]. Therefore, while a low-carbohydrate diet may be beneficial in patients with isolated HTG, patients with ASCVD, obesity, diabetes, and hypertension should exercise extreme caution when considering such a diet that incorporates a ketogenic component [65, 66].

Plant-Based Diets

Vegan, vegetarian, lacto-vegetarian, lacto-ovo-vegetarian, and pesco-vegetarian diets are examples of plant-based diets, which are defined by low frequency of consumption of animal foods [67]. Prospective observational studies have found that higher intake of animal protein is associated with higher cardiovascular mortality [68] and higher intake of plant protein correlates with lower all-cause and cardiovascular mortality [68, 69]. Furthermore, substitution of red meat for plant protein is associated with lower all-cause mortality and cardiovascular mortality, suggesting the importance of protein source for long-term health and longevity [68, 69]. However, meta-analyses of meat-restricted diets compared with omnivorous diets demonstrated no associated reduction in serum TGs [70, 71]. The Cardiovascular Prevention with Vegetarian Diet (CARDIVEG) was an RCT that found, when compared to a low-calorie lacto-ovo-vegetarian diet, the Mediterranean diet experienced greater reduction (~10%) in TG levels [72]. Overall, the literature on the beneficial effects of plant-based diets on TG levels has not been encouraging. Importantly, whole-food plant-based diets do not seem to raise triglycerides significantly.

Marine Omega-3 Fatty Acids

Fish oil supplements containing the marine omega-3 PUFAs eicosapentaenoic acid (EPA) and docosahexaenoic acid (DHA) can lower TGs by 20–50% [73]. Interestingly, marine omega-3 PUFAs can also be found in krill oil supplements, which were demonstrated in a meta-analysis of seven trials to reduce TGs [74]. The Japan EPA Lipid Intervention Study (JELIS), in which patients received a statin plus either EPA or a placebo, did not demonstrate a statistically significant ASCVD risk reduction in either baseline triglyceride subgroup (<151 or ≥151 mg/dL) [75]. However, a subgroup analysis of primary prevention patients in JELIS showed that, in patients with baseline triglyceride levels ≥150 mg/dL and HDL-C < 40 mg/dL, combination therapy with statin plus EPA reduced ASCVD risk by 53% that was not a primary triglyceride-mediated effect [76]. Mechanisms for lowering of TG levels include: reduced hepatic secretion of TG-rich lipoproteins, reduced expression of SREBP (sterol regulatory element binding protein)-1c, reduced-hepatic synthesis of very low-density lipoprotein cholesterol (VLDL-C), inhibition of esterification of other fatty acids, inhibition of phosphatidic acid phosphatase, and increased β-oxidation in the liver [20, 77]. While omega-3 PUFAs constitute only 30–50% of many fish oil supplements, prescription preparations of omega-3 ethyl esters, and icosapent ethyl (IPE), a purified ethyl ester of EPA, are 85% and ≥96% omega-3

PUFAs, respectively [78, 79]. The Reduction of Cardiovascular Events With EPA – Intervention Trial (REDUCE-IT) trial was a multicenter, double-blind RCT in patients with ASCVD or with T2DM and other risk factors. The trial demonstrated that in statin-treated patients with fasting TGs between 135–499 mg/dL high-dose IPE, a highly purified and stable EPA, 2 g twice daily significantly reduced the risk of ischemic events including cardiovascular death by approximately 25% over a median follow-up period of 4.9 years [80]. The importance of lowering TGs was further demonstrated in a multivariable meta-regression model that found the relative risk reduction (RRR) of major vascular events was 0.84 (95% CI 0.75–0.94) per 1-mmol/L reduction in TGs [81]. Of note, these findings were markedly attenuated by the REDUCE-IT trial and with REDUCE-IT excluded, the RRR was 0.91 (95% CI 0.81–1.006) per 1-mmol/L reduction in TGs [81]. The US Food and Drug Administration (FDA) recently approved IPE to reduce ASCVD risk in patients with ASCVD or T2DM and two or more ASCVD risk factors in association with TG levels ≥150 mg/dL [82]. A 2018 review found that, while marine omega-3 PUFAs supplementation reduces TG levels, there was no evidence ALA, EPA, and DHA reduce heart disease, stroke, or death [83]. The 2019 Vitamin D and Omega-3 Trial (VITAL) found that supplementation with n-3 PUFAs did not lower the incidence of the primary end points of major cardiovascular events (a composite of MI, stroke, or death from cardiovascular cause) compared to placebo [84]. Additionally, the STRENGTH (Outcomes Study to Assess Statin Residual Risk Reduction With Epanova in High Cardiovascular Risk Patients With Hypertriglyceridemia) trial (NCT02104817) examining omega-3 carboxylic acids was discontinued January 2020 due to its low likelihood of demonstrating a benefit in patients with mixed dyslipidemia and elevated ASCVD risk [85]. Emerging evidence suggests that higher EPA blood levels, not DHA, strongly correlate with lower rates of cardiovascular events perhaps due slowing the progression of coronary plaques [86]. The 2019 European Society of Cardiology (ESC)/European Atherosclerosis

Society EAS) Guidelines now recommend that in high-risk patients with TG levels between 135 and 499 mg/dL despite statin treatment, omega-3 PUFAs should be considered in combination with a statin [19]. There are validated concerns about toxin accumulation in seafood including polychlorinated biphenyls (PCBs), dioxins, heavy metals, and even microplastics. Further, the environmental impact of large-scale fish consumptions is considerable. In contrast to marine omega-3 PUFAs, plant-based omega-3 sources that are generally derived from α-linolenic acid (ALA) (e.g., flaxseed, soybeans, and walnuts) have no measurable effect on TG lowering and conversion rates to EPA/DHA are minimal [20]. Nonetheless, nuts that contain the polyphenol, proanthocyanidin (e.g., hazelnuts and walnuts) may reduce TG via inhibition of pancreatic lipase [87, 88]. Foods highest in proanthocyanidin content (mg/100 g) are ground cinnamon, unsweetened chocolate, chokeberries, red kidney beans, grape juice, hazelnuts, pecans, cranberries, blueberries, plums, and pistachios [89].

Other Dietary Supplements

In addition to losing weight, exercising, adopting a Mediterranean diet, and consuming omega-3 PUFAs, other dietary supplements are available to lower TG levels. Meta-analysis suggests glucomannan, nuts, cocoa products, cinnamon, curcumin, berberine, and spirulina also possess TG-lowering effects.

Fiber

Soluble fibers have been demonstrated to reduce both total cholesterol (TC) and LDL-C; however, TGs are not generally influenced by soluble fibers [90, 91] except, perhaps in patients with T2DM where fiber decreased TG levels [92]. Glucomannan, a soluble fiber that is a polysaccharide constituted by glucose and mannose, was demonstrated in a meta-analysis of RCTs to significantly reduce TGs by approximately 16 mg/dL compared to placebo [93]. Overall, additional

randomized controlled trials are needed to elucidate the role of fiber on TG levels [94].

Nuts

Intake of nuts is associated with decreased risk of fatal and non-fatal ASCVD, MI, and sudden death [95]. The mechanisms in which nuts protect against ASCVD include the improvement in lipid and apolipoprotein profile, reduction in oxidative stress and inflammation, and improvement in endothelial function [95]. Tree nuts consumed in moderation (1-oz serving/day) have been found to lower TG levels in non-randomized trials with a mean reduction of 2.2 mg/dL per serving [96]. A meta-analysis of RCTs found that almonds significantly reduced TG levels [97]. Another meta-analysis of RCTs found a diet rich in walnuts significantly reduced TG levels compared to control diets [98].

Cocoa Products

Cocoa products, which are a rich source of flavanols, were demonstrated in a meta-analysis of RCTs to significantly lower TGs by a weighted mean difference between treatment and placebo groups of 0.10 mmol/L or approximately 9 mg/dL [99]. Flavanol-containing tea, cocoa, and apple products have been demonstrated to have favorable changes in weight and lipid biomarkers including TG levels [100]. An RCT of 46 healthy subjects during a 4-week period showed that a flavanol-rich cocoa diet significantly lowered TG levels and significantly reduced arachidonic acid (AA)/EPA ratio in a dose-dependent manner, indicating flavonoids may influence the metabolism of PUFAs [101].

Cinnamon

A meta-analysis of RCTs that evaluated consumption of cinnamon in patients with T2DM found significantly reduced TG levels by approximately 30 mg/dL [102]. Another meta-analysis of RCTs found cinnamon statistically reduced TG levels by approximately 24 mg/dL [103]. Mechanisms of action to explain the triglyceride-lowering effect of cinnamon include pancreatic lipase inhibition (see below), increased glycogen synthesis and decreased glycogenolysis, and increased the expression of peroxisome proliferator-activated receptor (PPAR)-mediated metabolism [104].

Turmeric

Curcumin is a phenol found in the spice turmeric. A meta-analysis of RCTs found that turmeric and curcumin significantly reduced TG levels [105]. Mechanisms of action to explain the TG-lowering effect of curcumin include interactions with PPAR, LPL, and cholesteryl ester transfer protein (CETP) and effecting genes related to mitochondrial fatty acid β-oxidation [106].

Berberine

Berberine is an alkaloid found in plants that has been demonstrated to reduce serum cholesterol through reduction of intestinal cholesterol absorption [107], enhanced cholesterol excretion from the liver to the bile [108], upregulation of LDL receptors [109], and inhibition of proprotein convertase subtilisin/kexin 9 (PCSK9) [110]. Furthermore, berberine has been found to increase fatty oxidation and reduce the expression of lipogenic genes [111]. In a meta-analysis of six trials, berberine supplementation lowered TG levels by approximately 35 mg/dL when compared with placebo or lifestyle modification [112].

Red Yeast Rice

Red yeast rice (RYR) is a fermented rice product that contains naturally occurring substances called monacolin K (lovastatin) that have 3-hydroxy-3-methyl-glutaryl-coenzyme A (HMG CoA) reductase inhibitor activity as well as phytochemicals with lipid-lowering actions including sterols, isoflavones, monounsatu-

rated fatty acids, and niacin [113]. In an RCT of patients with ASCVD, RYR significantly decreased recurrent events by 45% [114]. A systematic review and meta-analysis found RYR reduced TG levels by 0.23 mmol/L or approximately 20.4 mg/dL [115]. A recent systematic review and meta-analysis found RYR reduced TG levels by 24.69 mg/dL in MI patients [116]. These findings suggest RYR may be useful for the primary and secondary prevention of heart disease. It is important to note that RYR is often not standardized in dosing across brands and can sometimes be more expensive than generic statins.

Spirulina

Spirulina is a filamentous, blue–green microalga (Cyanobacterium) with an unclear mechanism of action [117]. In a meta-analysis of seven RCTs, spirulina significantly lowered TGs by approximately 44 mg/dL [118]. Overall, further well-designed RCTs are needed to clarify the clinical value of spirulina for patients with HTG.

Conclusion

Lifestyle modification plays a major role in the management of HTG and is often the most effective way to reduce TGs. As shown in Table 14.1,

Table 14.1 Lifestyle approaches to triglyceride lowering. Reprinted with permission from Circulation. 2011;123:2292–2333 [20]. ©2011 American Heart Association, Inc.

Nutrition practice	Triglyceride-lowering
Weight loss (5–10% of body weight)	20%
Implement a Mediterranean-style diet vs. a low-fat diet	10–15%
Add marine-derived PUFAs (EPA/DHA) (per gram)	5–10%
Exercise (brisk 30-min walk three-times per week)	5–10%
Decrease carbohydrates (1% energy replacement with MUFA/PUFA)	1–2%
Eliminate *trans* fats (1% energy replacement with MUFA/PUFA)	1%

weight loss, dietary changes, and moderate-to-high aerobic may reduce TG levels by 50% or more when used in combination [19, 20]. Worthwhile dietary changes to reduce TG levels include elimination of TFAs, adopting a Mediterranean style diet, increasing consumption of omega-3 PUFAs, and replacing refined starchy foods and simple sugars with fiber-enriched whole food products (e.g., fruits, vegetables, nuts, and whole grains). Additional TG-lowering effects may also be obtained with cocoa products, cinnamon, curcumin, berberine, RYR, and spirulina.

References

1. Carroll M, Kit B, Lacher D. Trends in elevated triglyceride in adults: United States, 2001–2012. NCHS Data Brief. 2015;198:198.
2. Ford ES, Li C, Zhao G, Pearson WS, Mokdad AH. Hypertriglyceridemia and its pharmacologic treatment among US adults. Arch Intern Med. 2009;169(6):572–8.
3. Nichols GA, Horberg M, Koebnick C, et al. Cardiometabolic risk factors among 1.3 million adults with overweight or obesity, but not diabetes, in 10 geographically diverse regions of the United States, 2012–2013. Prev Chronic Dis. 2017;14:E22.
4. Berglund L, Brunzell JD, Goldberg AC, et al. Evaluation and treatment of hypertriglyceridemia: an Endocrine Society clinical practice guideline. J Clin Endocrinol Metab. 2012;97(9):2969–89.
5. Sarwar N, Danesh J, Eiriksdottir G, et al. Triglycerides and the risk of coronary heart disease: 10,158 incident cases among 262,525 participants in 29 Western prospective studies. Circulation. 2007;115(4):450–8.
6. Madsen CM, Varbo A, Nordestgaard BG. Unmet need for primary prevention in individuals with hypertriglyceridaemia not eligible for statin therapy according to European Society of Cardiology/European Atherosclerosis Society guidelines: a contemporary population-based study. Eur Heart J. 2018;39(7):610–9.
7. Triglyceride Coronary Disease Genetics Consortium, Emerging Risk Factors Collaboration, Sarwar N, et al. Triglyceride-mediated pathways and coronary disease: collaborative analysis of 101 studies. Lancet. 2010;375(9726):1634–9.
8. Varbo A, Benn M, Tybjaerg-Hansen A, Jorgensen AB, Frikke-Schmidt R, Nordestgaard BG. Remnant cholesterol as a causal risk factor for ischemic heart disease. J Am Coll Cardiol. 2013;61(4):427–36.
9. Holmes MV, Asselbergs FW, Palmer TM, et al. Mendelian randomization of blood lipids for coronary heart disease. Eur Heart J. 2015;36(9):539–50.
10. Myocardial Infarction Genetics and CARDIoGRAM Exome Consortia Investigators, Stitziel NO, et al. Coding variation in ANGPTL4, LPL, and SVEP1 and the risk of coronary disease. N Engl J Med. 2016;374(12):1134–44.
11. Dewey FE, Gusarova V, O'Dushlaine C, et al. Inactivating variants in ANGPTL4 and risk of coronary artery disease. N Engl J Med. 2016;374(12):1123–33.
12. Pollin TI, Damcott CM, Shen H, et al. A null mutation in human APOC3 confers a favorable plasma lipid profile and apparent cardioprotection. Science. 2008;322(5908):1702–5.
13. Nordestgaard BG. Triglyceride-rich lipoproteins and atherosclerotic cardiovascular disease: new insights from epidemiology, genetics, and biology. Circ Res. 2016;118(4):547–63.
14. Bittner V. Implications for REDUCE IT in clinical practice. Prog Cardiovasc Dis. 2019;62(5):395–400.
15. Ference BA, Kastelein JJP, Ray KK, et al. Association of triglyceride-lowering LPL variants and LDL-C-lowering LDLR variants with risk of coronary heart disease. JAMA. 2019;321(4):364–73.
16. Grundy SM, Stone NJ, Bailey AL, et al. 2018 AHA/ACC/AACVPR/AAPA/ABC/ACPM/ADA/AGS/APhA/ASPC/NLA/PCNA Guideline on the Management of Blood Cholesterol: Executive Summary: A Report of the American College of Cardiology/American Heart Association Task Force on Clinical Practice Guidelines. J Am Coll Cardiol. 2019;73(24): 3168–209.
17. Johnson RK, Appel LJ, Brands M, et al. Dietary sugars intake and cardiovascular health: a scientific statement from the American Heart Association. Circulation. 2009;120(11):1011–20.
18. Hegele RA, Ginsberg HN, Chapman MJ, et al. The polygenic nature of hypertriglyceridaemia: implications for definition, diagnosis, and management. Lancet Diabetes Endocrinol. 2014;2(8):655–66.
19. Mach F, Baigent C, Catapano AL, et al. 2019 ESC/EAS guidelines for the management of dyslipidaemias: lipid modification to reduce cardiovascular risk. Eur Heart J. 2020;41(1):111–88.
20. Miller M, Stone NJ, Ballantyne C, et al. Triglycerides and cardiovascular disease: a scientific statement from the American Heart Association. Circulation. 2011;123(20):2292–333.
21. Kraus WE, Houmard JA, Duscha BD, et al. Effects of the amount and intensity of exercise on plasma lipoproteins. N Engl J Med. 2002;347(19):1483–92.
22. Huffman KM, Hawk VH, Henes ST, et al. Exercise effects on lipids in persons with varying dietary patterns-does diet matter if they exercise? Responses in studies of a targeted risk reduction intervention through defined exercise I. Am Heart J. 2012;164(1):117–24.
23. Byrne A, Makadia S, Sutherland A, Miller M. Optimizing non-pharmacologic management of hypertriglyceridemia. Arch Med Res. 2017;48(6):483–7.
24. Van Gaal LF, Mertens IL, Ballaux D. What is the relationship between risk factor reduction and degree of weight loss? Eur Heart J Suppl. 2005;7(L):L21–6.

25. Jensen MD, Ryan DH, Apovian CM, et al. 2013 AHA/ACC/TOS guideline for the management of overweight and obesity in adults: a report of the American College of Cardiology/American Heart Association Task Force on Practice Guidelines and the Obesity Society. Circulation. 2014;129(25 Suppl 2): S102–38.

26. Kraus WE, Slentz CA. Exercise training, lipid regulation, and insulin action: a tangled web of cause and effect. Obesity. 2009;17(SUPPL. 3):S21–6.

27. Vogel JH, Bolling SF, Costello RB, et al. Integrating complementary medicine into cardiovascular medicine. A report of the American College of Cardiology Foundation Task Force on Clinical Expert Consensus Documents (Writing Committee to Develop an Expert Consensus Document on Complementary and Integrative Medicine). J Am Coll Cardiol. 2005;46(1): 184–221.

28. Varady KA, Jones PJ. Combination diet and exercise interventions for the treatment of dyslipidemia: an effective preliminary strategy to lower cholesterol levels? J Nutr. 2005;135(8):1829–35.

29. Catapano AL, Graham I, De Backer G, et al. 2016 ESC/EAS guidelines for the management of dyslipidaemias. Eur Heart J. 2016;37(39):2999–3058.

30. Taskinen MR, Soderlund S, Bogl LH, et al. Adverse effects of fructose on cardiometabolic risk factors and hepatic lipid metabolism in subjects with abdominal obesity. J Intern Med. 2017;282(2):187–201.

31. Stanhope KL, Medici V, Bremer AA, et al. A dose-response study of consuming high-fructose corn syrup-sweetened beverages on lipid/lipoprotein risk factors for cardiovascular disease in young adults. Am J Clin Nutr. 2015;101(6):1144–54.

32. Parks EJ, Skokan LE, Timlin MT, Dingfelder CS. Dietary sugars stimulate fatty acid synthesis in adults. J Nutr. 2008;138(6):1039–46.

33. Chong MF, Fielding BA, Frayn KN. Mechanisms for the acute effect of fructose on postprandial lipemia. Am J Clin Nutr. 2007;85(6):1511–20.

34. Stanhope KL, Havel PJ. Endocrine and metabolic effects of consuming beverages sweetened with fructose, glucose, sucrose, or high-fructose corn syrup. Am J Clin Nutr. 2008;88(6):1733S–7S.

35. Welsh JA, Sharma A, Abramson JL, Vaccarino V, Gillespie C, Vos MB. Caloric sweetener consumption and dyslipidemia among US adults. JAMA. 2010;303(15):1490–7.

36. Mensink RP, Zock PL, Kester AD, Katan MB. Effects of dietary fatty acids and carbohydrates on the ratio of serum total to HDL cholesterol and on serum lipids and apolipoproteins: a meta-analysis of 60 controlled trials. Am J Clin Nutr. 2003;77(5):1146–55.

37. Lichtenstein AH, Appel LJ, Brands M, et al. Diet and lifestyle recommendations revision 2006: a scientific statement from the American Heart Association Nutrition Committee. Circulation. 2006;114(1):82–96.

38. Mozaffarian D, Aro A, Willett WC. Health effects of trans-fatty acids: experimental and observational evidence. Eur J Clin Nutr. 2009;63:S5–S21.

39. De Souza RJ, Mente A, Maroleanu A, et al. Intake of saturated and trans unsaturated fatty acids and risk of all cause mortality, cardiovascular disease, and type 2 diabetes: Systematic review and meta-analysis of observational studies. BMJ (Online). 2015;351.

40. Lichtenstein AH, Ausman LM, Jalbert SM, Schaefer EJ. Effects of different forms of dietary hydrogenated fats on serum lipoprotein cholesterol levels. N Engl J Med. 1999;340(25):1933–40.

41. Rimm EB, Williams P, Fosher K, Criqui M, Stampfer MJ. Moderate alcohol intake and lower risk of coronary heart disease: meta-analysis of effects on lipids and haemostatic factors. Br Med J. 1999;319(7224):1523–8.

42. Brien SE, Ronksley PE, Turner BJ, Mukamal KJ, Ghali WA. Effect of alcohol consumption on biological markers associated with risk of coronary heart disease: systematic review and meta-analysis of interventional studies. BMJ. 2011;342(7795):480.

43. Foerster M, Marques-Vidal P, Gmel G, et al. Alcohol drinking and cardiovascular risk in a population with high mean alcohol consumption. Am J Cardiol. 2009;103(3):361–8.

44. Pownall HJ, Ballantyne CM, Kimball KT, Simpson SL, Yeshurun D, Gotto AM Jr. Effect of moderate alcohol consumption on hypertriglyceridemia: a study in the fasting state. Arch Intern Med. 1999;159(9): 981–7.

45. Ewald N, Hardt PD, Kloer HU. Severe hypertriglyceridemia and pancreatitis: presentation and management. Curr Opin Lipidol. 2009;20(6):497–504.

46. Martínez-González MÁ, Hershey MS, Zazpe I, Trichopoulou A. Transferability of the Mediterranean diet to non-Mediterranean countries. What is and what is not the Mediterranean diet. Nutrients. 2017;9(11).

47. Sofi F, Macchi C, Abbate R, Gensini GF, Casini A. Mediterranean diet and health status: an updated meta-analysis and a proposal for a literature-based adherence score. Public Health Nutr. 2013;17(12):2769–82.

48. Grosso G, Marventano S, Yang J, et al. A comprehensive meta-analysis on evidence of Mediterranean diet and cardiovascular disease: are individual components equal? Crit Rev Food Sci Nutr. 2017;57(15):3218–32.

49. Estruch R, Ros E, Salas-Salvado J, et al. Primary prevention of cardiovascular disease with a Mediterranean diet supplemented with extra-virgin olive oil or nuts. N Engl J Med. 2018;378(25):e34.

50. Rees K, Takeda A, Martin N, et al. Mediterranean-style diet for the primary and secondary prevention of cardiovascular disease. Cochrane Database Syst Rev. 2019;3:CD009825.

51. Salas-Salvado J, Diaz-Lopez A, Ruiz-Canela M, et al. Effect of a lifestyle intervention program with energy-restricted Mediterranean diet and exercise on weight loss and cardiovascular risk factors: one-year results of the PREDIMED-plus trial. Diabetes Care. 2019;42(5):777–88.

52. Huo R, Du T, Xu Y, et al. Effects of Mediterranean-style diet on glycemic control, weight loss and

cardiovascular risk factors among type 2 diabetes individuals: a meta-analysis. Eur J Clin Nutr. 2015;69(11):1200–8.

53. Moore TJ, Vollmer WM, Appel LJ, et al. Effect of dietary patterns on ambulatory blood pressure: results from the dietary approaches to stop hypertension (DASH) trial. Hypertension. 1999;34(3):472–7.

54. Obarzanek E, Sacks FM, Vollmer WM, et al. Effects on blood lipids of a blood pressure-lowering diet: the dietary approaches to stop hypertension (DASH) trial. Am J Clin Nutr. 2001;74(1):80–9.

55. Azadbakht L, Fard NR, Karimi M, et al. Effects of the dietary approaches to stop hypertension (DASH) eating plan on cardiovascular risks among type 2 diabetic patients: a randomized crossover clinical trial. Diabetes Care. 2011;34(1):55–7.

56. Chiavaroli L, Viguiliouk E, Nishi SK, et al. DASH dietary pattern and cardiometabolic outcomes: an umbrella review of systematic reviews and meta-analyses. Nutrients. 2019;11(2):338.

57. Appel LJ, Sacks FM, Carey VJ, et al. Effects of protein, monounsaturated fat, and carbohydrate intake on blood pressure and serum lipids: results of the OmniHeart randomized trial. JAMA. 2005;294(19): 2455–64.

58. Naude CE, Schoonees A, Nguyen KA, et al. Low carbohydrate versus balanced carbohydrate diets for reducing weight and cardiovascular risk. Cochrane Database Syst Rev. 2019;2019(5):CD013334.

59. Naude CE, Schoonees A, Senekal M, Young T, Garner P, Volmink J. Low carbohydrate versus isoenergetic balanced diets for reducing weight and cardiovascular risk: a systematic review and meta-analysis. PLoS One. 2014;9(7):e100652.

60. Mansoor N, Vinknes KJ, Veierod MB, Retterstol K. Effects of low-carbohydrate diets v. low-fat diets on body weight and cardiovascular risk factors: a meta-analysis of randomised controlled trials. Br J Nutr. 2016;115(3):466–79.

61. Bueno NB, de Melo IS, de Oliveira SL, da Rocha Ataide T. Very-low-carbohydrate ketogenic diet v. low-fat diet for long-term weight loss: a meta-analysis of randomised controlled trials. Br J Nutr. 2013;110(7):1178–87.

62. Kwiterovich PO Jr, Vining EP, Pyzik P, Skolasky R Jr, Freeman JM. Effect of a high-fat ketogenic diet on plasma levels of lipids, lipoproteins, and apolipoproteins in children. JAMA. 2003;290(7):912–20.

63. Azevedo de Lima P, Baldini Prudencio M, Murakami DK, Pereira de Brito Sampaio L, Figueiredo Neto AM, Teixeira Damasceno NR. Effect of classic ketogenic diet treatment on lipoprotein subfractions in children and adolescents with refractory epilepsy. Nutrition. 2017;33:271–7.

64. Ference BA, Ginsberg HN, Graham I, et al. Low-density lipoproteins cause atherosclerotic cardiovascular disease. 1. Evidence from genetic, epidemiologic, and clinical studies. A consensus statement from the European Atherosclerosis Society Consensus Panel. Eur Heart J. 2017;38(32):2459–72.

65. Kinoshita M, Yokote K, Arai H, et al. Japan Atherosclerosis Society (JAS) guidelines for prevention of atherosclerotic cardiovascular diseases 2017. J Atheroscler Thromb. 2018;25(9):846–984.

66. O'Neill B, Raggi P. The ketogenic diet: pros and cons. Atherosclerosis. 2020;292:119–26.

67. Satija A, Hu FB. Plant-based diets and cardiovascular health. Trends Cardiovasc Med. 2018;28(7):437–41.

68. Song M, Fung TT, Hu FB, et al. Association of animal and plant protein intake with all-cause and cause-specific mortality. JAMA Intern Med. 2016;176(10):1453–63.

69. Budhathoki S, Sawada N, Iwasaki M, et al. Association of animal and plant protein intake with all-cause and cause-specific mortality in a Japanese cohort. JAMA Intern Med. 2019;179(11):1509–18.

70. Wang F, Zheng J, Yang B, Jiang J, Fu Y, Li D. Effects of vegetarian diets on blood lipids: a systematic review and meta-analysis of randomized controlled trials. J Am Heart Assoc. 2015;4(10):e002408.

71. Yokoyama Y, Levin SM, Barnard ND. Association between plant-based diets and plasma lipids: a systematic review and meta-analysis. Nutr Rev. 2017;75(9):683–98.

72. Sofi F, Dinu M, Pagliai G, et al. Low-calorie vegetarian versus Mediterranean diets for reducing body weight and improving cardiovascular risk profile: CARDIVEG study (cardiovascular prevention with vegetarian diet). Circulation. 2018;137(11):1103–13.

73. Harris WS, Bulchandani D. Why do omega-3 fatty acids lower serum triglycerides? Curr Opin Lipidol. 2006;17(4):387–93.

74. Ursoniu S, Sahebkar A, Serban MC, et al. Lipid-modifying effects of krill oil in humans: systematic review and meta-analysis of randomized controlled trials. Nutr Rev. 2017;75(5):361–73.

75. Yokoyama M, Origasa H, Matsuzaki M, et al. Effects of eicosapentaenoic acid on major coronary events in hypercholesterolaemic patients (JELIS): a randomised open-label, blinded endpoint analysis. Lancet. 2007;369(9567):1090–8.

76. Saito Y, Yokoyama M, Origasa H, et al. Effects of EPA on coronary artery disease in hypercholesterolemic patients with multiple risk factors: sub-analysis of primary prevention cases from the Japan EPA Lipid Intervention Study (JELIS). Atherosclerosis. 2008;200(1):135–40.

77. Skulas-Ray AC, Wilson PWF, Harris WS, et al. Omega-3 fatty acids for the management of hypertriglyceridemia: a science advisory from the American Heart Association. Circulation. 2019;140(12): e673–91.

78. Ballantyne CM, Bays HE, Kastelein JJ, et al. Efficacy and safety of eicosapentaenoic acid ethyl ester (AMR101) therapy in statin-treated patients with persistent high triglycerides (from the ANCHOR study). Am J Cardiol. 2012;110(7):984–92.

79. Harris WS, Ginsberg HN, Arunakul N, et al. Safety and efficacy of Omacor in severe hypertriglyceridemia. J Cardiovasc Risk. 1997;4(5–6):385–91.

80. Bhatt DL, Steg PG, Miller M, et al. Cardiovascular risk reduction with icosapent ethyl for hypertriglyceridemia. N Engl J Med. 2019;380(1):11–22.

81. Marston NA, Giugliano RP, Im K, et al. Association between triglyceride lowering and reduction of cardiovascular risk across multiple lipid-lowering therapeutic classes: a systematic review and meta-regression analysis of randomized controlled trials. Circulation. 2019;140(16):1308–17.

82. U.S. Food and Drug Administration. FDA approves use of drug to reduce risk of cardiovascular events in certain adult patient groups. https://www.fda.gov/news-events/press-announcements/fda-approves-use-drug-reduce-risk-cardiovascular-events-certain-adult-patient-groups. Published 2019, December 13. Accessed.

83. Abdelhamid AS, Brown TJ, Brainard JS, et al. Omega-3 fatty acids for the primary and secondary prevention of cardiovascular disease. Cochrane Database Syst Rev. 2018;7:CD003177.

84. Manson JE, Cook NR, Lee IM, et al. Marine n-3 fatty acids and prevention of cardiovascular disease and cancer. N Engl J Med. 2019;380(1):23–32.

85. AstraZeneca. Update on Phase III STRENGTH trial for Epanova in mixed dyslipidaemia. https://www.astrazeneca.com/media-centre/press-releases/2020/update-on-phase-iii-strength-trial-for-epanova-in-mixed-dyslipidaemia-13012020.html. Published 2020, January 13. Accessed.

86. Mason RP, Libby P, Bhatt DL. Emerging mechanisms of cardiovascular protection for the omega-3 fatty acid eicosapentaenoic acid. Arterioscler Thromb Vasc Biol. 2020;40(5):1135–47.

87. Mercanligil SM, Arslan P, Alasalvar C, et al. Effects of hazelnut-enriched diet on plasma cholesterol and lipoprotein profiles in hypercholesterolemic adult men. Eur J Clin Nutr. 2007;61(2):212–20.

88. Torabian S, Haddad E, Cordero-MacIntyre Z, Tanzman J, Fernandez ML, Sabate J. Long-term walnut supplementation without dietary advice induces favorable serum lipid changes in free-living individuals. Eur J Clin Nutr. 2010;64(3):274–9.

89. Gu L, Kelm MA, Hammerstone JF, et al. Concentrations of proanthocyanidins in common foods and estimations of normal consumption. J Nutr. 2004;134(3):613–7.

90. Brown L, Rosner B, Willett WW, Sacks FM. Cholesterol-lowering effects of dietary fiber: a meta-analysis. Am J Clin Nutr. 1999;69(1):30–42.

91. Hollaender PL, Ross AB, Kristensen M. Whole-grain and blood lipid changes in apparently healthy adults: a systematic review and meta-analysis of randomized controlled studies. Am J Clin Nutr. 2015;102(3):556–72.

92. Anderson JW, Randles KM, Kendall CWC, Jenkins DJA. Carbohydrate and fiber recommendations for individuals with diabetes: a quantitative assessment and meta-analysis of the evidence. J Am Coll Nutr. 2004;23(1):5–17.

93. Sood N, Baker WL, Coleman CI. Effect of glucomannan on plasma lipid and glucose concentrations, body weight, and blood pressure: systematic review and meta-analysis. Am J Clin Nutr. 2008;88(4):1167–75.

94. Pirro M, Vetrani C, Bianchi C, Mannarino MR, Bernini F, Rivellese AA. Joint position statement on "Nutraceuticals for the treatment of hypercholesterolemia" of the Italian Society of Diabetology (SID) and of the Italian Society for the Study of Arteriosclerosis (SISA). Nutr Metab Cardiovasc Dis. 2017;27(1):2–17.

95. Bitok E, Sabate J. Nuts and cardiovascular disease. Prog Cardiovasc Dis. 2018;61(1):33–7.

96. Del Gobbo LC, Falk MC, Feldman R, Lewis K, Mozaffarian D. Effects of tree nuts on blood lipids, apolipoproteins, and blood pressure: systematic review, meta-analysis, and dose-response of 61 controlled intervention trials. Am J Clin Nutr. 2015;102(6):1347–56.

97. Musa-Veloso K, Paulionis L, Poon T, Lee HY. The effects of almond consumption on fasting blood lipid levels: a systematic review and meta-analysis of randomised controlled trials. J Nutr Sci. 2016;5:e34.

98. Guasch-Ferre M, Li J, Hu FB, Salas-Salvado J, Tobias DK. Effects of walnut consumption on blood lipids and other cardiovascular risk factors: an updated meta-analysis and systematic review of controlled trials. Am J Clin Nutr. 2018;108(1):174–87.

99. Lin X, Zhang I, Li A, et al. Cocoa flavanol intake and biomarkers for cardiometabolic health: a systematic review and meta-analysis of randomized controlled trials. J Nutr. 2016;146(11):2325–33.

100. González-Sarrías A, Combet E, Pinto P, et al. A systematic review and meta-analysis of the effects of flavanol-containing tea, cocoa and apple products on body composition and blood lipids: exploring the factors responsible for variability in their efficacy. Nutrients. 2017;9(7):746.

101. Davinelli S, Corbi G, Zarrelli A, et al. Short-term supplementation with flavanol-rich cocoa improves lipid profile, antioxidant status and positively influences the AA/EPA ratio in healthy subjects. J Nutr Biochem. 2018;61:33–9.

102. Allen RW, Schwartzman E, Baker WL, Coleman CI, Phung OJ. Cinnamon use in type 2 diabetes: an updated systematic review and meta-analysis. Ann Fam Med. 2013;11(5):452–9.

103. Maierean SM, Serban MC, Sahebkar A, et al. The effects of cinnamon supplementation on blood lipid concentrations: a systematic review and meta-analysis. J Clin Lipidol. 2017;11(6):1393–406.

104. Medagama AB. The glycaemic outcomes of Cinnamon, a review of the experimental evidence and clinical trials. Nutr J. 2015;14:108.

105. Qin S, Huang L, Gong J, et al. Efficacy and safety of turmeric and curcumin in lowering blood lipid levels in patients with cardiovascular risk factors: a meta-analysis of randomized controlled trials. Nutr J. 2017;16(1):68.

106. Panahi Y, Ahmadi Y, Teymouri M, Johnston TP, Sahebkar A. Curcumin as a potential candidate for treating hyperlipidemia: a review of cellular and metabolic mechanisms. J Cell Physiol. 2018;233(1):141–52.

107. Wang Y, Yi X, Ghanam K, Zhang S, Zhao T, Zhu X. Berberine decreases cholesterol levels in rats through multiple mechanisms, including inhibition of cholesterol absorption. Metabolism. 2014;63(9):1167–77.

108. Li XY, Zhao ZX, Huang M, et al. Effect of berberine on promoting the excretion of cholesterol in high-fat diet-induced hyperlipidemic hamsters. J Transl Med. 2015;13:278.

109. Kong W, Wei J, Abidi P, et al. Berberine is a novel cholesterol-lowering drug working through a unique mechanism distinct from statins. Nat Med. 2004;10(12):1344–51.

110. Li H, Dong B, Park SW, Lee HS, Chen W, Liu J. Hepatocyte nuclear factor 1alpha plays a critical role in PCSK9 gene transcription and regulation by the natural hypocholesterolemic compound berberine. J Biol Chem. 2009;284(42):28885–95.

111. Kim WS, Lee YS, Cha SH, et al. Berberine improves lipid dysregulation in obesity by controlling central and peripheral AMPK activity. Am J Physiol Endocrinol Metab. 2009;296(4):E812–9.

112. Lan J, Zhao Y, Dong F, et al. Meta-analysis of the effect and safety of berberine in the treatment of type 2 diabetes mellitus, hyperlipemia and hypertension. J Ethnopharmacol. 2015;161:69–81.

113. Heber D, Yip I, Ashley JM, Elashoff DA, Elashoff RM, Go VL. Cholesterol-lowering effects of a proprietary Chinese red-yeast-rice dietary supplement. Am J Clin Nutr. 1999;69(2):231–6.

114. Lu Z, Kou W, Du B, et al. Effect of Xuezhikang, an extract from red yeast Chinese rice, on coronary events in a Chinese population with previous myocardial infarction. Am J Cardiol. 2008;101(12):1689–93.

115. Li Y, Jiang L, Jia Z, et al. A meta-analysis of red yeast rice: an effective and relatively safe alternative approach for dyslipidemia. PLoS ONE. 2014;9(6):e98611.

116. Sungthong B, Yoothaekool C, Promphamorn S, Phimarn W. Efficacy of red yeast rice extract on myocardial infarction patients with borderline hypercholesterolemia: a meta-analysis of randomized controlled trials. Sci Rep. 2020;10(1):2769.

117. Cicero AFG, Colletti A, Bajraktari G, et al. Lipid lowering nutraceuticals in clinical practice: position paper from an International Lipid Expert Panel. Arch Med Sci. 2017;13(5):965–1005.

118. Serban MC, Sahebkar A, Dragan S, et al. A systematic review and meta-analysis of the impact of Spirulina supplementation on plasma lipid concentrations. Clin Nutr. 2016;35(4):842–51.

Role of the Microbiome in Cardiovascular Disease

15

Thanat Chaikijurajai, Jennifer Wilcox, and W. H. Wilson Tang

Introduction

Cardiovascular disease (CVD) remains the leading cause of morbidity and mortality worldwide, and especially in developed countries, despite the consistent development of novel treatment modalities and recommendations leading toward the reduction of a global burden of CVD. During the past decade, research has focused on discovering new pathways contributing to the development and progression of CVD. One of the most promising targets for future CVD treatment is the role of human gut microbiota in CVD and in metabolic disorders, like obesity and insulin resistance, that are known CVD risk factors [1]. Recent evidence suggests that gut microbiota can modulate host physiology and play a crucial role in the pathogenesis and natural history of cardiometabolic diseases. The ability of gut microbiota to filter and metabolize dietary nutrients, and then produce metabolites as signaling molecules, makes it a major endocrine organ influenced by dietary intake, which is itself one of the greatest environmental exposures in daily life. Therefore, we here discuss the physiology of gut microbiota, the alterations in the composition of gut microbiota in different cardiometabolic diseases, the association between gut microbiota-derived metabolites and cardiometabolic diseases, and the potential of gut microbiota to be a novel therapeutic target for the future treatment of CVD.

T. Chaikijurajai
Department of Cardiovascular Medicine, Heart, Vascular and Thoracic Institute, Cleveland Clinic, Cleveland, OH, USA

Department of Internal Medicine, Faculty of Medicine Ramathibodi Hospital, Mahidol University, Bangkok, Thailand

J. Wilcox
Center for Microbiome and Human Health, Department of Cardiovascular and Metabolic Sciences, Lerner Research Institute, Cleveland Clinic, Cleveland, OH, USA
e-mail: kirsopj@ccf.org

W. H. W. Tang (✉)
Department of Cardiovascular Medicine, Heart, Vascular and Thoracic Institute, Cleveland Clinic, Cleveland, OH, USA

Center for Microbiome and Human Health, Department of Cardiovascular and Metabolic Sciences, Lerner Research Institute, Cleveland Clinic, Cleveland, OH, USA
e-mail: tangw@ccf.org

Physiology of Gut Microbiota

The term "microbiota" is often used to describe the complex communities of microbial cells, including different species of bacteria, fungi, archaea, and virus, living inside the human body, whereas the term "microbiome" commonly refers to the genome of these microbiota. The human gastrointestinal tract is populated by trillions of microbial cells, mostly bacteria, as a

© Springer Nature Switzerland AG 2021
M. J. Wilkinson et al. (eds.), *Prevention and Treatment of Cardiovascular Disease*, Contemporary Cardiology, https://doi.org/10.1007/978-3-030-78177-4_15

result of continuous environmental exposure and dietary intake starting at birth. The majority of gut microbiota colonizes in the colon, which provides the perfect environment for their metabolism in terms of nutrients and relatively depleted oxygen compared to the stomach and small intestine. Based on the available methods to assess the composition of gut microbiota, five main phyla of bacteria have been identified, *Bacteroidetes*, *Firmicutes*, *Proteobacteria*, *Verrucomicrobia*, and *Actinobacteria* [2]. Of note, in healthy people *Bacteroidetes* and *Firmicutes* combine for more than 90% of the total amount of gut microbiota [3]. Even though the composition of gut microbiota is relatively stable over time within each individual, there is significant variation between individuals, indicating that different host genetics and environmental exposures can alter microbial communities within the gastrointestinal tract [4], resulting in different metabolic profiles and susceptibility to cardiometabolic diseases in each person.

Gut microbiota have been shown to be involved in the development and homeostasis of humans as a symbiotic relationship. Starting at birth, environmental exposure to microbial cells stimulates both innate and adaptive immune responses mainly through the mucosal-associated lymphatic tissue. This results in the differentiation and activation of different mature lymphocytes and the secretion of immunoglobulin A for an effective mucosal protection, as well as promoting an anti-inflammatory response from regulatory T cells in order to maintain the physiologic inflammatory tone within the intestinal mucosa [5]. Interestingly, gut microbiota can also aid the human host by suppressing the growth and colonization of some intestinal pathogens through competitive exclusion and the production of antimicrobial compounds. Furthermore, gut microbiota also regulate the integrity of the intestinal mucosa by maintaining the structure and function of tight junctions found in intestinal epithelial cells [6].

Gut microbiota are also responsible for the synthesis of a variety of substances and metabolites found in the human body. It has been known for almost a century that gut microbiota mediate the synthesis of a wide range of vitamins, including vitamin K and eight different members of the vitamin B group. In addition to synthesizing essential products for humans, the gut microbiota also participates in the metabolism of our dietary nutrients and produces several metabolites, such as short-chain fatty acids (SCFA), bile acids, trimethylamine *N*-oxide (TMAO), and phenylacetylglutamine (PAGln), that can contribute to the pathogenesis of CVD and metabolic diseases.

Alterations in the Composition of Gut Microbiota

The development and progression of cardiometabolic diseases have been associated with subsequent changes in the gut microbial composition, resulting in significantly different bacterial communities between patients with cardiometabolic diseases and healthy individuals. This shift in gut microbiota is referred to as dysbiosis. Atherosclerosis, hypertension (HTN), heart failure (HF), obesity, and type 2 diabetes mellitus (T2DM) are all associated with different patterns of gut microbial dysbiosis.

Atherosclerosis

The mechanistic link between altered gut microbial communities and atherosclerosis was first suggested by Koren et al. [7] in 2011. They demonstrated that bacterial DNA from gut-associated bacteria can be found in atherosclerotic plaques and the amount of DNA correlated with the plaque size, which may contribute to plaque instability and rupture. Subsequent case–control studies revealed several patterns of an altered gut microbiome in patients with atherosclerosis. Karlsson et al. [8] analyzed stool samples from 12 patients with symptomatic carotid artery disease undergoing carotid endarterectomy compared with 13 healthy controls using whole metagenomic shotgun sequencing. They revealed that patients with carotid artery disease had a higher proportion of the genus *Collinsella* and a lower proportion of *Roseburia* and *Eubacterium*. Yin et al.

[9] showed that 141 patients with cerebrovascular disease, either stroke or transient ischemic attack, had an increase in the relative abundance of pathogenic bacteria, such as *Enterobacter, Proteobacteria, Megasphera, Oscillibacter,* and *Desulfovibrio,* and a decrease in beneficial and commensal genera like *Bacteroides, Prevotella,* and *Faecalibacterium.* Importantly, the extent of the observed dysbiosis was correlated with stroke severity.

In studies of patients with coronary artery disease (CAD), some common patterns of changes in the gut microbial composition have been described across different cohorts of CAD patients. An increased ratio of *Firmicutes* to *Bacteroidetes* [10, 11] and a lower abundance of the SCFA (butyrate)-producing bacteria *Roseburia* and *Faecalibacterium* [12, 13] were observed in patients with CAD undergoing coronary angiography. Normally, butyrate serves as an energy source for epithelial cells in the intestinal mucosa and suppresses the inflammatory response within the intestinal mucosa by stimulating colonic regulatory T cells [14], resulting in an intact gut mucosal barrier that prevents the escape of gut microbiota and their endotoxins, such as lipopolysaccharide (LPS), from the gut lumen. Leakage of gut microbiota and LPS stimulates the innate immune response, leading to inflammation and atherosclerosis [6, 15]. However, all of these findings still need to be confirmed in larger cohorts of patients with different stages and phenotypes of atherosclerosis.

Hypertension

HTN is a major risk factor for the development of a variety forms of CVD. Some studies have suggested a possible role of gut microbiota in regulating blood pressure and the contribution of gut microbiota dysbiosis in the development of HTN. Similar to what was seen in atherosclerosis, Yang et al. [16] observed an increased *Firmicutes/Bacteroidetes* ratio and a decreased relative amount of SCFA-producing bacteria in animal models of HTN and some hypertensive patients. Another study of the alteration of the gut microbial composition and HTN also revealed that decreased SCFA-producing bacteria was associated with HTN accompanied by an increase in the abundance of *Prevotella* and *Klebsiella* [17]. Similarly, depletion of a SCFA-producing genus, *Odoribacter,* was found to be associated with higher blood pressure in obese pregnant women [18]. Interestingly , high sodium intake, which can cause elevated blood pressure [19], decreases the abundance of *Lactobacillus murinus* in mice and shortens the survival of *Lactobacillus* spp. in humans [20]. Furthermore, supplementation of *Lactobacillus murinus* in mice was shown to prevent the development of salt-sensitive HTN [20].

Despite the evidence suggesting the association between the alteration of gut microbial composition and HTN, most of the results are from animal models or in relatively small cohorts of hypertensive patients. Future research is needed to verify these findings in larger cohorts of patients with HTN.

Heart Failure

The association between HF and intestinal mucosal dysfunction with gut microbial dysbiosis, known as the gut hypothesis of HF, has been widely described. It is believed that decreased cardiac output and systemic venous congestion cause edema and ischemic injury in the intestinal mucosa, resulting in increased intestinal permeability, overgrowth and translocation of some pathogenic strains of gut microbiota, increased blood levels of their endotoxins and metabolites, and subsequent promotion of inflammation throughout the natural course of HF, ultimately creating a deleterious cycle of accelerated worsening HF [6, 21].

Changes in the composition of gut microbiota in patients with HF have been demonstrated recently in different cohorts of HF patients [6]. Mamic et al. [22] revealed that the higher incidence of *Clostridium difficile* infection (CDI) was independently associated with HF even after adjusting for known risk factors of CDI. This finding led to the hypothesis that HF patients may have a relative depletion of gut microbiota, which is a widely known risk factor for CDI. Subsequent studies corroborated this hypothesis by demonstrating that patients with HF had significantly decreased diversity of gut microbiota including SCFA producers as assessed by 16S rRNA sequencing [23–26]. In addition, an increase in some pathogenic bacteria, such as *Campylobacter, Shigella, Salmonella*, and *Yersinia enterocolitica*, was also found to be associated with HF [27]. Nevertheless, there are discrepancies in the specific characteristic genera of gut microbiota in HF patients, suggesting significant interindividual variations. Cui et al. [24] found that HF patients had elevated levels of *Ruminococcus gnavus*, whereas Kummen et al. [26] found an increase in the abundance of *Prevotella, Hungatella*, and *Succinclasticum*. Recent findings from Mayerhofer et al. [28] suggest that HF patients have a lower *Firmicutes* to *Bacteroidetes* ratio compared with healthy controls. Therefore, future research needs to focus on finding and validating specific microbes that have causal relationships with HF and adverse clinical outcomes.

Obesity and Insulin Resistance

Obesity is one of the most common traditional risk factors for CVD and insulin resistance, which can lead to the development of T2DM. Although genetic susceptibility, increased caloric intake, and energy-balance dysregulation are important contributors to obesity, alteration in the composition of gut microbiota has also been shown to be associated with obesity. The same elevated ratio of *Firmicutes* to *Bacteroidetes* found in atherosclerosis and HTN, it is also associated with obesity [29–31]. Interestingly, Ley et al. [29] demonstrated that weight reduction and low-calorie diets decreased the *Firmicutes/Bacteroidetes* ratio in mice.

There is increasing evidence suggesting that insulin resistance and T2DM are affected by altered gut microbial composition [1, 15]. Zeevi et al. [32] suggested that gut microbiota might play an important role in postprandial glycemic control. In patients with insulin resistance,

elevated serum levels of branched chain amino acids were seen as well as an increased proportion of *Prevotella corpi* and *Bacteroides vulgaris* [33]. Meanwhile, other studies have observed different patterns of alteration in gut microbial composition in patients with T2DM. For example, in a metagenomic study a decreased abundance of butyrate-producing genera, especially *Faecalibacterium prausnitzii* and *Roseburia intestinalis*, was associated with T2DM whereas a higher abundance of some bacteria, such as *Akkermansia muciniphila, Clostridium* species, and *Escherichia coli*, were found in patients with T2DM [34].

Gut Microbiota-Derived Metabolites and CVD

There are several metabolites from gut microbial fermentation of dietary intake that affect human physiology and metabolism, and alter susceptibility to cardiometabolic diseases (Fig. 15.1). Some metabolites can be absorbed directly into the systemic circulation, while others need to be chemically modified by host enzymes before becoming active substances that can accumulate or communicate with target organs, meaning that gut microbial metabolites serve as both hormones and prohormones. Measuring gut microbiota-derived metabolites is a promising approach to gain insights into metabolic function of microbial communities that can be associated with many forms of CVD and metabolic disturbances in human.

Short-Chain Fatty Acids

SCFAs, such as acetate, propionate, and butyrate, are products from the fermentation of undigested dietary nutrients, including fiber, resistant starch, and complex carbohydrates. As mentioned earlier, SCFAs, especially butyrate, serve as protectors of, and an energy source for, intestinal mucosa. SCFAs also modulate proper immune response and capacity of postinfarction cardiac repair [35]. And, at the same time, they

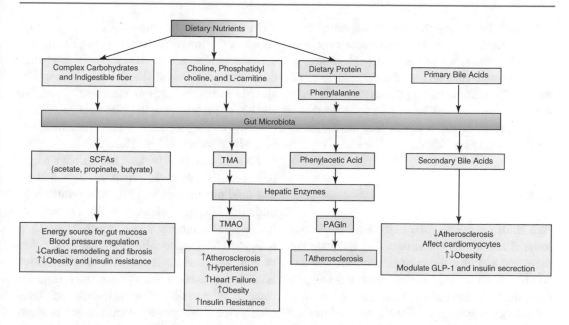

Fig. 15.1 Associations between each gut microbiota-related metabolite and cardiometabolic diseases. The gut microbiota serves as an intestinal filter of dietary nutrients and primary bile acids, which are metabolized into signaling molecules that contribute to the development and pro-

gression of CVD and metabolic disturbances. *GLP-1* Glucagon-like peptide-1, *PAGln* Phenylacetylglutamine, *SCFAs* Short chain fatty acids, *TMA* Trimethylamine, *TMAO* Trimethylamine *N*-oxide

are also actively and passively absorbed into the bloodstream via enterohepatic circulation, and subsequently act as signaling molecules by binding to specific G-protein-coupled receptors. For example, by binding to olfactory receptor 78 (Olfr78) and G-protein receptor 41 (GRP41), SCFAs can impact blood pressure regulation. Olfr78 is expressed in the renal juxtaglomerular apparatus and in vascular smooth muscle cells, and its activation, mainly by acetate and propionate, results in increased blood pressure by stimulating renin secretion and increasing vascular tone [36]. In contrast, GRP41 is only found in vascular endothelium and, following activation by acetate or propionate, negatively affects vascular tone, causing lower blood pressure [37]. Therefore, an alteration in the relative amount of SCFA-producing microbes may lead to imbalanced signaling of these two pathways, resulting in impaired blood pressure regulation and HTN.

Additional evidence for the importance of SCFAs in modulating blood pressure comes from an observational study on more than 4600 people

where an increase in the abundance of SCFA-producing microbes was shown to be associated with lower blood pressure [38]. Moreover, additional studies have demonstrated the potential therapeutic effect of SCFA supplements on blood pressure reduction [39, 40]. Recently, Marques et al. [41] developed a hypertensive animal model and demonstrated that a high-fiber diet and acetate supplementation significantly decreased blood pressure and attenuated cardiac hypertrophy and fibrosis. Interestingly, acetate was also shown to reduce renal fibrosis.

However, dysregulation and overproduction of SCFAs may also lead to metabolic disturbances. Higher fecal SCFA levels have been associated with altered gut microbial composition, intestinal mucosal permeability, HTN, obesity, and dyslipidemia [42, 43]. However, Senna et al. [44] revealed that increased gut microbial production of butyrate was associated with improved insulin sensitivity, whereas higher propionate production resulted in insulin resistance, thus showing the importance of the balance of specific SCFAs in the ultimate response. Another study also corroborated the finding that dysregulation of propionate production by gut microbiota may lead to insulin resistance and T2DM [45]. Hence, it is conceivable that finding the optimal level of each SCFA and elucidating the mechanistic links between individual SCFAs and cardiometabolic diseases could be key to developing dietary interventions targeting SCFAs.

Bile Acids

Bile acids are synthesized in the liver from cholesterol and act as emulsifiers that facilitate the digestion and absorption of dietary fats and fat-soluble vitamins. Primary bile acids are secreted from the liver into the small intestine to emulsify fat-soluble substances before being reabsorbed via enterohepatic circulation, with less than 10% left in the intestinal lumen. Unabsorbed primary bile acids are metabolized by gut microbiota in the colon by bile salt hydrolase enzymes, resulting in numerous secondary bile acids, which are less toxic to gut microbial communities. Similar to primary bile acids, secondary bile acids are also reabsorbed into the bloodstream through enterohepatic circulation.

In addition to the role of bile acids as emulsifiers in the intestinal lumen, both primary and secondary bile acids also serve as signaling molecules affecting different target organs with specific receptors, such as farnesoid X receptor (FXR), G-protein coupled bile acid receptor 1 (TGR5), and sphingosine 1-phosphate receptors [46, 47], as shown in Fig. 15.2.

FXR is the most widely known physiologic bile acid receptor. It regulates carbohydrate and lipid metabolism and bile acid synthesis by inhibiting hepatic cholesterol 7α-hydroxylase indirectly through fibroblast growth factor 15 as a negative feedback control. FXR has been linked to both atherosclerosis and HF. FXR activation is able to attenuate the inflammatory response through suppression of nuclear factor-κB (NF-κB), which subsequently stabilizes and prevents the progression of atherosclerotic lesions [48, 49]. The link between FXR and HF is more controversial. Since NF-κB mediates cardiac hypertrophy and remodeling [50], one would expect the activation of FXR to exhibit protective effects against the development of HF following cardiomyocyte injury. However, there is evidence suggesting that FXR activation actually impairs myocardial structure and function. For example,

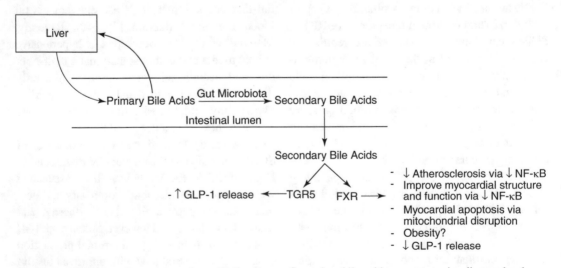

Fig. 15.2 Bile acids pathway and cardiometabolic effects mediated through FXR and TGR5 signaling. Primary bile acids are synthesized and released by the liver into the intestinal lumen, where they can be either reabsorbed or converted into secondary bile acids by gut microbiota.

Secondary bile acids can act as signaling molecules on farsenoid X receptor (FXR) and G-protein coupled bile acid receptor 1 (TGR5), resulting in different cardiometabolic effects. *GLP-1* Glucagon-like peptide-1, *NF-κB* Nuclear factor-κB

Pu et al. [51] revealed that FXR activation promoted myocardial apoptosis through disruption of mitochondria. Therefore, the role of bile acids and FXR in the pathogenesis of HF still needs to be addressed by further investigation.

Despite the unclear mechanism for the effects of bile acids on cardiomyocytes, there is strong evidence showing the association between bile acids and HF. In a case–control study on 142 HF patients and 20 sex-matched healthy individuals, reduced levels of primary bile acids were found in HF patients while the total level of secondary bile acids did not significantly differ between cohorts [52]. Interestingly, Von Haehling et al. [53] conducted a double-blind, randomized, placebo-controlled trial investigating the effects of 4-week supplementation with ursodeoxycholic acid (UDCA) , a secondary bile acid, on endothelial function in patients with chronic HF and demonstrated that UDCA administration was associated with improved peripheral blood flow. These results raise the possibility that bile acids supplementation or modification may be interesting therapeutic approach for HF.

Bile acids have also been implicated in the development of obesity. In obese patients, elevated fasting serum bile acid levels were associated with increased body mass index (BMI) [54], which may be attributed by increased bile acid synthesis and impaired bile salt transport. However, studies in animal models showed conflicting results on the role of FXR in obesity. Li et al. [55] demonstrated that inhibition of FXR signaling in mice fed with high-fat diet results in decreased diet-induced obesity, whereas Fang et al. [56] found that activation of FXR signaling was associated with decreased obesity. Therefore, it is necessary for future research to investigate the physiologic effects of bile acids on metabolism and obesity, as they have the potential to become a therapeutic target in the future.

The effects of bile acids on glucose homeostasis have been described in a variety of studies demonstrating the roles of both FXR and TGR5 signaling in regulating glucagon-like peptide-1 (GLP-1) secretion and stimulating insulin secretion [57, 58]. Interestingly, elevated serum bile acid levels have consistently been shown to be associated with T2DM [55, 59–61] and positively correlated with insulin resistance in humans [55, 61, 62]. Furthermore , treatment with bile acid sequestrants was shown to improve glycemic control in patients with T2DM by attenuating FXR signaling, resulting in increased GLP-1 [63].

Thus, there is a complex relationship between bile acids and human physiology, including metabolism and disease susceptibilities, that represents another aspect of the impact of gut microbiota on human health and cardiometabolic diseases. Targeting bile acids could be a promising therapeutic approach for a variety of CVD, such as atherosclerosis, HF, obesity, and T2DM.

Trimethylamine *N*-oxide (TMAO)

TMAO has been increasingly recognized as one of the most interesting gut microbiota-derived metabolites and reflects the complex interactions between diet, gut microbiota, and cardiometabolic diseases (Fig. 15.3) [1, 15]. TMAO is a gut microbiota-dependent metabolite of specific dietary nutrients, especially choline, L-carnitine, and phosphatidylcholine, found in dairy products, eggs, red meat, some shellfish, and finfish. Interestingly, deep sea fish contain a significantly higher amount of TMAO than fish living in shallow water, supporting a hypothesis that TMAO is used in fish for freeze tolerance and different water temperatures at different times of year may affect the TMAO levels in fish [1]. Some specific gut microbiota strains, such as *Firmicutes*, *Proteobacteria* [64] and *Emergencia timonensis* [65], produce trimethylamine (TMA) from choline and phosphatidylcholine as a waste product by the enzyme TMA lyase, whereas L-carnitine needs to be converted into γ-butyrobetaine before being metabolized into TMA by TMA lyase [66]. Notably, the capability of TMA production can be transmitted between humans through fecal microbiota transplantation (FMT) [67]. TMA is absorbed into systemic circulation before being oxidized and converted into TMAO by hepatic flavin monooxygenases (FMO) , especially the FMO3 isoform [68]. TMAO has been shown to

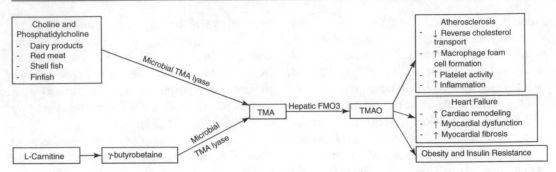

Fig. 15.3 TMA/TMAO pathway and mechanistic links to cardiometabolic diseases. Dietary choline, phosphatidylcholine, and L-carnitine are converted into trimethylamine (TMA) by microbial TMA lyase. TMA is then absorbed into systemic circulation and metabolized in the liver by flavin monooxygenase 3 (FMO3), resulting in the formation of trimethylamine N-oxide (TMAO), which increases host susceptibility to cardiometabolic diseases

promote atherosclerosis by inhibiting reverse cholesterol transport [69], enhancing macrophage foam cell formation [70], platelet aggregation [71, 72], endothelial dysfunction [73], vascular inflammation [74], the inflammatory response within atherosclerotic plaques [75], and plaque vulnerability [76]. In addition, TMAO can cause renal fibrosis and dysfunction, leading to decreased TMAO clearance, increased serum TMAO levels, and further worsening of kidney function in a vicious cycle [77].

The association between TMAO and atherosclerotic CVD was discovered by Wang et al. [70] in 2011 using untargeted metabolomics analysis in a cohort of more than 1800 subjects where they showed that TMAO levels were able to predict subsequent major adverse cardiovascular events (MACE), including death, myocardial infarction, and stroke. Another study on approximately 4000 patients undergoing elective coronary angiography revealed that elevated plasma TMAO levels were associated with increased risk of MACE during a 3-year follow-up period [78]. TMAO was also shown to be independently associated with atherosclerotic burden within coronary arteries as assessed by the number of coronary arteries with significant obstruction and SYNTAX (Synergy between PCI with Taxus and Cardiac Surgery) score in patients with stable CAD [79] and acute myocardial infarction [80]. Moreover, there is evidence suggesting that TMAO is associated with plaque vulnerability and risk of plaque rupture, which can lead to acute coronary syndrome and myocardial infarction [81, 82]. The prognostic implications of TMAO for MACE have recently been validated by several meta-analyses [83–85], and persistently elevated TMAO levels over 10 years are associated with a high risk of developing CAD in healthy individuals [86]. These findings suggest that baseline and serial TMAO measurement can be used as risk predictors for atherosclerotic CVD in addition to traditional cardiovascular risk models.

Some evidence suggests that TMAO may also be associated with the development and progression of HTN. In animal models, TMAO was found to prolong the hypertensive effect of angiotensin-II [87], high salt intake was associated with increased plasma TMAO levels [88], and high blood pressure was associated with intestinal permeability to TMA [89]. And while the mechanistic links between TMAO and HTN in humans remain unclear, a recent meta-analysis of clinical studies revealed that elevated TMAO was associated with increased prevalence of HTN in a dose-dependent manner [90]. Thus, it is conceivable that TMAO may contribute to high blood pressure, and the pathogenic role of TMAO in HTN needs to be elucidated.

TMAO has also been shown to play a role in the pathogenesis of HF. In animal models, TMAO has been associated with adverse cardiac remodeling [91, 92], increased myocardial inflammation [92], impaired energy metabolism [93], calcium regulation, and mitochondrial dysfunction within myocytes [94], while attenuation of TMAO production prevents myocardial dysfunction and fibrosis [95]. In addition to the accumulating evidence on the mechanistic links between TMAO and HF, many clinical studies have demonstrated the diagnostic and prognostic implications of TMAO in patients with chronic and acute HF. Tang et al. [96] studied a cohort of 720 patients with HF with reduced ejection fraction (HFrEF) and found that serum TMAO levels were significantly higher in patients with HFrEF compared to healthy controls and elevated TMAO was associated with a more than three-fold increase in 5-year mortality risk. The prognostic value of TMAO in patients with chronic HF was also shown in a number of subsequent studies [97–102]. Notably, in patients with chronic systolic HF, increased TMAO is associated with higher plasma N-terminal pro-B-type natriuretic peptide, diastolic dysfunction [97], and HF severity [98] that cannot be reduced by guideline-directed medical therapy for HFrEF. Furthermore, TMAO was also shown to be associated with mortality and HF rehospitalization in patients with acute HF [103]. However, conflicting results on the prognostic value of TMAO were observed in patients with HF with preserved ejection fraction (HFpEF) [99, 104] and further investigation on the prognostic utility of TMAO in the setting of HFpEF is needed. Therefore, beyond neurohormonal activation in HFrEF, TMAO may serve as another important residual risk factor for the development and progression of HF, and might be useful as a novel therapeutic target for HF.

Recently, TMAO was also linked to obesity in a study demonstrating that FMO3 deletion protected mice against high-fat-diet-induced obesity, while elevated TMAO was associated with adipose tissue dysfunction [105]. However, human studies report conflicting results. Several studies suggest that elevated TMAO is associated with increased BMI [106–109], including a recent meta-analysis [110], while other studies did not observe a significant correlation between BMI and TMAO [111, 112]. Interestingly, despite the discrepancies on the correlation between TMAO and BMI, hypocaloric diet and exercise are able to reduce plasma TMAO levels in obese patients

[113]. Therefore, future investigations are necessary to verify the association between TMAO and obesity and clarify the mechanisms by which TMAO contributes to the development of obesity.

Meanwhile, the role of TMAO in insulin resistance and T2DM has been demonstrated in a variety of both animal and clinical studies. Gao et al. [114] revealed that dietary TMAO was associated with impaired glucose tolerance, increased fasting insulin levels, and insulin resistance in mice fed with high-fat diet. Interestingly, a study from Miao et al. [115] on the role of FMO3 in glucose homeostasis revealed that FMO3 was increased in mice and humans with insulin resistance, while knocking down FMO3 in insulin-resistant mice could prevent hyperglycemia. Results from clinical studies, including a recent meta-analysis [116], have consistently revealed that elevated serum TMAO levels are associated with T2DM in different cohorts of patients [109, 117, 118]. Of note, TMAO was also shown to be independently associated with 3-year MACE and 5-year mortality in patients with T2DM after adjusting for traditional risk factors, history of CVD, inflammation, renal function, and glycemic control [118].

Nonetheless, findings from a relatively fewer number of studies contradict the above-described roles of TMAO in CVD. For instance, Collin et al. [119] showed that mice fed a high-dose of L-carnitine had significantly higher TMAO levels but lower atherosclerotic lesion size compared to controls, suggesting that TMAO might be a protective factor against atherosclerosis. These findings, however, need to be interpreted cautiously, since TMAO levels in the treatment group were much lower than values reported in other studies and the inverse correlation between TMAO and atherosclerotic plaque size was modest. Additionally, TMAO was found to be significantly lower in 322 patients with stroke or transient ischemic attack compared to 141 asymptomatic controls [9]. Of note, the range of TMAO levels in both groups was much lower than those reported in previous studies [78]. Lastly, Huc et al. [120] showed that TMAO supplementation was associated with attenuated diastolic dysfunction and myocardial fibrosis in a mouse model, which supports the hypothesis that TMA might be more responsible for adverse hemodynamic effects than TMAO.

Taken together, the TMA/TMAO pathway, which has been widely investigated over the past decade, provides substantial insights into the complex interactions between dietary exposure and the development of cardiometabolic diseases. There is lots of evidence suggesting that TMAO has potential to become the gut microbiota-derived biomarker of choice for risk stratification, and a promising therapeutic target in patients with cardiometabolic diseases, especially atherosclerosis and HF.

Phenylacetylglutamine (PAGln)

Recently, Nemet et al. [121] discovered PAGln as a novel gut microbiota-derived metabolite that can contribute to the development and progression of atherosclerotic CVD. Gut microbiota convert phenylalanine from dietary protein into phenylacetic acid, which is then absorbed into the bloodstream and subsequently conjugated with glutamine in the liver, resulting in the formation of PAGln [121]. PAGln was shown to promote atherosclerosis by activating platelet adrenergic receptors, which caused increased platelet responsiveness and thrombotic risk [121]. Interestingly, Nemet and colleagues also demonstrated that after adjusting for traditional risk factors of CVD, PAGln was independently associated with the probability of 3-year MACE in a cohort of 4000 individuals undergoing elective coronary angiography [121]. These findings shed light on the possibility that there are still other, as yet unknown, gut microbiota-derived metabolites that play a role in the pathogenesis of cardiometabolic diseases.

Gut Microbiota as a Novel Therapeutic Target for CVD

Given the relationship between gut microbiota and susceptibility for cardiometabolic diseases, there have been efforts to target gut microbiota structure and function to reduce morbidity and mortality in patients with CVD, including using probiotics, prebiotics, FMT, dietary modifications and interventions, traditional Chinese medicine (TCM), and pharmacologic interventions.

Probiotics and Prebiotics

Probiotics are live microorganisms that, when administered in adequate amounts, provide health benefits by creating and maintaining an appropriate balance of gut microbiota. There have been a variety of preclinical studies that demonstrate the benefits of probiotics on CVD and metabolism. For example, Lam et al. [122] showed that administration of *Lactobacillus plantarum 299v* in rats 24 h before coronary artery ligation resulted in decreased infarct sizes and greater recovery of LV function. Similarly, Gan et al. [123] studied rats undergoing coronary artery occlusion and showed that treatment with *Lactobacillus rhamnosus* GR-1 during the occlusion period was associated with attenuated LV hypertrophy and improved LV function. Subsequent studies on animal models also revealed that probiotic supplementation was associated with reduced atherosclerotic burden [124, 125], changes in fecal levels of some SCFAs [126], and decreased serum TMAO levels [127, 128]. In addition, results from human studies showed that probiotics exhibit cardioprotective effects and have the ability to improve the metabolic profile. *Lactobacillis platarum 299v* was shown to reduce inflammation and improve endothelial function in patients with stable CAD [129], Matsumoto et al. [130] demonstrated that Bifidobacterium animalis subsp. lactis LKM512 supplementation decreased TMA production in healthy individuals, and a pilot study from Costanza et al. [131] revealed that treatment with *Sacharomyces Boulardii* in 20 patients with chronic HF for 3 months significantly improved LV ejection fraction and reduced serum creatinine and inflammatory biomarkers. However, a subsequent randomized controlled trial investigating the cardioprotective effects of *Sacharomyces Boulardii* in a larger cohort of chronic HF patients failed to show significant cardiovascular benefits

[132]. Furthermore, there have been other clinical studies suggesting that probiotic supplementation cannot alter TMAO levels [133–135]. Nonetheless, while there is limited evidence for probiotics having a direct therapeutic effect on atherosclerosis and HF, they may reduce cardiovascular risk indirectly through their demonstrated ability to prevent obesity and improve lipid profiles and insulin sensitivity [136–139].

Prebiotics , such as insulin, lactulose, fructo-, transgalacto- and galacto-oligosaccharides, are indigestible dietary substances that can be fermented by gut microbiota and subsequently alter gut microbial composition and function [140]. Treatment with prebiotics has been associated with improved diversity and metabolic function of gut microbiota [141], blood pressure reduction [142], weight loss [143], decreased fat mass [144], and improved glycemic control [143, 145, 146], but no changes in TMAO [147] or cardiac remodeling have been observed [148]. Moreover, results from animal models have expanded the potential benefits of prebiotics in cardiometabolic diseases. Everard et al. [149] demonstrated that prebiotics were associated with reduced gut permeability , inflammation, and metabolic endotoxemia. Another study from Catry et al. [150] showed that supplementation with prebiotics resulted in attenuated endothelial dysfunction via several mechanisms, such as activation of the nitric oxide (NO) synthase/NO pathway, increased NO-producing microbes, and reduced secondary bile acid synthesis. However, interindividual variation, especially differences in the composition and function of gut microbiota, is an important factor that may contribute to variable responses to prebiotics and needs to be taken into account when examining their potential therapeutic effects.

Fecal Microbiota Transplantation

FMT has been the most definitive therapeutic intervention for modifying the composition of gut microbiota by using fecal contents from healthy individuals to replace pathogenic microbes in the gastrointestinal tract of diseased patients. FMT

has been used successfully as a treatment for both recurrent CDI and inflammatory bowel disease. There is also some evidence suggesting the potential benefits of FMT on cardiometabolic diseases. Vrieze et al. [151] and Kootte et al. [152] both demonstrated that FMT from lean donors could improve insulin sensitivity in patients with metabolic syndrome, but conflicting results on changes in the abundance of *Roseburia* from both studies were also reported. A recent study showed that FMT from vegan donors was able to shift gut microbial composition of patients with metabolic syndrome toward a vegan profile compared with autologous FMT [153]. Interestingly, there was no significant change in TMAO levels in both groups [153]. Even though FMT has the potential to be a therapeutic approach for CVD, there are associated risks that need to be carefully considered, such as gastrointestinal complications and possible transmitted infections. Therefore, the use of FMT is still limited and further investigation is needed on both the benefits and risks of FMT.

Dietary Modifications and Intervention

Dietary Habits and Circadian Rhythms

Recent evidence suggests that not only does the content of dietary intake affect gut microbiota, but the timing of food consumption and circadian rhythms also have a significant impact on the composition and function of gut microbiota, which may link the effects of dietary changes and misaligned circadian rhythms with the development of cardiometabolic diseases. For example, disruption of circadian rhythms in mice is associated with gut microbial derangement and poor postinfarction myocardial repair [154], while early preclinical studies have demonstrated that the composition and metabolism of gut microbiota change over the course of a day and feeding/fasting cycle [155–157]. Zarrinpar et al. [155] showed that *Firmicutes* and *Bacteroidetes* exhibited diurnal variations, with the abundance of *Firmicutes* peaking during the night, while the highest abundance of *Bacteroidetes* was found during daytime, and that time-restricted feeding was significantly associated with specific patterns of gut microbial composition in mice that may be protective against obesity and improve metabolism. Interestingly, an interventional study that disrupted the circadian rhythm in mice by reversing the 12-h light/dark cycle for 12 weeks showed that in mice fed a high-fat, high-sugar diet, cycle disruption was associated with higher *Firmicutes/Bacteroidetes* ratio compared to controls [158]. However, there is limited evidence for the same relationships in humans. A clinical study from Kaczmarek et al. [159] on 28 healthy individuals revealed that the levels of SCFAs and the relative abundances of SCFA-producing bacteria in fecal samples decreased throughout the day. Furthermore, eating frequency, early energy consumption, and overnight-fast duration were also associated with changes in the composition of gut microbiota [159]. Meanwhile, Washburn et al. [160] showed that 24-h intermittent fasting significantly reduced TMAO levels, which subsequently returned to baseline at the end of the nonfasting day. Additional research needs to focus on investigating the interactions between eating habits, circadian rhythms , and gut microbiota.

Dietary Intervention

Changes in diet can modify the composition and metabolism of gut microbiota and, therefore, dietary intervention is a promising therapeutic approach for CVD [161–163]. This approach is considered one of the safest and simplest methods to prevent the development of cardiometabolic diseases. There are some specific diets and dietary components that have been shown to be able to influence both the composition of gut microbiota and their ability to produce metabolites, which may be helpful in reducing the risk of CVD.

Dietary Fiber

Dietary fiber is a general term for indigestible carbohydrate polymers found in foods like nuts, fruits, vegetables, legumes, cereals, and grains, including isolated and synthetic forms that escape digestion and absorption in the small intestine. Once fermented by gut microbiota, dietary fiber can promote microbial growth and

increased production of SCFAs and other metabolites [164]. Theoretically, prebiotics, discussed earlier, can be considered dietary fiber that can be selectively metabolized by gut microbiota and provide health benefits to the host. This section, however, discusses the impact of general dietary fiber intervention on the composition and function of gut microbiota.

Many studies have demonstrated the impact of dietary fiber on gut microbiota. In 2007, Duncan et al. [165] demonstrated that decreased dietary fiber intake for 3 days was associated with reduced abundances of the butyrate-producing microbes *Roseburia* spp. and *Eubacterium rectale*. These findings were corroborated by Desai et al. [166], who demonstrated that in mice colonized with human microbiota, a low-fiber diet promoted the growth of intestinal mucus-degrading microbes, resulting in dysfunction of the intestinal barrier. Furthermore, real-world data from observational studies in two different human cohorts revealed that a high-fiber diet was associated with increased abundance of *Prevotella*, whereas animal protein and fat consumption was shown to enrich *Bacteroides* [167, 168], suggesting the long-term effects of different amounts of fiber intake on the composition of gut microbiota. Interestingly, some randomized controlled trials on healthy individuals have revealed the effects of general dietary fiber intervention on the composition and function of other various microbes, such as increased abundances of *Bifidobacterium* spp. [169, 170], *Lactobacillus* spp. [169–171], and *Feacalibacterium prausnitzii* [172], including increased fecal SCFAs, especially butyrate [171–173]. However, these trials were conducted on a relatively small number of participants, and the results need to be validated by future large randomized controlled trials.

A high-fiber diet has also been shown to provide cardiovascular benefits through modification of gut microbial composition. Marques et al. [41] demonstrated that mice fed a high-fiber diet had increased amounts of *Bacteroides acidifaciens*, which has been previously shown to prevent obesity and insulin resistance [174]. They also showed that a decreased *Firmicutes* to *Bacteroidetes* ratio, blood pressure, cardiac fibrosis, and hypertrophy were all observed in mice fed with the high-fiber diet. Moreover, a recent cross-sectional study on cohorts of HF patients and healthy controls revealed that low-fiber intake was associated with a decreased abundance of microbes in the Firmicutes phylum [28]. However, these findings need to be validated in future prospective studies on CVD patients and healthy individuals to elucidate the complex interactions between dietary fiber, gut microbiota, and CVD risk.

Mediterranean Diet

The Mediterranean diet is inspired by the eating habits of countries surrounding the Mediterranean sea and consists mainly of olive oil, nuts, fresh fruits, vegetables, whole grains, and lower-fat or fat-free dairy products. It is also lower in red meat and high-fat dairy products than a traditional western diet. The Mediterranean diet is high in fiber and polyunsaturated fatty acids, but low in unsaturated fatty acids [175], which may explain the cardiovascular benefits associated with this diet observed in many different studies and meta-analyses [176–180]. For example, in a relatively small study on 27 healthy subjects, greater adherence to the Mediterranean diet was associated with a lower *Firmicutes/Bacteroidetes* ratio [181]. Furthermore, in the PREDIMED study, a randomized controlled trial of more than 7400 participants at high risk for CVD, Estruch et al. [162] demonstrated that subjects following a Mediterranean diet supplemented with either extra-virgin olive oil or nuts had a reduced risk of MACE compared to a control group assigned to a simple low-fat diet.

Similar to dietary fiber, the Mediterranean diet has also been linked to gut microbiota, SCFAs [182, 183], and TMAO production [182, 184, 185]. In 2015, Vazquez-Freson et al. [186] studied a small cohort of 98 participants enrolled in the PREDIMED study, and revealed that subjects randomly assigned to Mediterranean diet group had significantly lower TMAO than the subjects assigned to the low-fat diet. Subsequently, De Filippis et al. [182] demonstrated that high adherence to the Mediterranean diet was associated with lower urinary TMAO levels and Barrea et al. [185] found that adherence to the

Mediterranean diet was inversely correlated with plasma TMAO levels. These beneficial findings might be explained by the presence of 3,3-dimethyl-1-butanol (DMB) in extra-virgin olive oil, which has been shown to inhibit TMA lyase [187]. Nonetheless, several studies have observed conflicting results on the impact of the Mediterranean diet on the composition and function of gut microbiota, including an observational study [188] and two randomized controlled trials [184, 189]. So, although some evidence suggests that adherence to a Mediterranean diet could be a promising therapeutic approach for lowering TMAO levels, mixed results from clinical studies create the need for future interventional studies that directly demonstrate the effect of the Mediterranean diet on the composition of gut microbiota and TMAO production.

Dietary Interventions Targeting TMAO

In addition to studies on probiotics, prebiotics, and the Mediterranean diet, TMAO has, itself, been used as a surrogate endpoint in clinical trials investigating the relationship between different dietary interventions and gut microbiota in recent years (Table 15.1). Some dietary interventions were shown to reduce plasma TMAO levels. For instance, Erickson et al. [113] demonstrated that a hypocaloric diet combined with exercise was associated with lower TMAO levels at 12 weeks, which the authors believed to be secondary to a reduced dietary intake of the TMAO precursors usually found in high-caloric diets. In addition, Tenore et al. [190] showed that lacto-fermented Annurca apple puree containing polyphenols with antimicrobial and antioxidant properties could reduce TMAO production at 8 weeks. Interestingly, even though pistachios contain a significant amount of choline, 4-month pistachio consumption was associated with lower urinary TMAO levels in prediabetic patients, suggesting that gut microbial modifications by the dietary fiber in pistachios outweighs the effects of increased choline intake [191]. Finally, Obeid et al. [192] revealed that vitamin B and D supplementation was associated with decreased plasma TMAO levels at 12 months, which supports the hypothesis that vitamin D may promote the formation of dimethyglycerine

Table 15.1 Clinical studies investigating the effects of dietary interventions on trimethylamine N-oxide

Publication	Dietary intervention	Subjects	Duration	Changes in TMAO
Wang et al. [193]	Red meat	113 healthy subjects	4 weeks	↑
Mitchell et al. [194]	Protein intake at twice the RDA	29 elderly, healthy men	10 weeks	↑
Griffin et al. [189]	Mediterranean diet	115 healthy people at risk of colon cancer	6 months	↔
Washburn et al. [160]	24-h intermittent fasting	30 healthy subjects	48 h	↓
Erickson et al. [113]	Hypocaloric diet	16 obese patients	12 weeks	↓
Annunziata et al. [190]	Grape pomace extract	20 healthy subjects	4 weeks	↓
Tenore et al. [190]	Lacto-fermented Annurca apple puree	90 subjects with dyslipidemia	8 weeks	↓
Koeth et al. [65]	L-carnitine	72 healthy subjects (40 omnivores and 32 vegans/vegetarians	24 h	↑↑ in omnivores ↑ in vegans/ vegetarians
Genoni et al. [201]	Paleolithic diet containing resistant starch	39 healthy women	4 weeks	↔
Malik et al. [129]	*Lactobacillus plantarum 299v*	20 men with stable coronary artery disease	6 weeks	↔
Angiletta et al. [202]	Flavanol	20 obese patients	5 days	↔
Baugh et al. [147]	Insulin	18 overweight/obese patients	6 weeks	↔
Heianza et al. [203]	Hypocaloric diet	510 overweight/obese patients	6 months	↔
Schmedes et al. [195]	Lean-seafood diet	20 healthy subjects	4 weeks	↑
Borges et al. [135]	Probiotics	21 patients undergoing hemodialysis	3 months	↔
Missimer et al. [204]	Oatmeal breakfast and 2 eggs/day	50 healthy subjects	4 weeks	↔
Iannotti et al. [197]	1 egg/day	163 infants aged 6–9 months	6 months	↑
Guash-Ferre et al. [184]	Mediterranean diet	980 participants from PREDIMED study	1 year	↔
Hernandez-Alonso et al. [191]	Pistachio	39 prediabetic subjects	4 months	↓
Obeid et al. [192]	Vitamin B and D	25 healthy subjects	1 year	↓
Cho et al. [196]	Fish	40 healthy men	1 time	↑
Bergeron et al. [200]	Low carbohydrate/ high-resistant starch	52 healthy subjects	2 weeks	↑
Boutagy et al. [134]	Probiotics	19 healthy subjects	2 weeks	↔
Vazquez-Fresno et al. [186]	Mediterranean diet	98 participants from PREDIMED study	3 year	↓
Tripolt et al. [133]	Lactobacillus casei Shirota	30 patients with metabolic syndrome	12 weeks	↔
Barton et al. [199]	Low glycemic load diet	19 healthy subjects	4 weeks	↑
Miller et al. [198]	More than 2 eggs/day	6 healthy subjects	1 day	↑

RDA Recommended daily allowances, *TMAO* Trimethylamine *N*-oxide

instead of TMA from dietary choline by modifying the gut microbial community. The mechanism of vitamin B and the TMA/TMAO pathway is still unclear.

In contrast, there have also been studies suggesting that some diets may increase TMAO levels and therefore should be limited or avoided, including diets high in red meat [65, 193], protein

[194], L-carnitine [65], seafood [195, 196], eggs [197, 198], low glycemic load foods [199], and resistant starches [200]. In addition, a number of studies have demonstrated neutral results on changes in TMAO levels following dietary interventions [201–204], leading to the conclusion that more research needs to be done on this topic.

It is worth noting that there are some important factors that need to be considered when interpreting results from studies demonstrating the impact of dietary interventions on TMAO. Firstly, TMAO itself has significant intra- and inter-personal variations, so the generalizability of each study might be limited. Secondly , the duration of dietary implementation required to significantly affect TMAO has never been standardized, which may explain the neutral findings from some previous studies. Lastly, it is widely known that clinical nutrition studies have numerous challenges and limitations, for example, unreliable dietary recall and noncompliance, that can affect the validity or wide applicability of the results.

Traditional Chinese Medicine (TCM)

Interestingly, recent evidence from preclinical studies suggests that TCM confers cardiometabolic benefits through modulation of the composition and function of gut microbiota. For instance, berberine is one of the phyto-alkaloids found in Huang-lian (*Coptis chinensis*), which is a common herbal treatment used in TCM for infectious diarrhea [205]. Berberine has been shown to reduce atherosclerotic burden in mice through an increase in the abundance of SCFA-producing bacteria (*Akkermansia* spp.) [206], reduced FMO3 expression, and reduced TMAO levels [207]. Similarly, the increase in SCFA producers following berberine supplementation is also associated with reduced obesity and insulin resistance [208–210]. In addition, Chang et al. [211] demonstrated that Ling Zhi (*Ganoderma lucidum*), a medicinal mushroom used in TCM [212], was associated with decreased body weight and insulin resistance, along with a reduced *Firmicutes/Bacteroidetes* ratio and less metabolic endotoxemia. Therefore, alterations

to the composition and/or metabolism of the gut microbial community may be responsible for the cardiovascular benefits offered by TCM. Future research is warranted to uncover the direct mechanistic links between TCM and changes in gut microbiota profiles and metabolites in humans.

TMA Lyase Inhibitors

Now that the TMA/TMAO pathway has been identified and widely studied, there have been efforts to target certain microbial enzymes with the goal of reducing their ability to produce TMAO from diets with choline, phosphatidylcholine, and carnitine. One of the promising approaches to reducing TMAO production is to target microbial TMA lyase, which consists of catalytic and regulatory polypeptides, including choline TMA lyase (CutC), CutC-activating protein (CutD), and carnitine TMA lyase (CntA and CntB) [213, 214]. Recently, DMB was developed as the prototype of TMA lyase inhibitors by Wang et al. [187]. DMB can competitively inhibit CutC in mice, resulting in a reduction in TMAO levels, macrophage foam cell formation, atherosclerotic plaque development induced by a high-choline diet [187], and adverse cardiac remodeling from pressure overload [215]. DMB was also tested in human gut microbiota and was found to be effective in suppressing TMA production without an inhibitory effect on normal bacterial growth [187].

There are also some other interesting substances that have been shown to successfully reduce TMA and TMAO production. Roberts et al. [216] developed a suicide substrate inhibitor of TMA lyase from a choline analogue, including iodomethylcholine (IMC) and fluoromethylcholine (FMC), that can irreversibly inhibit TMA lyase and reduce TMAO-mediated platelet hyperresponsiveness without affecting gut microbial viability or increasing bleeding risk. Of note, IMC was also shown to be able to improve cardiac structure and function [217], reduce hepatic cholesterol accumulation, and upregulate hepatic bile acid synthesis [218]. Moreover, Kuka et al. [219] demonstrated in a mouse model that meldonium, an aza-analogue of carnitine and gamma-butyrobetaine, can decrease TMAO production from L-carnitine without affecting bacterial growth. Chen et al. [220] showed that a natural phytoalexin, resveratrol, was able to reduce TMA production and atherosclerotic burden in mice by modifying the composition of gut microbiota, which was subsequently demonstrated in a pilot study on 201 healthy subjects as well [190]. Similarly, allicin, a natural antimicrobial phytochemical compound found in garlic, is able to inhibit carnitine-derived TMAO production [221]. Thus, in addition to dietary modifications, these pharmacologic approaches can potentially be alternative interventions for reducing cardiovascular risk caused by gut microbiota.

Conclusions and Future Directions

Over the past decade, gut microbiota have been linked to dietary habits and cardiometabolic disease, including atherosclerosis, HTN, HF, obesity, and insulin resistance. Changes in the composi-

tion and metabolism of gut microbiota have been shown to be associated with CVD susceptibility, as summarized in Table 15.2. Since there are both inter- and intraindividual variability in the composition of the gut microbial community, and the utility of metagenomic sequencing is still limited by cost and availability, most of the studies to date have focused on metabolites produced from gut microbiota-dependent metabolism, such as SCFAs, bile acids, TMAO, and PAGln, which can mechanistically link gut microbes and CVD. However, since there are variations and diversity in the structure and metabolism of each gut microbial community, there may be other still undiscovered metabolic pathways and complex host-microbe interactions that could contribute to the development and progression of cardiometabolic diseases. Future longitudinal studies need to identify other potential metabolites and verify which can be used as biomarkers for cardiovascular risk stratification in clinical practice.

Given the high morbidity and mortality burden of CVD throughout the world, it is unsurprising that many efforts are underway to develop novel

Table 15.2 Cardiometabolic diseases and associated alterations in the composition of gut microbiota and gut microbiota-derived metabolites

	Altered composition of gut microbiota	Associated gut microbiota-derived metabolites
Atherosclerosis	↑ *Firmicutes/Bacteroidetes* ratio [9–11] ↓ SCFA-producing bacteria [8, 12, 13] ↑ *Collinsella* [8] ↑ *Enterobacteriaceae, Proteobacteria, Eschericia, Shigella* [9]	↑ TMAO [70, 78–82] ↑ PAGln [121]
HTN	↑ *Firmicutes/Bacteroidetes* ratio [16] ↓ SCFA-producing bacteria [16–18] ↓ *Lactobacillus* [20]	SCFAs [17, 39–43] ↑ TMAO [87–90]
HF	↑ *Clostidium difficile* [22] ↓ SCFA-producing bacteria [23–26] ↑ *Campylobacter, Shigella, Salmonella, Yersinia* [27] ↑ *Ruminocuccus* [24] ↑ *Lactobacillus* [25] ↑ *Prevotella, Hungatella, Succinclasticum* [26] ↓ *Firmicutes/Bacteroidetes* ratio [28]	↑ TMAO [91, 95–97, 103] ↓ Primary bile acids [52, 53]
Obesity and insulin resistance	↑ *Firmicutes/Bacteroidetes* ratio [29–31] ↓ SCFA-producing bacteria [34] ↑ *Prevotella, Bacteroides* [33]	↑ TMAO [105–109, 114, 115, 117, 118] SCFAs [42–45] ↑ Bile acids [55, 59–63]

HF Heart failure; *HTN* Hypertension; *PAGln* Phenylacetyl glutamine; *SCFA* Short-chain fatty acid; *TMAO* Trimethylamine *N*-oxide

treatment strategies for the prevention and treatment of CVD. One promising strategy is to modify the composition and function of gut microbiota through the use of probiotics, prebiotics, FMT, dietary modifications and interventions, and/or TCM, all of which seem to have potential as alternative or adjunctive treatments for CVD. A popular focus of recent research has been the TMA/TMAO pathway, which has been shown to be a promising target for both dietary interventions, such as the Mediterranean diet and extra-virgin olive oil, and microbial enzyme inhibitors, such as DMB. Although there are still questions about the effects of TMAO modification on CVD risk, previous findings suggest the possibility of a future with personalized dietary interventions based on an individual's gut microbial composition and plasma TMAO levels, as well as the development of sequestrants that can inhibit microbial TMA lyase in the intestinal lumen without suppressing the growth of gut microbes in order to maintain the physiologic function of a healthy gut microbiota and reduce the risk of microbial resistance and opportunistic infections.

Disclosure Dr. Tang is a consultant for Sequana Medical A.G., Owkin Inc., Relypsa Inc., proCARDIA Inc, Cardiol Therapeutics, and Genomics plc, and has received honorarium from Springer Nature for authorship/editorship and American Board of Internal Medicine for exam writing committee, all unrelated to the contents of this paper. All other authors have no relationships to disclose.

Funding Dr. Tang is partially supported by grants from the National Institutes of Health and the Office of Dietary Supplements (R01HL103931, R01DK106000, R01HL126827).

References

1. Tang WHW, Backhed F, Landmesser U, Hazen SL. Intestinal microbiota in cardiovascular health and disease: JACC state-of-the-art review. J Am Coll Cardiol. 2019;73(16):2089–105.
2. Yang X, Xie L, Li Y, Wei C. More than 9,000,000 unique genes in human gut bacterial community: estimating gene numbers inside a human body. PLoS One. 2009;4(6):0006074.
3. Qin J, Li R, Raes J, Arumugam M, Burgdorf KS, Manichanh C, et al. A human gut microbial gene catalogue established by metagenomic sequencing. Nature. 2010;464(7285):59–65.
4. Lloyd-Price J, Mahurkar A, Rahnavard G, Crabtree J, Orvis J, Hall AB, et al. Strains, functions and dynamics in the expanded human microbiome project. Nature. 2017;550(7674):61–6.
5. Cerf-Bensussan N, Gaboriau-Routhiau V. The immune system and the gut microbiota: friends or foes? Nat Rev Immunol. 2010;10(10):735–44.
6. Tang WHW, Li DY, Hazen SL. Dietary metabolism, the gut microbiome, and heart failure. Nat Rev Cardiol. 2019;16(3):137–54.
7. Koren O, Spor A, Felin J, Fak F, Stombaugh J, Tremaroli V, et al. Human oral, gut, and plaque microbiota in patients with atherosclerosis. Proc Natl Acad Sci U S A. 2011;1:4592–8.
8. Karlsson FH, Fak F, Nookaew I, Tremaroli V, Fagerberg B, Petranovic D, et al. Symptomatic atherosclerosis is associated with an altered gut metagenome. Nat Commun. 2012;3:1245.
9. Yin J, Liao SX, He Y, Wang S, Xia GH, Liu FT, et al. Dysbiosis of gut microbiota with reduced trimethylamine-N-oxide level in patients with large-artery atherosclerotic stroke or transient ischemic attack. J Am Heart Assoc. 2015;4(11):002699.
10. Emoto T, Yamashita T, Sasaki N, Hirota Y, Hayashi T, So A, et al. Analysis of gut microbiota in coronary artery disease patients: a possible link between gut microbiota and coronary artery disease. J Atheroscler Thromb. 2016;23(8):908–21.
11. Cui L, Zhao T, Hu H, Zhang W, Hua X. Association study of gut Flora in coronary heart disease through high-throughput sequencing. Biomed Res Int. 2017;2017(10):3796359.
12. Jie Z, Xia H, Zhong SL, Feng Q, Li S, Liang S, et al. The gut microbiome in atherosclerotic cardiovascular disease. Nat Commun. 2017;8(1):017–00900.
13. Zhu Q, Gao R, Zhang Y, Pan D, Zhu Y, Zhang X, et al. Dysbiosis signatures of gut microbiota in coronary artery disease. Physiol Genomics. 2018;50(10):893–903.
14. Furusawa Y, Obata Y, Fukuda S, Endo TA, Nakato G, Takahashi D, et al. Commensal microbe-derived butyrate induces the differentiation of colonic regulatory T cells. Nature. 2013;504(7480):446–50.
15. Tang WH, Kitai T, Hazen SL. Gut microbiota in cardiovascular health and disease. Circ Res. 2017;120(7):1183–96.
16. Yang T, Santisteban MM, Rodriguez V, Li E, Ahmari N, Carvajal JM, et al. Gut Dysbiosis is linked to hypertension. Hypertension. 2015;65(6):1331–40.
17. Li J, Zhao F, Wang Y, Chen J, Tao J, Tian G, et al. Gut microbiota dysbiosis contributes to the development of hypertension. Microbiome. 2017;5(1):14.
18. Gomez-Arango LF, Barrett HL, McIntyre HD, Callaway LK, Morrison M, Dekker NM. Increased systolic and diastolic blood pressure is associated with altered gut microbiota composition and butyrate production in early pregnancy. Hypertension. 2016;68(4):974–81.

19. Mozaffarian D, Fahimi S, Singh GM, Micha R, Khatibzadeh S, Engell RE, et al. Global sodium consumption and death from cardiovascular causes. N Engl J Med. 2014;371(7):624–34.

20. Wilck N, Matus MG, Kearney SM, Olesen SW, Forslund K, Bartolomaeus H, et al. Salt-responsive gut commensal modulates TH17 axis and disease. Nature. 2017;551(7682):585–9.

21. Yuzefpolskaya M, Bohn B, Nasiri M, Zuver AM, Onat DD, Royzman EA, et al. Gut microbiota, endotoxemia, inflammation, and oxidative stress in patients with heart failure, left ventricular assist device, and transplant. J Heart Lung Transplant. 2020;39(9):880–90.

22. Mamic P, Heidenreich PA, Hedlin H, Tennakoon L, Staudenmayer KL. Hospitalized patients with heart failure and common bacterial infections: a Nationwide analysis of concomitant Clostridium Difficile infection rates and in-hospital mortality. J Card Fail. 2016;22(11):891–900.

23. Luedde M, Winkler T, Heinsen FA, Ruhlemann MC, Spehlmann ME, Bajrovic A, et al. Heart failure is associated with depletion of core intestinal microbiota. ESC Heart Fail. 2017;4(3):282–90.

24. Cui X, Ye L, Li J, Jin L, Wang W, Li S, et al. Metagenomic and metabolomic analyses unveil dysbiosis of gut microbiota in chronic heart failure patients. Sci Rep. 2018;8(1):017–18756.

25. Kamo T, Akazawa H, Suda W, Saga-Kamo A, Shimizu Y, Yagi H, et al. Dysbiosis and compositional alterations with aging in the gut microbiota of patients with heart failure. PLoS One. 2017;12(3):e0174099.

26. Kummen M, Mayerhofer CCK, Vestad B, Broch K, Awoyemi A, Storm-Larsen C, et al. Gut microbiota signature in heart failure defined from profiling of 2 independent cohorts. J Am Coll Cardiol. 2018;71(10):1184–6.

27. Pasini E, Aquilani R, Testa C, Baiardi P, Angioletti S, Boschi F, et al. Pathogenic gut Flora in patients with chronic heart failure. JACC Heart Fail. 2016;4(3):220–7.

28. Mayerhofer CCK, Kummen M, Holm K, Broch K, Awoyemi A, Vestad B, et al. Low fibre intake is associated with gut microbiota alterations in chronic heart failure. ESC Heart Fail. 2020;24(10):12596.

29. Turnbaugh PJ, Ley RE, Mahowald MA, Magrini V, Mardis ER, Gordon JI. An obesity-associated gut microbiome with increased capacity for energy harvest. Nature. 2006;444(7122):1027–31.

30. Turnbaugh PJ, Hamady M, Yatsunenko T, Cantarel BL, Duncan A, Ley RE, et al. A core gut microbiome in obese and lean twins. Nature. 2009;457(7228):480–4.

31. Ley RE, Backhed F, Turnbaugh P, Lozupone CA, Knight RD, Gordon JI. Obesity alters gut microbial ecology. Proc Natl Acad Sci U S A. 2005;102(31):11070–5.

32. Zeevi D, Korem T, Zmora N, Israeli D, Rothschild D, Weinberger A, et al. Personalized nutrition by prediction of glycemic responses. Cell. 2015;163(5):1079–94.

33. Pedersen HK, Gudmundsdottir V, Nielsen HB, Hyotylainen T, Nielsen T, Jensen BAH, et al. Human gut microbes impact host serum metabolome and insulin sensitivity. Nature. 2016;535(7612):376–81.

34. Qin J, Li Y, Cai Z, Li S, Zhu J, Zhang F, et al. A metagenome-wide association study of gut microbiota in type 2 diabetes. Nature. 2012;490(7418):55–60.

35. Tang TWH, Chen HC, Chen CY, Yen CYT, Lin CJ, Prajnamitra RP, et al. Loss of gut microbiota alters immune system composition and cripples Postinfarction cardiac repair. Circulation. 2019;139(5):647–59.

36. Pluznick JL, Protzko RJ, Gevorgyan H, Peterlin Z, Sipos A, Han J, et al. Olfactory receptor responding to gut microbiota-derived signals plays a role in renin secretion and blood pressure regulation. Proc Natl Acad Sci U S A. 2013;110(11):4410–5.

37. Natarajan N, Hori D, Flavahan S, Steppan J, Flavahan NA, Berkowitz DE, et al. Microbial short chain fatty acid metabolites lower blood pressure via endothelial G protein-coupled receptor 41. Physiol Genomics. 2016;48(11):826–34.

38. Verhaar BJH, Collard D, Prodan A, Levels JHM, Zwinderman AH, Bäckhed F, et al. Associations between gut microbiota, faecal short-chain fatty acids, and blood pressure across ethnic groups: the HELIUS study. Eur Heart J. 2020;41(44):4259–67.

39. Pluznick JL. Microbial short-chain fatty acids and blood pressure regulation. Curr Hypertens Rep. 2017;19(4):25.

40. Pagel MD, Ahmad S, Vizzo JE, Scribner BH. Acetate and bicarbonate fluctuations and acetate intolerance during dialysis. Kidney Int. 1982;21(3):513–8.

41. Marques FZ, Nelson E, Chu PY, Horlock D, Fiedler A, Ziemann M, et al. High-Fiber diet and acetate supplementation change the gut microbiota and prevent the development of hypertension and heart failure in hypertensive mice. Circulation. 2017;135(10):964–77.

42. de la Cuesta-Zuluaga J, Mueller NT, Alvarez-Quintero R, Velasquez-Mejia EP, Sierra JA, Corrales-Agudelo V, et al. Higher fecal short-chain fatty acid Levels are associated with gut microbiome Dysbiosis, obesity, hypertension and Cardiometabolic disease risk factors. Nutrients. 2018;11(1):51.

43. Teixeira TF, Grzeskowiak L, Franceschini SC, Bressan J, Ferreira CL, Peluzio MC. Higher level of faecal SCFA in women correlates with metabolic syndrome risk factors. Br J Nutr. 2013;109(5):914–9.

44. Sanna S, van Zuydam NR, Mahajan A, Kurilshikov A, Vich Vila A, Vosa U, et al. Causal relationships among the gut microbiome, short-chain fatty acids and metabolic diseases. Nat Genet. 2019;51(4):600–5.

45. Tirosh A, Calay ES, Tuncman G, Claiborn KC, Inouye KE, Eguchi K, et al. The short-chain fatty acid propionate increases glucagon and FABP4 production, impairing insulin action in mice and humans. Sci Transl Med. 2019;11(489):eaav0120.

46. Kawamata Y, Fujii R, Hosoya M, Harada M, Yoshida H, Miwa M, et al. A G protein-coupled

receptor responsive to bile acids. J Biol Chem. 2003;278(11):9435–40.

47. Rosen H, Gonzalez-Cabrera PJ, Sanna MG, Brown S. Sphingosine 1-phosphate receptor signaling. Annu Rev Biochem. 2009;78:743–68.

48. Li YTY, Swales KE, Thomas GJ, Warner TD, Bishop-Bailey D. Farnesoid x receptor ligands inhibit vascular smooth muscle cell inflammation and migration. Arterioscler Thromb Vasc Biol. 2007;27(12):2606–11.

49. Mencarelli A, Renga B, Distrutti E, Fiorucci S. Antiatherosclerotic effect of farnesoid X receptor. Am J Physiol Heart Circ Physiol. 2009;296(2):H272–81.

50. Gordon JW, Shaw JA, Kirshenbaum LA. Multiple facets of NF-kappaB in the heart: to be or not to NF-kappaB. Circ Res. 2011;108(9):1122–32.

51. Pu J, Yuan A, Shan P, Gao E, Wang X, Wang Y, et al. Cardiomyocyte-expressed farnesoid-X-receptor is a novel apoptosis mediator and contributes to myocardial ischaemia/reperfusion injury. Eur Heart J. 2012;34(24):1834–45.

52. Mayerhofer CCK, Ueland T, Broch K, Vincent RP, Cross GF, Dahl CP, et al. Increased secondary/primary bile acid ratio in chronic heart failure. J Card Fail. 2017;23(9):666–71.

53. von Haehling S, Schefold JC, Jankowska EA, Springer J, Vazir A, Kalra PR, et al. Ursodeoxycholic acid in patients with chronic heart failure: a double-blind, randomized, placebo-controlled, crossover trial. J Am Coll Cardiol. 2012;59(6):585–92.

54. Prinz P, Hofmann T, Ahnis A, Elbelt U, Goebel-Stengel M, Klapp BF, et al. Plasma bile acids show a positive correlation with body mass index and are negatively associated with cognitive restraint of eating in obese patients. Front Neurosci. 2015;9:199.

55. Haeusler RA, Astiarraga B, Camastra S, Accili D, Ferrannini E. Human insulin resistance is associated with increased plasma levels of 12alpha-hydroxylated bile acids. Diabetes. 2013;62(12):4184–91.

56. Fang S, Suh JM, Reilly SM, Yu E, Osborn O, Lackey D, et al. Intestinal FXR agonism promotes adipose tissue browning and reduces obesity and insulin resistance. Nat Med. 2015;21(2):159–65.

57. Chávez-Talavera O, Tailleux A, Lefebvre P, Staels B. Bile acid control of metabolism and inflammation in obesity, type 2 diabetes, dyslipidemia, and nonalcoholic fatty liver disease. Gastroenterology. 2017;152(7):1679–1694.e3.

58. Ahmad TR, Haeusler RA. Bile acids in glucose metabolism and insulin signalling — mechanisms and research needs. Nat Rev Endocrinol. 2019;15(12):701–12.

59. Sonne DP, van Nierop FS, Kulik W, Soeters MR, Vilsbøll T, Knop FK. Postprandial plasma concentrations of individual bile acids and FGF-19 in patients with type 2 diabetes. J Clin Endocrinol Metabol. 2016;101(8):3002–9.

60. Wewalka M, Patti M-E, Barbato C, Houten SM, Goldfine AB. Fasting serum taurine-conjugated bile acids are elevated in type 2 diabetes and do not change

61. Cariou B, Chetiveaux M, Zaïr Y, Pouteau E, Disse E, Guyomarc'h-Delasalle B, et al. Fasting plasma chenodeoxycholic acid and cholic acid concentrations are inversely correlated with insulin sensitivity in adults. Nutr Metab. 2011;8(1):48.

62. Legry V, Francque S, Haas JT, Verrijken A, Caron S, Chavez-Talavera O, et al. Bile acid alterations are associated with insulin resistance, but not with NASH, in obese subjects. J Clin Endocrinol Metab. 2017;102(10):3783–94.

63. Smushkin G, Sathananthan M, Piccinini F, Dalla Man C, Law JH, Cobelli C, et al. The effect of a bile acid Sequestrant on glucose metabolism in subjects with type 2 diabetes. Diabetes. 2013;62(4):1094–101.

64. Romano KA, Vivas EI, Amador-Noguez D, Rey FE. Intestinal microbiota composition modulates choline bioavailability from diet and accumulation of the Proatherogenic metabolite trimethylamine->N-oxide. MBio. 2015;6(2):e02481-14.

65. Koeth RA, Lam-Galvez BR, Kirsop J, Wang Z, Levison BS, Gu X, et al. l-Carnitine in omnivorous diets induces an atherogenic gut microbial pathway in humans. J Clin Invest. 2019;129(1):373–87.

66. Koeth RA, Levison BS, Culley MK, Buffa JA, Wang Z, Gregory JC, et al. Gamma-Butyrobetaine is a proatherogenic intermediate in gut microbial metabolism of L-carnitine to TMAO. Cell Metab. 2014;20(5):799–812.

67. Skye SM, Zhu W, Romano KA, Guo CJ, Wang Z, Jia X, et al. Microbial transplantation with human gut commensals containing CutC is sufficient to transmit enhanced platelet reactivity and thrombosis potential. Circ Res. 2018;123(10):1164–76.

68. Bennett BJ, de Aguiar Vallim TQ, Wang Z, Shih DM, Meng Y, Gregory J, et al. Trimethylamine-N-oxide, a metabolite associated with atherosclerosis, exhibits complex genetic and dietary regulation. Cell Metab. 2013;17(1):49–60.

69. Koeth RA, Wang Z, Levison BS, Buffa JA, Org E, Sheehy BT, et al. Intestinal microbiota metabolism of l-carnitine, a nutrient in red meat, promotes atherosclerosis. Nat Med. 2013;19(5):576–85.

70. Wang Z, Klipfell E, Bennett BJ, Koeth R, Levison BS, Dugar B, et al. Gut flora metabolism of phosphatidylcholine promotes cardiovascular disease. Nature. 2011;472(7341):57–63.

71. Zhu W, Wang Z, Tang WHW, Hazen SL. Gut microbe-generated trimethylamine N-oxide from dietary choline is Prothrombotic in subjects. Circulation. 2017;135(17):1671–3.

72. Zhu W, Gregory JC, Org E, Buffa JA, Gupta N, Wang Z, et al. Gut microbial metabolite TMAO enhances platelet Hyperreactivity and thrombosis risk. Cell. 2016;165(1):111–24.

73. Boini KM, Hussain T, Li PL, Koka S. Trimethylamine-N-oxide instigates NLRP3 Inflammasome activation and endothelial dysfunction. Cell Physiol Biochem. 2017;44(1):152–62.

74. Chen ML, Zhu XH, Ran L, Lang HD, Yi L, Mi MT. Trimethylamine-N-oxide induces vascular inflammation by activating the NLRP3 Inflammasome through the SIRT3-SOD2-mtROS signaling pathway. J Am Heart Assoc. 2017;6(9):006347.

75. Seldin MM, Meng Y, Qi H, Zhu W, Wang Z, Hazen SL, et al. Trimethylamine N-oxide promotes vascular inflammation through signaling of mitogen-activated protein kinase and nuclear factor-kappaB. J Am Heart Assoc. 2016;5(2):002767.

76. Liu X, Xie Z, Sun M, Wang X, Li J, Cui J, et al. Plasma trimethylamine N-oxide is associated with vulnerable plaque characteristics in CAD patients as assessed by optical coherence tomography. Int J Cardiol. 2018;265:18–23.

77. Gupta N, Buffa JA, Roberts AB, Sangwan N, Skye SM, Li L, et al. Targeted inhibition of gut microbial trimethylamine N-oxide production reduces renal Tubulointerstitial fibrosis and functional impairment in a murine model of chronic kidney disease. Arterioscler Thromb Vasc Biol. 2020;40(5):1239–55.

78. Tang WH, Wang Z, Levison BS, Koeth RA, Britt EB, Fu X, et al. Intestinal microbial metabolism of phosphatidylcholine and cardiovascular risk. N Engl J Med. 2013;368(17):1575–84.

79. Senthong V, Li XS, Hudec T, Coughlin J, Wu Y, Levison B, et al. Plasma trimethylamine N-oxide, a gut microbe-generated phosphatidylcholine metabolite, is associated with atherosclerotic burden. J Am Coll Cardiol. 2016;67(22):2620–8.

80. Sheng Z, Tan Y, Liu C, Zhou P, Li J, Zhou J, et al. Relation of circulating trimethylamine N-oxide with coronary atherosclerotic burden in patients with ST-segment elevation myocardial infarction. Am J Cardiol. 2019;123(6):894–8.

81. Fu Q, Zhao M, Wang D, Hu H, Guo C, Chen W, et al. Coronary plaque characterization assessed by optical coherence tomography and plasma trimethylamine-N-oxide Levels in patients with coronary artery disease. Am J Cardiol. 2016;118(9):1311–5.

82. Tan Y, Sheng Z, Zhou P, Liu C, Zhao H, Song L, et al. Plasma trimethylamine N-oxide as a novel biomarker for plaque rupture in patients with ST-segment-elevation myocardial infarction. Circ Cardiovasc Interv. 2019;12(1):007281.

83. Heianza Y, Ma W, Manson JE, Rexrode KM, Qi L. Gut microbiota metabolites and risk of major adverse cardiovascular disease events and death: a systematic review and Meta-analysis of prospective studies. J Am Heart Assoc. 2017;6(7):004947.

84. Schiattarella GG, Sannino A, Toscano E, Giugliano G, Gargiulo G, Franzone A, et al. Gut microbe-generated metabolite trimethylamine-N-oxide as cardiovascular risk biomarker: a systematic review and dose-response meta-analysis. Eur Heart J. 2017;38(39):2948–56.

85. Qi J, You T, Li J, Pan T, Xiang L, Han Y, et al. Circulating trimethylamine N-oxide and the risk of cardiovascular diseases: a systematic review and meta-analysis of 11 prospective cohort studies. J Cell Mol Med. 2018;22(1):185–94.

86. Heianza Y, Ma W, DiDonato JA, Sun Q, Rimm EB, Hu FB, et al. Long-term changes in gut microbial metabolite trimethylamine N-oxide and coronary heart disease risk. J Am Coll Cardiol. 2020;75(7):763–72.

87. Ufnal M, Jazwiec R, Dadlez M, Drapala A, Sikora M, Skrzypecki J. Trimethylamine-N-oxide: a carnitine-derived metabolite that prolongs the hypertensive effect of angiotensin II in rats. Can J Cardiol. 2014;30(12):1700–5.

88. Bielinska K, Radkowski M, Grochowska M, Perlejewski K, Huc T, Jaworska K, et al. High salt intake increases plasma trimethylamine N-oxide (TMAO) concentration and produces gut dysbiosis in rats. Nutrition. 2018;54:33–9.

89. Jaworska K, Huc T, Samborowska E, Dobrowolski L, Bielinska K, Gawlak M, et al. Hypertension in rats is associated with an increased permeability of the colon to TMA, a gut bacteria metabolite. PLoS One. 2017;12(12):e0189310.

90. Ge X, Zheng L, Zhuang R, Yu P, Xu Z, Liu G, et al. The gut microbial metabolite trimethylamine N-oxide and hypertension risk: a systematic review and dose–response Meta-analysis. Adv Nutr. 2019;11(1):66–76.

91. Organ CL, Otsuka H, Bhushan S, Wang Z, Bradley J, Trivedi R, et al. Choline diet and its gut microbe-derived metabolite, trimethylamine N-oxide, exacerbate pressure overload-induced heart failure. Circ Heart Fail. 2016;9(1):23.

92. Zhang H, Meng J, Yu H. Trimethylamine N-oxide supplementation abolishes the Cardioprotective effects of voluntary exercise in mice fed a Western diet. Front Physiol. 2017;8:944.

93. Makrecka-Kuka M, Volska K, Antone U, Vilskersts R, Grinberga S, Bandere D, et al. Trimethylamine N-oxide impairs pyruvate and fatty acid oxidation in cardiac mitochondria. Toxicol Lett. 2017;267: 32–8.

94. Savi M, Bocchi L, Bresciani L, Falco A, Quaini F, Mena P, et al. Trimethylamine-N-Oxide (TMAO)-induced impairment of cardiomyocyte function and the protective role of urolithin B-glucuronide. Molecules. 2018;23(3):549.

95. Chen K, Zheng X, Feng M, Li D, Zhang H. Gut microbiota-dependent metabolite trimethylamine N-oxide contributes to cardiac dysfunction in Western diet-induced obese mice. Front Physiol. 2017;8:139.

96. Tang WH, Wang Z, Fan Y, Levison B, Hazen JE, Donahue LM, et al. Prognostic value of elevated levels of intestinal microbe-generated metabolite trimethylamine-N-oxide in patients with heart failure: refining the gut hypothesis. J Am Coll Cardiol. 2014;64(18):1908–14.

97. Tang WH, Wang Z, Shrestha K, Borowski AG, Wu Y, Troughton RW, et al. Intestinal microbiota-dependent phosphatidylcholine metabolites, diastolic dysfunction, and adverse clinical outcomes in chronic systolic heart failure. J Card Fail. 2015;21(2):91–6.

98. Trøseid M, Ueland T, Hov JR, Svardal A, Gregersen I, Dahl CP, et al. Microbiota-dependent metabolite trimethylamine-N-oxide is associated with disease severity and survival of patients with chronic heart failure. J Intern Med. 2015;277(6):717–26.

99. Schuett K, Kleber ME, Scharnagl H, Lorkowski S, März W, Niessner A, et al. Trimethylamine-N-oxide and heart failure with reduced versus preserved ejection fraction. J Am Coll Cardiol. 2017;70(25):3202–4.

100. Suzuki T, Yazaki Y, Voors AA, Jones DJL, Chan DCS, Anker SD, et al. Association with outcomes and response to treatment of trimethylamine N-oxide in heart failure: results from BIOSTAT-CHF. Eur J Heart Fail. 2019;21(7):877–86.

101. Huang Y, Zheng S, Zhu H, Lu J, Li W, Hu Y. Gut microbe-generated metabolite trimethylamine-n-oxide and risk of major adverse cardiovascular events in patients with heart failure. J Am Coll Cardiol. 2020;75(11 Supplement 1):834.

102. Li W, Huang A, Zhu H, Liu X, Huang X, Huang Y, et al. Gut microbiota-derived trimethylamine N-oxide is associated with poor prognosis in patients with heart failure. Med J Aust. 2020;213(8):374–9.

103. Suzuki T, Heaney LM, Bhandari SS, Jones DJ, Ng LL. Trimethylamine N-oxide and prognosis in acute heart failure. Heart. 2016;102(11):841–8.

104. Salzano A, Israr MZ, Yazaki Y, Heaney LM, Kanagala P, Singh A, et al. Combined use of trimethylamine N-oxide with BNP for risk stratification in heart failure with preserved ejection fraction: findings from the DIAMONDHFpEF study. Eur J Prev Cardiol. 2019;14:2047487319870355.

105. Schugar RC, Shih DM, Warrier M, Helsley RN, Burrows A, Ferguson D, et al. The TMAO-producing enzyme Flavin-containing monooxygenase 3 regulates obesity and the Beiging of white adipose tissue. Cell Rep. 2017;19(12):2451–61.

106. Mente A, Chalcraft K, Ak H, Davis AD, Lonn E, Miller R, et al. The relationship between trimethylamine-N-oxide and prevalent cardiovascular disease in a multiethnic population living in Canada. Can J Cardiol. 2015;31(9):1189–94.

107. Krüger R, Merz B, Rist MJ, Ferrario PG, Bub A, Kulling SE, et al. Associations of current diet with plasma and urine TMAO in the KarMeN study: direct and indirect contributions. Mol Nutr Food Res. 2017;61(11):1700363.

108. Barrea L, Annunziata G, Muscogiuri G, Di Somma C, Laudisio D, Maisto M, et al. Trimethylamine-N-oxide (TMAO) as novel potential biomarker of early predictors of metabolic syndrome. Nutrients. 2018;10(12):1971.

109. Dambrova M, Latkovskis G, Kuka J, Strele I, Konrade I, Grinberga S, et al. Diabetes is associated with higher trimethylamine-N-oxide plasma levels. Exp Clin Endocrinol Diabetes. 2016;124(4):251–6.

110. Dehghan P, Farhangi MA, Nikniaz L, Nikniaz Z, Asghari-Jafarabadi M. Gut microbiota-derived metabolite trimethylamine N-oxide (TMAO) poten-tially increases the risk of obesity in adults: an exploratory systematic review and dose-response meta-analysis. Obes Rev. 2020;21(5):3.

111. Meyer KA, Benton TZ, Bennett BJ, Jacobs DR Jr, Lloyd-Jones DM, Gross MD, et al. Microbiota-dependent metabolite trimethylamine N-oxide and coronary artery calcium in the coronary artery risk development in Young adults study (CARDIA). J Am Heart Assoc. 2016;5(10):003970.

112. Stubbs JR, House JA, Ocque AJ, Zhang S, Johnson C, Kimber C, et al. Serum trimethylamine-N-oxide is elevated in CKD and correlates with coronary atherosclerosis burden. J Am Soc Nephrol. 2016;27(1):305–13.

113. Erickson ML, Malin SK, Wang Z, Brown JM, Hazen SL, Kirwan JP. Effects of lifestyle intervention on plasma trimethylamine N-oxide in obese adults. Nutrients. 2019;11(1):179.

114. Gao X, Liu X, Xu J, Xue C, Xue Y, Wang Y. Dietary trimethylamine N-oxide exacerbates impaired glucose tolerance in mice fed a high fat diet. J Biosci Bioeng. 2014;118(4):476–81.

115. Miao J, Ling AV, Manthena PV, Gearing ME, Graham MJ, Crooke RM, et al. Flavin-containing monooxygenase 3 as a potential player in diabetes-associated atherosclerosis. Nat Commun. 2015;6(1): 6498.

116. Zhuang R, Ge X, Han L, Yu P, Gong X, Meng Q, et al. Gut microbe-generated metabolite trimethylamine N-oxide and the risk of diabetes: a systematic review and dose-response meta-analysis. Obes Rev. 2019;20(6):883–94.

117. Shan Z, Sun T, Huang H, Chen S, Chen L, Luo C, et al. Association between microbiota-dependent metabolite trimethylamine-N-oxide and type 2 diabetes. Am J Clin Nutr. 2017;106(3):888–94.

118. Tang WHW, Wang Z, Li XS, Fan Y, Li DS, Wu Y, et al. Increased trimethylamine N-oxide portends high mortality risk independent of glycemic control in patients with type 2 diabetes mellitus. Clin Chem. 2020;63(1):297–306.

119. Collins HL, Drazul-Schrader D, Sulpizio AC, Koster PD, Williamson Y, Adelman SJ, et al. L-Carnitine intake and high trimethylamine N-oxide plasma levels correlate with low aortic lesions in ApoE(−/−) transgenic mice expressing CETP. Atherosclerosis. 2016;244:29–37.

120. Huc T, Drapala A, Gawrys M, Konop M, Bielinska K, Zaorska E, et al. Chronic, low-dose TMAO treatment reduces diastolic dysfunction and heart fibrosis in hypertensive rats. Am J Physiol Heart Circ Physiol. 2018;315(6):H1805–H20.

121. Nemet I, Saha PP, Gupta N, Zhu W, Romano KA, Skye SM, et al. A cardiovascular disease-linked gut microbial metabolite acts via adrenergic receptors. Cell. 2020;180(5):862–877.e22.

122. Lam V, Su J, Koprowski S, Hsu A, Tweddell JS, Rafiee P, et al. Intestinal microbiota determine severity of myocardial infarction in rats. FASEB J. 2012;26(4):1727–35.

123. Gan XT, Ettinger G, Huang CX, Burton JP, Haist JV, Rajapurohitam V, et al. Probiotic administration attenuates myocardial hypertrophy and heart failure after myocardial infarction in the rat. Circ Heart Fail. 2014;7(3):491–9.

124. Chan YK, El-Nezami H, Chen Y, Kinnunen K, Kirjavainen PV. Probiotic mixture VSL#3 reduce high fat diet induced vascular inflammation and atherosclerosis in ApoE(-/-) mice. AMB Express. 2016;6(1):016–0229.

125. Mizoguchi T, Kasahara K, Yamashita T, Sasaki N, Yodoi K, Matsumoto T, et al. Oral administration of the lactic acid bacterium Pediococcus acidilactici attenuates atherosclerosis in mice by inducing tolerogenic dendritic cells. Heart Vessel. 2017;32(6):768–76.

126. Karlsson C, Ahrne S, Molin G, Berggren A, Palmquist I, Fredrikson GN, et al. Probiotic therapy to men with incipient arteriosclerosis initiates increased bacterial diversity in colon: a randomized controlled trial. Atherosclerosis. 2010;208(1):228–33.

127. Qiu L, Tao X, Xiong H, Yu J, Wei H. Lactobacillus plantarum ZDY04 exhibits a strain-specific property of lowering TMAO via the modulation of gut microbiota in mice. Food Funct. 2018;9(8):4299–309.

128. Qiu L, Yang D, Tao X, Yu J, Xiong H, Wei H. Enterobacter aerogenes ZDY01 attenuates choline-induced trimethylamine N-oxide Levels by remodeling gut microbiota in mice. J Microbiol Biotechnol. 2017;27(8):1491–9.

129. Malik M, Suboc TM, Tyagi S, Salzman N, Wang J, Ying R, et al. Lactobacillus plantarum 299v supplementation improves vascular endothelial function and reduces inflammatory biomarkers in men with stable coronary artery disease. Circ Res. 2018;123(9):1091–102.

130. Matsumoto M, Kitada Y, Shimomura Y, Naito Y. Bifidobacterium animalis subsp. lactis LKM512 reduces levels of intestinal trimethylamine produced by intestinal microbiota in healthy volunteers: a double-blind, placebo-controlled study. J Funct Foods. 2017;36:94–101.

131. Costanza AC, Moscavitch SD, Faria Neto HCC, Mesquita ET. Probiotic therapy with Saccharomyces boulardii for heart failure patients: a randomized, double-blind, placebo-controlled pilot trial. Int J Cardiol. 2015;179:348–50.

132. Mayerhofer CCK, Awoyemi AO, Moscavitch SD, Lappegard KT, Hov JR, Aukrust P, et al. Design of the GutHeart-targeting gut microbiota to treat heart failure-trial: a phase II, randomized clinical trial. ESC Heart Fail. 2018;5(5):977–84.

133. Tripolt NJ, Leber B, Triebl A, Köfeler H, Stadlbauer V, Sourij H. Effect of Lactobacillus casei Shirota supplementation on trimethylamine-N-oxide levels in patients with metabolic syndrome: an open-label, randomized study. Atherosclerosis. 2015;242(1):141–4.

134. Boutagy NE, Neilson AP, Osterberg KL, Smithson AT, Englund TR, Davy BM, et al. Probiotic supple-

mentation and trimethylamine-N-oxide production following a high-fat diet. Obesity. 2015;23(12): 2357–63.

135. Borges NA, Stenvinkel P, Bergman P, Qureshi AR, Lindholm B, Moraes C, et al. Effects of probiotic supplementation on trimethylamine-N-oxide plasma Levels in hemodialysis patients: a pilot study. Probiotics Antimicrob Proteins. 2019;11(2):648–54.

136. Chen Z, Guo L, Zhang Y, Walzem RL, Pendergast JS, Printz RL, et al. Incorporation of therapeutically modified bacteria into gut microbiota inhibits obesity. J Clin Invest. 2014;124(8):3391–406.

137. Madjd A, Taylor MA, Mousavi N, Delavari A, Malekzadeh R, Macdonald IA, et al. Comparison of the effect of daily consumption of probiotic compared with low-fat conventional yogurt on weight loss in healthy obese women following an energy-restricted diet: a randomized controlled trial1. Am J Clin Nutr. 2015;103(2):323–9.

138. Bernini LJ, Simao AN, Alfieri DF, Lozovoy MA, Mari NL, de Souza CH, et al. Beneficial effects of Bifidobacterium lactis on lipid profile and cytokines in patients with metabolic syndrome: a randomized trial. Effects of probiotics on metabolic syndrome. Nutrition. 2016;32(6):716–9.

139. Tao YW, Gu YL, Mao XQ, Zhang L, Pei YF. Effects of probiotics on type II diabetes mellitus: a meta-analysis. J Transl Med. 2020;18(1):020–02213.

140. Wang S, Xiao Y, Tian F, Zhao J, Zhang H, Zhai Q, et al. Rational use of prebiotics for gut microbiota alterations: specific bacterial phylotypes and related mechanisms. J Funct Foods. 2020;66:103838.

141. Johnson LP, Walton GE, Psichas A, Frost GS, Gibson GR, Barraclough TG. Prebiotics modulate the effects of antibiotics on gut microbial diversity and functioning in vitro. Nutrients. 2015;7(6):4480–97.

142. Kaye DM, Shihata WA, Jama HA, Tsyganov K, Ziemann M, Kiriazis H, et al. Deficiency of prebiotic Fiber and insufficient signaling through gut metabolite-sensing receptors leads to cardiovascular disease. Circulation. 2020;141(17):1393–403.

143. Parnell JA, Reimer RA. Weight loss during oligofructose supplementation is associated with decreased ghrelin and increased peptide YY in overweight and obese adults. Am J Clin Nutr. 2009;89(6): 1751–9.

144. Dewulf EM, Cani PD, Claus SP, Fuentes S, Puylaert PG, Neyrinck AM, et al. Insight into the prebiotic concept: lessons from an exploratory, double blind intervention study with inulin-type fructans in obese women. Gut. 2013;62(8):1112–21.

145. Cani PD, Neyrinck AM, Fava F, Knauf C, Burcelin RG, Tuohy KM, et al. Selective increases of bifidobacteria in gut microflora improve high-fat-diet-induced diabetes in mice through a mechanism associated with endotoxaemia. Diabetologia. 2007;50(11):2374–83.

146. Robertson MD, Bickerton AS, Dennis AL, Vidal H, Frayn KN. Insulin-sensitizing effects of dietary

resistant starch and effects on skeletal muscle and adipose tissue metabolism. Am J Clin Nutr. 2005;82(3):559–67.

147. Baugh ME, Steele CN, Angiletta CJ, Mitchell CM, Neilson AP, Davy BM, et al. Inulin supplementation does not reduce plasma trimethylamine N-oxide concentrations in individuals at risk for type 2 diabetes. Nutrients. 2018;10(6):793.

148. Jama HA, Fiedler A, Tsyganov K, Nelson E, Horlock D, Nakai ME, et al. Manipulation of the gut microbiota by the use of prebiotic fibre does not override a genetic predisposition to heart failure. Sci Rep. 2020;10(1):17919.

149. Everard A, Lazarevic V, Derrien M, Girard M, Muccioli GG, Neyrinck AM, et al. Responses of gut microbiota and glucose and lipid metabolism to prebiotics in genetic obese and diet-induced leptin-resistant mice. Diabetes. 2011;60(11):2775–86.

150. Catry E, Bindels LB, Tailleux A, Lestavel S, Neyrinck AM, Goossens JF, et al. Targeting the gut microbiota with inulin-type fructans: preclinical demonstration of a novel approach in the management of endothelial dysfunction. Gut. 2018;67(2):271–83.

151. Vrieze A, Van Nood E, Holleman F, Salojarvi J, Kootte RS, Bartelsman JF, et al. Transfer of intestinal microbiota from lean donors increases insulin sensitivity in individuals with metabolic syndrome. Gastroenterology. 2012;143(4):913–6.

152. Kootte RS, Levin E, Salojarvi J, Smits LP, Hartstra AV, Udayappan SD, et al. Improvement of insulin sensitivity after lean donor feces in metabolic syndrome is driven by baseline intestinal microbiota composition. Cell Metab. 2017;26(4):611–9.

153. Smits LP, Kootte RS, Levin E, Prodan A, Fuentes S, Zoetendal EG, et al. Effect of vegan fecal microbiota transplantation on carnitine- and choline-derived trimethylamine-N-oxide production and vascular inflammation in patients with metabolic syndrome. J Am Heart Assoc. 2018;7(7):008342.

154. Mistry P, Reitz CJ, Khatua TN, Rasouli M, Oliphant K, Young ME, et al. Circadian influence on the microbiome improves heart failure outcomes. J Mol Cell Cardiol. 2020;149:54–72.

155. Zarrinpar A, Chaix A, Yooseph S, Panda S. Diet and feeding pattern affect the diurnal dynamics of the gut microbiome. Cell Metab. 2014;20(6):1006–17.

156. Thaiss CA, Levy M, Korem T, Dohnalová L, Shapiro H, Jaitin DA, et al. Microbiota diurnal rhythmicity programs host transcriptome oscillations. Cell. 2016;167(6):1495–1510.e12.

157. Paulose JK, Wright JM, Patel AG, Cassone VM. Human gut Bacteria are sensitive to melatonin and express endogenous circadian rhythmicity. PLoS One. 2016;11(1):e0146643.

158. Voigt RM, Forsyth CB, Green SJ, Mutlu E, Engen P, Vitaterna MH, et al. Circadian disorganization alters intestinal microbiota. PLoS One. 2014;9(5):e97500.

159. Kaczmarek JL, Musaad SM, Holscher HD. Time of day and eating behaviors are associated with the composition and function of the human gastrointestinal microbiota. Am J Clin Nutr. 2017;106(5): 1220–31.

160. Washburn RL, Cox JE, Muhlestein JB, May HT, Carlquist JF, Le VT, et al. Pilot study of novel intermittent fasting effects on Metabolomic and trimethylamine N-oxide changes during 24-hour water-only fasting in the FEELGOOD trial. Nutrients. 2019;11(2):246.

161. Appel LJ, Moore TJ, Obarzanek E, Vollmer WM, Svetkey LP, Sacks FM, et al. A clinical trial of the effects of dietary patterns on blood pressure. DASH collaborative research group. N Engl J Med. 1997;336(16):1117–24.

162. Estruch R, Ros E, Salas-Salvadó J, Covas M-I, Corella D, Arós F, et al. Primary prevention of cardiovascular disease with a Mediterranean diet supplemented with extra-virgin olive oil or nuts. N Engl J Med. 2018;378(25):e34.

163. David LA, Maurice CF, Carmody RN, Gootenberg DB, Button JE, Wolfe BE, et al. Diet rapidly and reproducibly alters the human gut microbiome. Nature. 2014;505(7484):559–63.

164. Kaczmarek JL, Thompson SV, Holscher HD. Complex interactions of circadian rhythms, eating behaviors, and the gastrointestinal microbiota and their potential impact on health. Nutr Rev. 2017;75(9):673–82.

165. Duncan SH, Belenguer A, Holtrop G, Johnstone AM, Flint HJ, Lobley GE. Reduced dietary intake of carbohydrates by obese subjects results in decreased concentrations of butyrate and butyrate-producing Bacteria in feces. Appl Environ Microbiol. 2007;73(4):1073–8.

166. Desai MS, Seekatz AM, Koropatkin NM, Kamada N, Hickey CA, Wolter M, et al. A dietary Fiber-deprived gut microbiota degrades the colonic mucus barrier and enhances pathogen susceptibility. Cell. 2016;167(5):1339–1353.e21.

167. Wu GD, Chen J, Hoffmann C, Bittinger K, Chen YY, Keilbaugh SA, et al. Linking long-term dietary patterns with gut microbial enterotypes. Science. 2011;334(6052):105–8.

168. De Filippo C, Cavalieri D, Di Paola M, Ramazzotti M, Poullet JB, Massart S, et al. Impact of diet in shaping gut microbiota revealed by a comparative study in children from Europe and rural Africa. Proc Natl Acad Sci U S A. 2010;107(33):14691–6.

169. Calame W, Weseler AR, Viebke C, Flynn C, Siemensma AD. Gum arabic establishes prebiotic functionality in healthy human volunteers in a dose-dependent manner. Br J Nutr. 2008;100(6):1269–75.

170. Wu WT, Cheng HC, Chen HL. Ameliorative effects of konjac glucomannan on human faecal beta-glucuronidase activity, secondary bile acid levels and faecal water toxicity towards Caco-2 cells. Br J Nutr. 2011;105(4):593–600.

171. Fernando WM, Hill JE, Zello GA, Tyler RT, Dahl WJ, Van Kessel AG. Diets supplemented with chick-

pea or its main oligosaccharide component raffinose modify faecal microbial composition in healthy adults. Benefic Microbes. 2010;1(2):197–207.

172. Francois IE, Lescroart O, Veraverbeke WS, Marzorati M, Possemiers S, Evenepoel P, et al. Effects of a wheat bran extract containing arabinoxylan oligosaccharides on gastrointestinal health parameters in healthy adult human volunteers: a double-blind, randomised, placebo-controlled, cross-over trial. Br J Nutr. 2012;108(12):2229–42.

173. Salden BN, Troost FJ, Wilms E, Truchado P, Vilchez-Vargas R, Pieper DH, et al. Reinforcement of intestinal epithelial barrier by arabinoxylans in overweight and obese subjects: a randomized controlled trial: Arabinoxylans in gut barrier. Clin Nutr. 2018;37(2):471–80.

174. Yang JY, Lee YS, Kim Y, Lee SH, Ryu S, Fukuda S, et al. Gut commensal Bacteroides acidifaciens prevents obesity and improves insulin sensitivity in mice. Mucosal Immunol. 2017;10(1):104–16.

175. Eckel RH, Jakicic JM, Ard JD, de Jesus JM, Houston Miller N, Hubbard VS, et al. 2013 AHA/ACC guideline on lifestyle management to reduce cardiovascular risk: a report of the American College of Cardiology/American Heart Association task force on practice guidelines. J Am Coll Cardiol. 2014;63(25, Part B):2960–84.

176. Sofi F, Cesari F, Abbate R, Gensini GF, Casini A. Adherence to Mediterranean diet and health status: meta-analysis. BMJ. 2008;11(337):a1344.

177. Rosato V, Temple NJ, La Vecchia C, Castellan G, Tavani A, Guercio V. Mediterranean diet and cardiovascular disease: a systematic review and meta-analysis of observational studies. Eur J Nutr. 2019;58(1):173–91.

178. Kastorini CM, Milionis HJ, Esposito K, Giugliano D, Goudevenos JA, Panagiotakos DB. The effect of Mediterranean diet on metabolic syndrome and its components: a meta-analysis of 50 studies and 534,906 individuals. J Am Coll Cardiol. 2011;57(11):1299–313.

179. Liyanage T, Ninomiya T, Wang A, Neal B, Jun M, Wong MG, et al. Effects of the Mediterranean diet on cardiovascular outcomes-a systematic review and Meta-analysis. PLoS One. 2016;11(8):e0159252.

180. Miró Ò, Estruch R, Martín-Sánchez FJ, Gil V, Jacob J, Herrero-Puente P, et al. Adherence to Mediterranean diet and all-cause mortality after an episode of acute heart failure: results of the MEDIT-AHF study. JACC Heart Fail. 2018;6(1):52–62.

181. Garcia-Mantrana I, Selma-Royo M, Alcantara C, Collado MC. Shifts on gut microbiota associated to Mediterranean diet adherence and specific dietary intakes on general adult population. Front Microbiol. 2018;9:890.

182. De Filippis F, Pellegrini N, Vannini L, Jeffery IB, La Storia A, Laghi L, et al. High-level adherence to a Mediterranean diet beneficially impacts the gut microbiota and associated metabolome. Gut. 2016;65(11):1812–21.

183. Mitsou EK, Kakali A, Antonopoulou S, Mountzouris KC, Yannakoulia M, Panagiotakos DB, et al. Adherence to the Mediterranean diet is associated with the gut microbiota pattern and gastrointestinal characteristics in an adult population. Br J Nutr. 2017;117(12):1645–55.

184. Guasch-Ferre M, Hu FB, Ruiz-Canela M, Bullo M, Toledo E, Wang DD, et al. Plasma metabolites from choline pathway and risk of cardiovascular disease in the PREDIMED (prevention with Mediterranean diet) study. J Am Heart Assoc. 2017;6(11):006524.

185. Barrea L, Annunziata G, Muscogiuri G, Laudisio D, Di Somma C, Maisto M, et al. Trimethylamine N-oxide, Mediterranean diet, and nutrition in healthy, normal-weight adults: also a matter of sex? Nutrition. 2019;62:7–17.

186. Vázquez-Fresno R, Llorach R, Urpi-Sarda M, Lupianez-Barbero A, Estruch R, Corella D, et al. Metabolomic pattern analysis after Mediterranean diet intervention in a nondiabetic population: a 1- and 3-year follow-up in the PREDIMED study. J Proteome Res. 2015;14(1):531–40.

187. Wang Z, Roberts AB, Buffa JA, Levison BS, Zhu W, Org E, et al. Non-lethal inhibition of gut microbial trimethylamine production for the treatment of atherosclerosis. Cell. 2015;163(7):1585–95.

188. Pignanelli M, Just C, Bogiatzi C, Dinculescu V, Gloor GB, Allen-Vercoe E, et al. Mediterranean diet score: associations with metabolic products of the intestinal microbiome, carotid plaque burden, and renal function. Nutrients. 2018;10(6):779.

189. Griffin LE, Djuric Z, Angiletta CJ, Mitchell CM, Baugh ME, Davy KP, et al. A Mediterranean diet does not alter plasma trimethylamine N-oxide concentrations in healthy adults at risk for colon cancer. Food Funct. 2019;10(4):2138–47.

190. Annunziata G, Maisto M, Schisano C, Ciampaglia R, Narciso V, Tenore GC, et al. Effects of grape pomace polyphenolic extract (Taurisolo(®)) in reducing TMAO serum Levels in humans: preliminary results from a randomized, placebo-controlled, cross-over study. Nutrients. 2019;11(1):139.

191. Hernández-Alonso P, Cañueto D, Giardina S, Salas-Salvadó J, Cañellas N, Correig X, et al. Effect of pistachio consumption on the modulation of urinary gut microbiota-related metabolites in prediabetic subjects. J Nutr Biochem. 2017;45:48–53.

192. Obeid R, Awwad HM, Kirsch SH, Waldura C, Herrmann W, Graeber S, et al. Plasma trimethylamine-N-oxide following supplementation with vitamin D or D plus B vitamins. Mol Nutr Food Res. 2017;61(2):10.

193. Wang Z, Bergeron N, Levison BS, Li XS, Chiu S, Jia X, et al. Impact of chronic dietary red meat, white meat, or non-meat protein on trimethylamine N-oxide metabolism and renal excretion in healthy men and women. Eur Heart J. 2019;40(7):583–94.

194. Mitchell SM, Milan AM, Mitchell CJ, Gillies NA, D'Souza RF, Zeng N, et al. Protein intake at twice the RDA in older men increases circulatory concentrations of the microbiome metabolite trimethylamine-N-oxide (TMAO). Nutrients. 2019;11(9):2207.

195. Schmedes M, Balderas C, Aadland EK, Jacques H, Lavigne C, Graff IE, et al. The effect of lean-seafood and non-seafood diets on fasting and postprandial serum metabolites and lipid species: results from a randomized crossover intervention study in healthy adults. Nutrients. 2018;10(5):598.

196. Cho CE, Taesuwan S, Malysheva OV, Bender E, Tulchinsky NF, Yan J, et al. Trimethylamine-N-oxide (TMAO) response to animal source foods varies among healthy young men and is influenced by their gut microbiota composition: a randomized controlled trial. Mol Nutr Food Res. 2017;61(1):3.

197. Iannotti LL, Lutter CK, Waters WF, Gallegos Riofrío CA, Malo C, Reinhart G, et al. Eggs early in complementary feeding increase choline pathway biomarkers and DHA: a randomized controlled trial in Ecuador. Am J Clin Nutr. 2017;106(6): 1482–9.

198. Miller CA, Corbin KD, da Costa KA, Zhang S, Zhao X, Galanko JA, et al. Effect of egg ingestion on trimethylamine-N-oxide production in humans: a randomized, controlled, dose-response study. Am J Clin Nutr. 2014;100(3):778–86.

199. Barton S, Navarro SL, Buas MF, Schwarz Y, Gu H, Djukovic D, et al. Targeted plasma metabolome response to variations in dietary glycemic load in a randomized, controlled, crossover feeding trial in healthy adults. Food Funct. 2015;6(9):2949–56.

200. Bergeron N, Williams PT, Lamendella R, Faghihnia N, Grube A, Li X, et al. Diets high in resistant starch increase plasma levels of trimethylamine-N-oxide, a gut microbiome metabolite associated with CVD risk. Br J Nutr. 2016;116(12):2020–9.

201. Genoni A, Lo J, Lyons-Wall P, Boyce MC, Christophersen CT, Bird A, et al. A Paleolithic diet lowers resistant starch intake but does not affect serum trimethylamine-N-oxide concentrations in healthy women. Br J Nutr. 2019;121(3):322–9.

202. Angiletta CJ, Griffin LE, Steele CN, Baer DJ, Novotny JA, Davy KP, et al. Impact of short-term flavanol supplementation on fasting plasma trimethylamine N-oxide concentrations in obese adults. Food Funct. 2018;9(10):5350–61.

203. Heianza Y, Sun D, Smith SR, Bray GA, Sacks FM, Qi L. Changes in gut microbiota-related metabolites and long-term successful weight loss in response to weight-loss diets: the POUNDS lost trial. Diabetes Care. 2018;41(3):413–9.

204. Missimer A, Fernandez ML, DiMarco DM, Norris GH, Blesso CN, Murillo AG, et al. Compared to an oatmeal breakfast, two eggs/day increased plasma carotenoids and choline without increasing Trimethyl amine N-oxide concentrations. J Am Coll Nutr. 2018;37(2):140–8.

205. Tang J, Feng Y, Tsao S, Wang N, Curtain R, Wang Y. Berberine and Coptidis rhizoma as novel antineoplastic agents: a review of traditional use and biomedical investigations. J Ethnopharmacol. 2009;126(1):5–17.

206. Zhu L, Zhang D, Zhu H, Zhu J, Weng S, Dong L, et al. Berberine treatment increases Akkermansia in the gut and improves high-fat diet-induced atherosclerosis in Apoe(-/-) mice. Atherosclerosis. 2018;268:117–26.

207. Shi Y, Hu J, Geng J, Hu T, Wang B, Yan W, et al. Berberine treatment reduces atherosclerosis by mediating gut microbiota in apoE-/- mice. Biomed Pharmacother. 2018;107:1556–63.

208. Zhang X, Zhao Y, Xu J, Xue Z, Zhang M, Pang X, et al. Modulation of gut microbiota by berberine and metformin during the treatment of high-fat diet-induced obesity in rats. Sci Rep. 2015;5(1):14405.

209. Zhang X, Zhao Y, Zhang M, Pang X, Xu J, Kang C, et al. Structural changes of gut microbiota during Berberine-mediated prevention of obesity and insulin resistance in high-fat diet-fed rats. PLoS One. 2012;7(8):e42529.

210. Xu J, Lian F, Zhao L, Zhao Y, Chen X, Zhang X, et al. Structural modulation of gut microbiota during alleviation of type 2 diabetes with a Chinese herbal formula. ISME J. 2015;9(3):552–62.

211. Chang C-J, Lin C-S, Lu C-C, Martel J, Ko Y-F, Ojcius DM, et al. Ganoderma lucidum reduces obesity in mice by modulating the composition of the gut microbiota. Nat Commun. 2015;6(1):7489.

212. Sanodiya BS, Thakur GS, Baghel RK, Prasad GB, Bisen PS. Ganoderma lucidum: a potent pharmacological macrofungus. Curr Pharm Biotechnol. 2009;10(8):717–42.

213. Zhu Y, Jameson E, Crosatti M, Schafer H, Rajakumar K, Bugg TD, et al. Carnitine metabolism to trimethylamine by an unusual Rieske-type oxygenase from human microbiota. Proc Natl Acad Sci U S A. 2014;111(11):4268–73.

214. Craciun S, Balskus EP. Microbial conversion of choline to trimethylamine requires a glycyl radical enzyme. Proc Natl Acad Sci. 2012;109(52):21307–12.

215. Wang G, Kong B, Shuai W, Fu H, Jiang X, Huang H. 3,3-Dimethyl-1-butanol attenuates cardiac remodeling in pressure-overload-induced heart failure mice. J Nutr Biochem. 2020;78:108341.

216. Roberts AB, Gu X, Buffa JA, Hurd AG, Wang Z, Zhu W, et al. Development of a gut microbe-targeted nonlethal therapeutic to inhibit thrombosis potential. Nat Med. 2018;24(9):1407–17.

217. Organ CL, Li Z, Sharp TE 3rd, Polhemus DJ, Gupta N, Goodchild TT, et al. Nonlethal inhibition of gut microbial trimethylamine N-oxide produc-

tion improves cardiac function and remodeling in a murine model of heart failure. J Am Heart Assoc. 2020;9(10):10.

218. Pathak P, Helsley RN, Brown AL, Buffa JA, Choucair I, Nemet I, et al. Small molecule inhibition of gut microbial choline trimethylamine lyase activity alters host cholesterol and bile acid metabolism. Am J Physiol Heart Circ Physiol. 2020;318(6):H1474–86.

219. Kuka J, Liepinsh E, Makrecka-Kuka M, Liepins J, Cirule H, Gustina D, et al. Suppression of intestinal microbiota-dependent production of pro-atherogenic trimethylamine N-oxide by shift-

ing L-carnitine microbial degradation. Life Sci. 2014;117(2):84–92.

220. Chen ML, Yi L, Zhang Y, Zhou X, Ran L, Yang J, et al. Resveratrol attenuates trimethylamine-N-oxide (TMAO)-induced atherosclerosis by regulating TMAO synthesis and bile acid metabolism via remodeling of the gut microbiota. MBio. 2016;7(2):e02210-15.

221. Wu W-K, Panyod S, Ho C-T, Kuo C-H, Wu M-S, Sheen L-Y. Dietary allicin reduces transformation of L-carnitine to TMAO through impact on gut microbiota. J Funct Foods. 2015;15:408–17.

Dietary and Nutritional Recommendations for the Prevention and Treatment of Heart Failure

16

Prerana Bhatia and Nicholas Wettersten

Introduction

The prevention and management of heart failure (HF) poses a unique challenge to clinicians practicing cardiovascular medicine. The prevalence of HF is expected to increase globally with an estimated 6.5 million Americans affected already [1], and HF places a substantial burden on the health-care system. Despite its marked prevalence and the frequency with which it is encountered in clinical practice, few advances have been made in reducing its incidence and prevalence likely because HF is a complex clinical syndrome that encompasses numerous pathophysiologic states and has significant overlap with various comorbidities. Medical management of HF is often determined by the degree of left ventricular systolic dysfunction as assessed by left ventricular ejection fraction (LVEF), with HF typically categorized as either heart failure with preserved ejection

fraction (HFpEF; LVEF $\geq$50%), heart failure with reduced ejection fraction (HFrEF; LVEF <40%), or heart failure with midrange ejection fraction (HFmrEF; LVEF 40–49%). Furthermore, the American College of Cardiology/American Heart Association (ACC/AHA) Heart Failure Guidelines now emphasize the stages of HF with Stage A being at risk patients where dietary modification may be critical to reduce the development of symptomatic HF. Regardless of the categorization or stage, there is no single guideline-based dietary or nutritional recommendation for patients with HF, outside of a controversial focus on salt and fluid restriction to minimize volume retention [2–4]. Dietary and nutritional modifications for HF patients should be highly individualized and focus on comorbidities that either have a complex interplay in the pathogenesis of HF or disproportionately affect HF patients. Modifications of these comorbidities—including hypertension, obesity, diabetes, and coronary artery disease—through diet is the primary aim to prevent the development of HF, reduce symptoms, and improve morbidity and mortality. This chapter will review the nutritional and dietary recommendations studied in HF patients with various comorbidities. Patient-specific dietary recommendations to be discussed include reducing sodium intake, fluid restriction, and nutritional supplementation for patients with advanced HF.

P. Bhatia (✉)
Division of Cardiology, University of California, San Diego, La Jolla, CA, USA
e-mail: p3bhatia@ucsd.edu

N. Wettersten
Division of Cardiology, University of California, San Diego, La Jolla, CA, USA

Section of Cardiology, San Diego Veterans Affairs Health System, San Diego, CA, USA
e-mail: nwettersten@health.ucsd.edu

© This is a U.S. government work and not under copyright protection in the U.S.;
foreign copyright protection may apply 2021
M. J. Wilkinson et al. (eds.), *Prevention and Treatment of Cardiovascular Disease*, Contemporary
Cardiology, https://doi.org/10.1007/978-3-030-78177-4_16

Metabolism in HF

With the development of HF, there is a complex and multifaceted alteration in metabolism. Recognition of this altered metabolism is a key first step in understanding how different diets and nutrients play an important role in preventing and treating HF. The core underlying pathophysiology in HF is a chronic inflammatory state, which not only interplays with altered cardiac function but is a systemic process which affects hepatic, renal, and gastrointestinal function among other organs. Neurohormonal regulation of appetite, satiety, and insulin resistance in HF exacerbates the energy imbalance during a hyperadrenergic state [5]. Anorexia, malabsorption, and pro-inflammatory cytokines lead to a decreased energy supply and malnutrition, which can trigger a maladaptive energy utilization and synthesis process (Fig. 16.1) [5].

Cardiac myocytes under normal circumstances derive the majority of their energy from mitochondrial oxidative phosphorylation via oxidation of fatty acids [6]. This energy is largely utilized for myocyte contraction and maintaining ion pumps, such as those responsible for main-

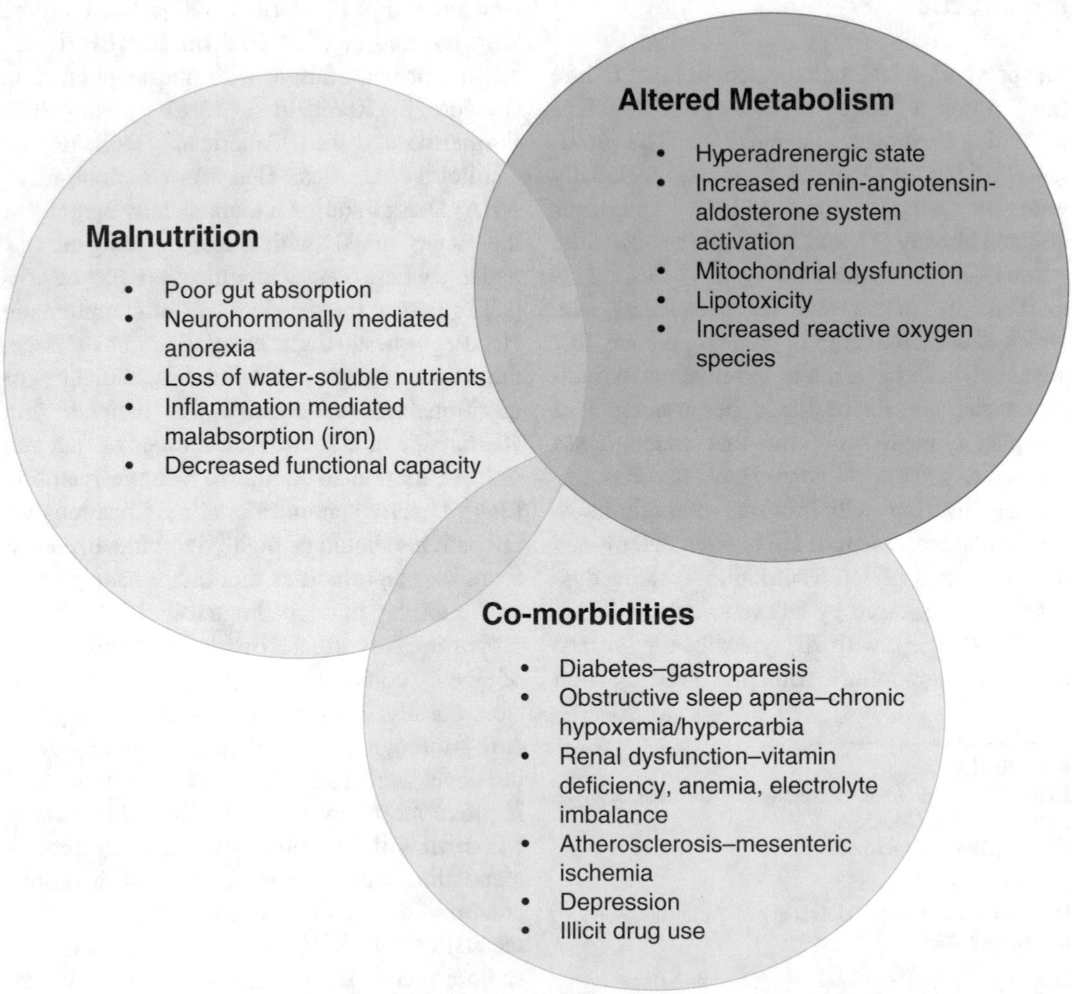

Altered Metabolism

- Hyperadrenergic state
- Increased renin-angiotensin-aldosterone system activation
- Mitochondrial dysfunction
- Lipotoxicity
- Increased reactive oxygen species

Malnutrition

- Poor gut absorption
- Neurohormonally mediated anorexia
- Loss of water-soluble nutrients
- Inflammation mediated malabsorption (iron)
- Decreased functional capacity

Co-morbidities

- Diabetes–gastroparesis
- Obstructive sleep apnea–chronic hypoxemia/hypercarbia
- Renal dysfunction–vitamin deficiency, anemia, electrolyte imbalance
- Atherosclerosis–mesenteric ischemia
- Depression
- Illicit drug use

Fig. 16.1 There is a complex interplay between altered metabolism, factors leading to malnutrition and comorbidities in heart failure. These different aspects overlap with each other in multiple different dimensions contributing to worse outcomes in heart failure. This also adds to the difficulty in treating heart failure patients, as attempting to control one aspect alone is inadequate given the interplay with the other two aspects

taining intracellular calcium in the sarcoplasmic reticulum. Due to the continuous work by the cardiac myocytes, the energy requirement in the myocardium is high and a constant supply of energy is required to maintain contractile function. Depending on the type, stage, and chronicity of HF, various alterations in cardiac metabolism have been observed in animal and human models [6]. In general, HF is associated with decreased fatty acid oxidation and energy production along with mitochondrial dysfunction. There is a shift to glucose oxidation and the citric acid cycle that is considered inadequate to produce the necessary energy. Additionally, increased reactive oxygen species in HF have been implicated in accelerating cardiac remodeling, lipotoxicity, mitochondrial damage, and autophagy [6]. Although altering energy utilization in the myocardium is a ripe area for pharmacotherapy research, dietary and nutritional interventions also have an important role in ensuring that adequate micro- and macronutrients are available to reduce reactive oxygen species, improve energy availability, and reduce remodeling.

A Heart Failure Diet?

There is no single "optimal" diet for HF, and specific recommendations for patients with HFrEF versus HFpEF do not exist. In fact, HFmrEF is another recently recognized category of HF for which pathogenesis, prognosis, and therapeutics are not clearly defined. Since each category of HF confers variable but overlapping risks and comorbidities, the mainstay of dietary and nutritional management of HF is an individualized assessment and modification of risk factors and comorbidities. This is reflected in a 2016 scientific statement by the AHA which highlights the need for dietary recommendations to be individualized to address comorbidities in each patient with HF [2]. The specific pathology and dietary recommendations associated with common comorbidities and risk factors are outlined in Table 16.1.

Due to the high prevalence of some common comorbidities in HFpEF and HFrEF patients, the Dietary Approaches to Stop Hypertension (DASH) and Mediterranean diets have been the most well studied diets in HF patients. Both DASH and Mediterranean diets have been shown to prevent HF in healthy or at-risk individuals and reduce symptoms and decrease mortality in patients with established HF [7–10]. The data for both of these findings though is highly variable. In terms of primary prevention, the DASH diet has been studied in large observational studies which included a range of 6814–38,987 study participants; these studies found a reduction in the development of clinical HF in both men and women as well as favorable echocardiographic findings associated with the DASH diet [8]. Data

Table 16.1 Pathophysiologic and dietary considerations for comorbidities and risk factors associated with heart failure

	Pathology	Dietary considerations
Obesity	Insulin resistance Chronic inflammatory state Obstructive sleep apnea	"U"-shaped association with BMI and mortality Mediterranean diet DASH diet Low-carb, low-fat, volumetric, high protein or vegetarian diet
Hypertension	RAAS activation Cardiac remodeling (LVH) Renal disease Contributing comorbidities—alcohol intake, obesity, obstructive sleep apnea	Avoiding high salt intake DASH diet
Diabetes	Microangiopathy Lipotoxicity Mitochondrial dysfunction	Low-calorie, low-fat diet DASH diet Plant-based diet
Atherosclerosis	Hyperlipidemia Ischemic cardiomyopathy	DASH diet Mediterranean diet

DASH Dietary Approaches to Stop Hypertension, *LVH* left ventricular hypertrophy, *RAAS* renin–angiotensin–aldosterone system

for the Mediterranean diet originates from slightly older studies, which includes the Lyon Diet Heart Study which was published in 1999 [8]. The Lyon Diet Heart study enrolled 604 individuals, of whom half were prospectively randomized to a Mediterranean Diet. This study showed that Mediterranean diet arm had a large reduction in a composite endpoint that included incident HF [11].

The evidence behind the favorable outcomes with the DASH and Mediterranean diets in patients who carry a diagnosis of HF comes from several small studies. The DASH diet was initially investigated in many small studies that included a range of 12–48 subjects with either unspecified HF or HFpEF [7, 8]. One of these studies had a 3-month follow-up period, with most follow-up periods less than 1 month [7, 8]. The only large study correlating adherence to the DASH diet with clinical outcomes is part of The Women's Health Initiative study which observed 3215 women in HF and found that DASH diet was associated with a lower mortality at 4.6 years [10]. Similarly, evidence for the benefit of the Mediterranean diet in patients with HF also stems from smaller studies. The Mediterranean Diet was studied in an overlapping cohort of 106–372 patients with HF over several studies and found that the Mediterranean Diet is associated with favorable echocardiographic findings and lower levels of circulating inflammatory cytokines [7]. The Women's Health Initiative study was the largest trial assessing benefits of the Mediterranean diet and found a trend toward decreased mortality in women adhering to a Mediterranean Diet [10].

More recently, there has been a focus on a plant-based diet which was studied in a 2019 publication [12]. This study included a large cohort of 16,068 individuals (59% women) followed for 8.7 years. The risk of developing HF (either HFrEF or HFpEF) was correlated with five different dietary patterns. Adherence to a plant-based diet high in vegetables, fruits, beans, and fish was associated with a reduced risk of HF development, even in individuals with baseline hypertension [12]. The proposed mechanism for benefit of a plant-based diet is the anti-inflammatory effects of ingesting higher amounts of foods rich in antioxidants leading to a reduction in reactive oxygen species which in turn changes cell signaling and function to reduce myocyte hypertrophy and interstitial fibrosis [12].

Comorbidities

Obesity

Measures of obesity , including body mass index (BMI) and waist circumference, are independently associated with the risk of HF development. The association between obesity and HF development appears to be multifactorial and related to not only excess body mass but also obesity-related hormonal abnormalities, insulin resistance, and a chronic inflammatory state. Obesity in HFpEF may have a significant association with obstructive sleep apnea which is another comorbidity that can exacerbate HFpEF. Obesity can also be seen in HFrEF patients and may overlap with metabolic syndrome which can increase the risk of ischemic cardiomyopathy.

Despite the increased risk of HF development in obese individuals, the severity of obesity is not always linearly correlated with risk for mortality in patients with established HF. In fact, a higher BMI in patients with known HFrEF and HFpEF is paradoxically associated with lower all-cause and cardiovascular mortality [13]. This is known as the "obesity paradox" [13]. Recent evidence suggests that the obesity paradox may only apply to older individuals, and younger patients with HF have a linear association between increasing obesity and worse clinical outcomes [14]. In fact, it has been noted that there is a "U shaped" association (Fig. 16.2) of BMI and clinical outcomes in older HF patients, where a BMI less than 18.5 kg/m^2 is also associated with worse prognosis [2, 13, 14]. Low BMI patients are likely to be experiencing malnutrition and/or cachexia related to a catabolic state in advanced HF. Additionally , the poor prognosis associated with a low BMI may be related to other underlying conditions

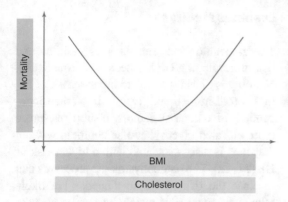

Fig. 16.2 The "U"-shaped association between body mass index (BMI) and total cholesterol with mortality in heart failure. Patients with high and low BMIs and total cholesterol levels experience the worst outcomes

leading to unintentional weight loss. Thus, management of obesity in patients with established HF is a complex topic with questionable benefit. Meanwhile, addressing obesity in patients at risk of HF has a very distinct role and benefit.

Weight loss in patients at risk of HF has several potential benefits including decreased blood pressure, cardiac mass, and filling pressures, and possibly improved diastolic and systolic cardiac function. Evidence for the potential benefits of weight loss in obese individuals is extrapolated from bariatric surgery studies. Weight loss through bariatric surgery has been shown to improve echocardiographic markers of diastolic function, with some evidence of improved systolic function as well [2]. Although no specific studies have prospectively assessed the effects of dietary weight loss for the prevention of HF, weight loss in obese individuals at risk for HF is recommended, and typically the Mediterranean, DASH, low-carb, low-fat, volumetric (low-calorie), high-protein, or vegetarian diets are recommended.

In contrast, the evidence for weight loss in patients with established HF and obesity is unclear. A pilot study of 14 individuals demonstrated that overweight patients with HFrEF and diabetes mellitus assigned to a high-protein diet lost more weight and had improved quality of life compared to those assigned a standard protein diet and conventional diet [15]. These results have yet to be demonstrated in large clinical trials

with sustained weight loss with measurement of core outcomes such as mortality or rehospitalizations. In fact, this finding is in contrast to another trial where 170 obese patients with HFrEF that experienced weight loss (not through a specified lifestyle modification recommendation) were observed to have a higher mortality [16]. It should be noted that patients in this study that had a higher mortality with weight loss may exemplify the obesity paradox discussed earlier; unintentional weight loss may be due to advanced HF and cardiac cachexia. Despite this study, there is an ongoing discussion about the potential benefits for weight loss in obese patients with HF when using structured interventions, which is evidenced by the positive data shown in bariatric surgery patients. In small studies (12–14 subjects) of obese patients with HFrEF undergoing bariatric surgery, weight loss was retrospectively associated with improved LVEF and functional capacity [2]. These studies suggest that the effects of weight loss on HF patients may be dependent on whether weight loss is actively and intentionally achieved (e.g., lifestyle, diet, or surgery) versus unintentional (e.g., related to malnutrition and cachexia).

Hypertension

Hypertension is a common comorbidity in both HFpEF and HFrEF patients, and it is also thought to be an underlying mechanism in the development of HFpEF as well a risk factor for HFrEF. There is an abundance of data suggesting that treatment of systolic and diastolic hypertension reduces the risk of developing HF [2]. Indeed, the Systolic Blood Pressure Intervention Trial (SPRINT) demonstrated the cardiovascular benefits of blood pressure lowering with HF being one of the most common incident cardiovascular diseases reduced [17]. Management of hypertension, however, is complex and requires consideration of secondary causes such as obesity, excess dietary sodium intake, sleep-disordered breathing, excess alcohol use, and progression of chronic kidney disease. Thus, there is some overlap in the dietary management of hypertension with these comorbid conditions. Much of the dietary management of hypertension tends to focus on limiting sodium intake as well as weight loss in the obese patient with obstructive sleep apnea. The benefits of limiting dietary sodium intake have been most well studied through the DASH diet. Adherence to the DASH diet has reproducibly led to decreased systolic and diastolic blood pressures [2, 18]. In the patients with Stage A HF, a low-sodium diet and specifically the DASH diet is the most commonly recommended diet for reducing the progression to HF.

For patients with established HF, management of hypertension is a cornerstone of treatment. Afterload reduction with agents that downregulate the renin–angiotensin–aldosterone system (RAAS) are often initial therapies because RAAS activation leads to the cycle of vasoconstriction, water retention, and increased blood pressure among other deleterious effects. Because of the potential benefits of blood pressure management in patients with HF and hypertension, the DASH diet has been extensively studied in patients with both HFrEF and HFpEF; however, results have been variable for the efficacy of the DASH diet. Specifically, in patients with hypertension and HFpEF, the DASH diet has been shown to improve diastolic function and decrease systemic vascular resistance [19]. More recently, the Geriatric Out-of-Hospital Randomized Meal Trial in heart failure investigators randomized 66 patients with HFpEF and HFrEF to receive home delivered DASH diet meals after hospital discharge [20]. The study showed a trend toward improved quality of life and reduction in 30-day readmission rates; however, it was underpowered and did not meet statistical significance when compared to the usual care group [20]. Although the DASH diet does limit sodium intake, it also encourages more consumption of fruits, vegetables, lean protein, and fiber which may have other beneficial effects through altering levels of other micronutrients and reducing systemic inflammation. Overall, dietary management of HF patients with HTN remains an active area of research.

Diabetes Mellitus

The association between diabetes mellitus and risk of developing HF has been well established. Not only is diabetes found to increase risk of HF by twofold in men and fivefold in women independent of other risk factors, insulin resistance (with elevated glycosylated hemoglobin without diabetes) is also associated with a higher risk of HF [21, 22]. The pathophysiologic processes that increase the risk of HF in diabetics are likely related to coexisting metabolic syndrome with concurrent obesity and hypertension in addition to the direct effects of hyperglycemia on microangiopathy, lipotoxicity, and mitochondrial dysfunction. Thus, it is not surprising that many HF patients also carry a diagnosis of diabetes. In patients with existing HF, diabetes is linked to higher rates of hospitalization and mortality [2].

Lifestyle modification for the prevention of diabetes in the at-risk population and management for those with known diabetes is a key component for the prevention of HF. Based on data by the Diabetes Prevention Program Research Group, lifestyle modification for the high-risk population has been shown to be more effective than metformin in preventing progression to diabetes. Specifically, this group showed that weight loss with a prescription of physical activity and a low-calorie, low-fat diet reduced the incidence of diabetes by 58% over 2.8 years in a cohort of 3243 nondiabetic individuals [23].

More recently, further analysis of the Look AHEAD (Action for Health in Diabetes) has been published [24]. The Look AHEAD trial was initially designed to assess the risk of developing cardiovascular disease in a cohort of obese and diabetic individuals randomized to lifestyle intervention and diet versus usual care. The aim was to sustain weight loss of at least 7% using a low-calorie diet, which included meal replacements, and moderate-intensity exercise for more than 175 min per week. The initial trial was stopped due to futility after a median follow-up of 9.6 years due to low cardiovascular events. With 5109 participants, this trial is one of the largest studies directly assessing the effects of diabetes and obesity management on the development of HF [24]. In the most recent analysis, which included follow-up of 12.4 years, investigators found that intensive lifestyle modification did not significantly reduce the risk of HF, despite sustained weight loss and lower glycosylated hemoglobin levels. Risk of HFpEF was lower in individuals with higher baseline functional capacity as determined by a maximal treadmill test [24]. Although there is not a specific diet recommended for individuals with diabetes and HF, the American Diabetes Association endorses the incorporation of Mediterranean, DASH, and plant-based diets into individualized meal planning for diabetics patients [25].

Atherosclerotic Heart Disease

Coronary artery disease has long been linked to the development of HF, with concern that the incidence and prevalence of HF will continue to rise as therapeutics improve survival after a myocardial infarction in the aging population. The dietary management of atherosclerotic heart disease to prevent HF has often focused on the management of dyslipidemia. In terms of specific diets, the Mediterranean diet is the most well studied. The initial trial showing the protective effects of adhering to the Mediterranean Diet was conducted from 1988 to 1992, and an extended follow-up of 46 months showed significantly lower rates of cardiovascular death, recurrent myocardial infarction, and HF in the group assigned the Mediterranean Diet [11]. The DASH diet and a vegetarian diet are also recommended for overall reducing atherosclerotic heart disease-related comorbidities [26]. Interestingly, there is some evidence that low total cholesterol levels in patients with known HF may be predictive of higher mortality [27]. This association is similar to the "U-shaped" relationship between BMI and mortality (Fig. 16.2), where an abnormally low cholesterol level likely reflects poor metabolic reserve in patients with advanced HF and cardiac cachexia. Conversely, elevated cholesterol levels are responsible for greater atherosclerotic cardiovascular disease burden.

Specific Dietary Recommendations in the Treatment and Prevention of Heart Failure

Sodium Restriction

Low sodium content is a major component of the DASH diet, which has an established role in reducing blood pressure and risk of HF development. Sodium restriction is also generally recommended for patients with Stage C or D HF as a means of preventing progression of disease, controlling symptoms, and reducing HF exacerbations. The data supporting sodium restriction is quite poor though, and the 2013 ACC/AHA Heart Failure Guidelines state there is "insufficient evidence" to suggest that lower sodium intake prevents HF or reduces symptoms [3]. Despite some evidence that low sodium diets in HF patients may reduce B-type natriuretic peptide (BNP) levels, improve QOL, and reduce risk of recurrent HF exacerbation [28, 29]; it is generally not well tolerated. An inpatient study where salt and fluid were restricted demonstrated that patients experienced increased sensation of thirst without an improvement in weight loss or clinical stability [30]. This raises the concern that the low-sodium diet recommendations likely are not adhered to and could potentially exacerbate malnutrition in patients with advanced HF who have limited appetite at baseline. Paradoxically, hypertonic saline has been used in patients with acute HF to assist in volume removal, which is contradictory to commonly held beliefs on sodium restriction [31]. Thus, sodium restriction is not a guideline-based recommendation for HF patients, and the implications on quality of life and nutrition should be considered for patients that are recommended to follow such a restriction.

Fluid Restriction

Limiting fluid intake in HF patients is another commonly employed strategy to help reduce diuretic requirements, especially in patients admitted with HF. The utility of fluid restriction in the management of HF remains unclear. As aforementioned, there is some evidence that salt and fluid restriction leads to increased perception of thirst without any clinical benefits [30]. It should be noted that some studies have found higher diuretic requirements in HF patients are associated with a worse mortality; however, other studies have not found this and it is often believed that the higher diuretic requirements reflect a more advanced HF patient population [27]. Regardless, fluid restrictions are often placed so as not to "feed the fire" with needing more diuretics to remove fluid. This recommendation is made despite a lack of evidence that fluid restriction alters the pathophysiology of HF or reduces mortality.

Nutrition in Advanced Heart Failure

Malnutrition in advanced HF is an incredibly common and multifaceted comorbidity. Malnutrition likely results from a complex interplay of a chronic hypercatabolic and inflammatory state, appetite suppression and malabsorption due to gut-edema, and muscle wasting due to cachexia or sarcopenia [4, 5]. The significance of malnutrition has been established over many studies that indicate low albumin, muscle mass, BMI, and cholesterol levels among other markers

of malnutrition are closely linked to poor survival in HF patients [5]. Although protein intake is commonly insufficient in this population, higher protein intake recommendations are not standardized since protein intake should be individualized based on a person's dietary pattern and renal function.

Inadequate consumption of several micronutrients is also commonly found in advanced HF patients, especially those adhering to a salt-restricted diet [32]. However, the clinical significance of these nutritional deficiencies is unclear. Thus, aside from the recent incorporation of iron replacement into the 2017 ACC/AHA Heart Failure Guidelines, replacement of other nutrients such as thiamine and coenzyme Q10 are not supported by major societies or guidelines (Table 16.2). In general, all HF patients should receive a comprehensive nutrition assessment either in the inpatient or outpatient setting, especially if there are signs of cardiac cachexia which includes edema-free weight loss of more than 6% over the preceding 6–12 months or BMI less than 20 kg/m^2 [4, 5]. Individualized assessment for possible malnutrition and specific nutritional deficiencies should guide clinical recommendations. Commonly encountered nutritional and vitamin deficiencies and the evidence of supplementation is outlined in Table 16.3.

Table 16.2 Dietary and supplement recommendations for patients with HF by guideline recommendations and indication class (when available)

	ACC/AHA/HFSA 2013 and 2017	ESC 2016
Salt intake	Reasonable to restrict sodium intake (<3 g/d) to reduce symptoms (Class IIa) [3]	Avoid high salt intake (>6 g/d) [44]
Fluid intake	Reasonable to restrict fluid intake (1.5–2 L/d) in stage D heart failure, especially with hyponatremia (Class IIa) [3]	Avoid excessive fluid intake [44] Restricting fluid intake to 1.5–2 L/d may be considered to relieve symptoms in severe heart failure [44]
Vitamin D	No recommendations	No recommendations
Iron	Reasonable to supplement with intravenous iron if iron deficient to improve symptoms and quality of life (Class IIa) [45]	No recommendations
Thiamine	No recommendations	No recommendations
Coenzyme Q10	No recommendations	No recommendations

ACC American College of Cardiology, *AHA* American Heart Association, *ESC* European Society of Cardiology, *HFSA* Heart Failure Society of North America

Table 16.3 Overview of some commonly encountered vitamin and nutritional deficiencies, their role in mediating cardiac function, and evidence of replacing these deficiencies

	Role in cardiac function	Evidence for replacement	Data
Vitamin D	Cardiac remodeling Calcium homeostasis	+/−	Several small studies with potential benefit Large WHI study with no difference in the incidence of HF
Iron	Mitochondrial function Oxygen transportation	+++	Good quality evidence for improved functional capacity and quality of life with intravenous ferric carboxymaltose and iron sucrose for individuals with iron deficiency with or without anemia No benefit from oral supplementation
Thiamine	Cardiac output	+/−	Theoretical benefit if high diuretic requirement or alcohol use No good evidence
Coenzyme Q10	Antioxidant	+	Small studies with fair evidence for improved functional capacity, reduction in HF admissions, and decreased mortality. Larger trials needed to confirm findings

HF heart failure, *WHI* Women's Health Initiative

Vitamin D

Vitamin D deficiency is thought to be very common in HF patients, but the evidence for vitamin D replacement for prevention of HF and treatment of HF is inconclusive. An observational study of 686 older adults (age 70–79 years) did not find any association between lower calcitriol levels and risk of HF over a period of 8.6 years [33], suggesting that vitamin D deficiency is not a major factor in development of HF. Another study of 227 patients with chronic kidney disease with moderate left ventricular hypertrophy and preserved ejection fraction showed that supplementation with an active vitamin D compound did not alter cardiac mass or change echocardiographic measurements of diastolic function over a 48-week follow-up period [34]. The largest trial on this topic comes from the Women's Health Initiative study which randomized 35,983 women to calcium and vitamin D supplementation versus placebo [35]. Over 7.1 years of follow-up, there was no difference in the incidence of HF in the overall population. The lack of benefit was seen in the subgroup of women with preexisting coronary artery disease, diabetes, and hypertension, but women without these risk factors did have a significantly lower incidence of HF (hazard ratio 0.63, CI 0.46–0.87) [35].

The hypothesized benefits of vitamin D supplementation are thought be from a direct receptor-mediated effect on intracellular calcium homeostasis in cardiac myocytes as well as downregulation of RAAS which may improve myocyte aerobic capacity and reduce water and salt retention. Although vitamin D deficient individuals with HFrEF have been shown to have lower aldosterone levels after 6 months of vitamin D supplementation, there is no clear improvement in cardiac function or functional status with vitamin D supplementation [36]. In another study of 94 patients with HFrEF and low vitamin D levels who were given vitamin D supplementation for 4 months, there was a statistically significant improvement in functional capacity measured by a 6-min walk test, reduction in biomarkers of HF, and improvement in LVEF as compared to baseline assessment [37]. These studies are small and benefits of vitamin D supplementation are not reproducible across all the studies, so vitamin D supplementation is not routinely recommended for all individuals with HF and remains an active area of interest.

Iron Deficiency

The ACC, AHA , and Heart Failure Society of North America (HFSA) recommend intravenous iron repletion for individuals with HF and iron deficiency regardless of ejection fraction [4]. Iron is well-known to be a major factor in providing oxygen carrying capacity and a core component of hemoglobin. Iron also plays an important role in supporting mitochondrial function and is actively involved in oxidative phosphorylation, citric acid cycle, and nitric oxide generation. Thus, when skeletal and cardiac muscles are operating under a state of high-energy consumption in HF, sarcomere structure and left ventricular function is particularly sensitive to iron deficiency even in the absence of anemia.

There are two major randomized clinical trials that have led to the widespread recognition and use of intravenous iron supplementation in HF patients with iron deficiency [38, 39]. The first major trial consisted of 459 HFrEF patients with iron deficiency (with and without anemia) who were randomized to intravenous ferric carboxymaltose versus placebo and followed for 24 weeks. Compared to individuals that received placebo, the ferric carboxymaltose group reported improvement in functional capacity and quality of life [38]. A more recent study of 304 ambulatory patients with HFrEF and iron deficiency showed that administration of ferric carboxymaltose resulted in sustained improvements in functional capacity and quality of life at 52 weeks [39]. There was also a reduction in HF admissions but no difference in mortality or adverse events in this study [39]. Similar beneficial effects have also been demonstrated with use of iron sucrose [40].

However, not all iron replacement strategies are equal. Other formulations of intravenous iron have either not been studied or failed to show benefit in HF patients. Furthermore, use of oral iron supplementation or dietary modification to increase oral iron intake in HF patients is not supported. The lack of benefit in oral iron supplementation was highlighted in a randomized clinical trial of 225 HFrEF patients with iron deficiency who had no benefits noted at the end of a 16-week follow-up period [41]. This is likely due to the chronic inflammatory state and gut edema in HF which can inhibit oral iron absorption.

Thiamine

Thiamine deficiency is a major concern in those with active alcohol use resulting in alcohol-induced cardiomyopathy. As a water-soluble nutrient, high-dose diuretics are also hypothesized to lead to thiamine deficiency [4]. Thiamine repletion has been suggested to improve left ventricular systolic function, but this evidence is not robust. Thus, thiamine repletion is not generally recommended for HF patients, unless there is a concern for active alcohol use or high doses of diuretics in the admitted patients at risk for water-soluble vitamin deficiencies [4, 42].

Coenzyme Q10

Deficiency in coenzyme Q10 (CoQ10) has been correlated with worsening symptoms and poor prognosis in HF patients. CoQ10 has been hypothesized to improve myocardial function by acting as an antioxidant, and it is one of the few micronutrients directly studied in randomized clinical trials in HF patients [42]. Although these studies are small and level of evidence is insufficient to translate to guidelines, CoQ10 supplementation has been associated with improved functional capacity, reduced HF admissions, and decreased cardiovascular and all-cause mortality in a randomized controlled trial of 420 patients with either HFrEF or HFpEF [43]. Although this trial had an extended follow-up period of up to 2 years, the predetermined study population was not enrolled and baseline patient population was healthier leading to a lower than expected mortality rate at 2 years [43]. Thus, these findings are largely hypothesis generating and larger trials are needed to confirm these findings.

Conclusion

Nutritional and dietary modification for the prevention and treatment of HF is a complex topic due to the various categories and stages of HF, the complex pathophysiology of HF, and constellation of accompanying comorbidities. To date, the DASH and Mediterranean diets have the most robust evidence for the prevention of HF and reducing mortality in patients with an existing HF diagnosis. More recently, there is growing evidence for the preventive benefits of a plant-based diet. However, specific guideline-based dietary and nutritional recommendations for HF patients are limited due to the heterogeneous patient populations and variability in published evidence. In general, clinicians are encouraged to individualize dietary and nutritional recommendations, which should include thorough assessment of comorbidities such as hypertension, obesity, diabetes mellitus, and atherosclerosis.

The evidence for specific dietary modification and nutritional supplementation in HF is even more variable. Salt and fluid restrictions are commonly recommended for HF patients for the management of symptoms and reduction in diuretic requirement; however, these generalized recommendations lack substantial evidence for benefit and may in fact exacerbate malnutrition in some patients. In paradox to these recommendations, recent publications on use of hypertonic saline to reduce fluid retention further raises questions about the benefits of these common practices. While an area of active interest, most nutritional supplementation lacks robust data and is not guideline recommended. Intravenous iron replacement, but not oral supplementation, is one of the few interventions that has robust evidence in improving symptoms and quality of life in iron deficient HF patients. For other vitamin and micronutrient deficiencies, benefits of replacement are less clear, and supplementation recommendations should be made based on an individualized assessment of patient factors and comorbidities. Overall, the variability in evidence and findings for different diets and nutritional supplementation in HF emphasize the need for large well-designed randomized trials. At this point, it is not a question if dietary modification is important in HF, but which specific modifications are most beneficial to potentially prevent and reverse HF.

References

1. Benjamin EJ, et al. Heart disease and stroke statistics'2017 update: a report from the American Heart Association. Circulation. 2017;135:e146–603.
2. Bozkurt B, et al. Contributory risk and management of comorbidities of hypertension, obesity, diabetes mellitus, hyperlipidemia, and metabolic syndrome in chronic heart failure: a scientific statement from the American Heart Association. Circulation. 2016;134:e535–78.
3. Eckel RH, et al. 2013 AHA/ACC guideline on lifestyle management to reduce cardiovascular risk: a report of the American College of cardiology/American Heart Association task force on practice guidelines. Circulation. 2014;129:76–99.
4. Vest AR, et al. Consensus statement nutrition, obesity, and cachexia in patients with heart failure: a consensus statement from the Heart Failure Society of America Scientific Statements Committee. J Card Fail. 2019;25:380–400.
5. Abu-Sawwa R, Dunbar SB, Quyyumi AA, Sattler ELP. Nutrition intervention in heart failure: should consumption of the DASH eating pattern be recommended to improve outcomes? Heart Fail Rev. 2019;24(4):565–73. https://doi.org/10.1007/s10741-019-09781-6.
6. Doenst T, Nguyen TD, Abel ED. Cardiac metabolism in heart failure: implications beyond atp production. Circ Res. 2013;113:709–24.
7. Dos Reis Padilha G, et al. Dietary patterns in secondary prevention of heart failure: a systematic review. Nutrients. 2018;10:828.
8. Kerley CP. A review of plant-based diets to prevent and treat heart failure. Card Fail Rev. 2018;4:1.
9. Miró Ò, et al. Adherence to mediterranean diet and all-cause mortality after an episode of acute heart failure: results of the MEDIT-AHF study. JACC Heart Fail. 2018;6:52–62.
10. Levitan EB, et al. Mediterranean and DASH diet scores and mortality in women with heart failure the women s health initiative. Circ Hear Fail. 2013;6:1116–23.
11. de Lorgeril M, et al. Mediterranean diet, traditional risk factors, and the rate of cardiovascular complications after myocardial infarction. Circulation. 1999;99:779–85.
12. Lara KM, et al. Dietary patterns and incident heart failure in U.S. adults without known coronary disease. J Am Coll Cardiol. 2019;73:2036–45.
13. Oreopoulos A, et al. Body mass index and mortality in heart failure: a meta-analysis. Am Heart J. 2008;156:13–22.
14. Regan JA, et al. Impact of age on comorbidities and outcomes in heart failure with reduced ejection fraction. JACC Heart Fail. 2019;7:1056–65.
15. Evangelista LS, et al. Reduced body weight and adiposity with a high-protein diet improves functional

status, lipid profiles, glycemic control, and quality of life in patients with heart failure. J Cardiovasc Nurs. 2009;24:207–15.

16. Zamora E, et al. Weight loss in obese patients with heart failure. J Am Heart Assoc. 2015;5(3):e002468.

17. Wright JT, et al. A randomized trial of intensive versus standard blood-pressure control. N Engl J Med. 2015;373:2103–16.

18. Moore TJ, Conlin PR, Ard J, Svetkey LP. DASH (dietary approaches to stop hypertension) diet is effective treatment for stage 1 isolated systolic hypertension. Hypertension. 2001;38:155–8.

19. Hummel SL, et al. Low-sodium DASH diet improves diastolic function and ventricular arterial coupling in hypertensive heart failure with preserved ejection fraction. Circ Hear Fail. 2013;6:1165–71.

20. Hummel SL, et al. Home-delivered meals postdischarge from heart failure hospitalization. Circ Heart Fail. 2018;11:e004886.

21. Kannel WB, McGee DL. Diabetes and cardiovascular disease: the Framingham study. JAMA J Am Med Assoc. 1979;241:2035–8.

22. Matsushita K, et al. The association of hemoglobin A1c with incident heart failure among people without diabetes: the atherosclerosis risk in communities study. Diabetes. 2010;59:2020–6.

23. Knowler WC, et al. Reduction in the incidence of type 2 diabetes with lifestyle intervention or metformin. N Engl J Med. 2002;346:393–403.

24. Pandey A, et al. Association of Intensive Lifestyle Intervention, fitness, and body mass index with risk of heart failure in overweight or obese adults with type 2 diabetes mellitus. Circulation. 2020;141:1295–306.

25. American Diabetes Association. Lifestyle management: standards of medical care in Diabetesd. Diabetes Care. 2018;41:S38–50.

26. Pallazola VA, et al. A Clinician's guide to healthy eating for cardiovascular disease prevention. Mayo Clin Proc Innov Qual Outcomes. 2019;3:251–67.

27. Levy WC, et al. The Seattle heart failure model prediction of survival in heart failure. Circulation. 2006;113(11):1424–33. https://doi.org/10.1161/CIRCULATIONAHA.105.584102.

28. Arcand J, et al. A high-sodium diet is associated with acute decompensated heart failure in ambulatory heart failure patients: a prospective follow-up study. Am J Clin Nutr. 2011;93:332–7.

29. Colin-Ramirez E, et al. The long-term effects of dietary sodium restriction on clinical outcomes in patients with heart failure. The SODIUM-HF (Study of Dietary Intervention under 100 mmol in Heart Failure): a pilot study. Am Heart J. 2015;169:274–81, e1.

30. Aliti GB, et al. Aggressive fluid and sodium restriction in acute decompensated heart failure: a randomized clinical trial. JAMA Intern Med. 2013;173:1058–64.

31. Griffin M, et al. Real world use of hypertonic saline in refractory acute decompensated heart failure: a U.S. center's experience. JACC Heart Fail. 2020;8:199–208.

32. Bilgen F, et al. Insufficient calorie intake worsens post-discharge quality of life and increases readmission burden in heart failure. JACC Heart Fail. 2020;8(9):756–64. https://doi.org/10.1016/j.jchf.2020.04.004.

33. Selamet U, et al. Serum calcitriol concentrations and kidney function decline, heart failure, and mortality in elderly community-living adults: the health, aging, and body composition study. Am J Kidney Dis. 2018;72:419–28.

34. Thadhani R, et al. Vitamin D therapy and cardiac structure and function in patients with chronic kidney disease: the PRIMO randomized controlled trial. JAMA. 2012;307:674–84.

35. Donneyong MM, et al. Risk of heart failure among postmenopausal women a secondary analysis of the randomized trial of vitamin D plus calcium of the women's health initiative. Circ Hear Fail. 2015;8:49–56.

36. Boxer RS, et al. The effect of vitamin D on aldosterone and health status in patients with heart failure. J Card Fail. 2014;20:334–42.

37. Amin A, et al. Can vitamin D supplementation improve the severity of congestive heart failure? Congest Hear Fail. 2013;19:E22–8.

38. Anker SD, et al. Ferric carboxymaltose in patients with heart failure and iron deficiency. N Engl J Med. 2009;17:2436–84.

39. Ponikowski P. Beneficial effects of long-term intravenous iron therapy with ferric carboxymaltose in patients with symptomatic heart failure and iron deficiency. Eur Heart J. 2015;36:657–68.

40. Okonko DO, et al. Effect of intravenous iron sucrose on exercise tolerance in anemic and nonanemic patients with symptomatic chronic heart failure and iron deficiency FERRIC-HF: a randomized, controlled, observer-blinded trial. J Am Coll Cardiol. 2008;51(2):103–12. https://doi.org/10.1016/j.jacc.2007.09.036.

41. Lewis GD, et al. Effect of oral iron repletion on exercise capacity in patients with heart failure with reduced ejection fraction and iron deficiency the IRONOUT HF randomized clinical trial. JAMA. 2017;317:1958–66.

42. Aggarwal M, et al. Lifestyle modifications for preventing and treating heart failure. J Am Coll Cardiol. 2018;72:2391–405.

43. Mortensen SA, et al. The effect of coenzyme Q10 on morbidity and mortality in chronic heart failure: results from Q-SYMBIO: a randomized double-blind trial. JACC Heart Fail. 2014;2:641–9.

44. Ponikowski P, et al. ESC guidelines for the diagnosis and treatment of acute and chronic heart failure: the task force for the diagnosis and treatment of acute and chronic heart failure of the European Society of Cardiology (ESC). Developed with the special contri-

bution of the Heart Failure Association (HFA) of the ESC. Eur J Heart Fail. 2016;18:891–975.

45. Yancy CW, et al. 2017 ACC/AHA/HFSA focused update of the 2013 ACCF/AHA guideline for the Management of Heart Failure: a report of the American College of Cardiology/American Heart Association Task Force on Clinical Practice Guidelines and the Heart Failure Society of America. Circulation. 2017;136:e137–61.

Dietary Considerations for the Prevention and Treatment of Arrhythmia

17

Marin Nishimura and Jonathan C. Hsu

Atrial Fibrillation and Obesity

Atrial fibrillation (AF) is the most common cardiac arrhythmia and results in significant morbidity and mortality worldwide [1, 2]. The lifetime risk of AF is estimated to be 1 in 6, and its prevalence is expected to increase further with aging of the population [1, 3]. Prevention is the most effective way to reduce the burden of disease, and given the high prevalence and significant societal burden of AF, greater understanding of modifiable risk factors contributing to the development and progression of AF is paramount.

Studies have established multiple cardiovascular risk factors for AF, including advanced age, diabetes, and hypertension, in addition to intrinsic cardiac pathologies such as congestive heart failure, coronary artery disease, and valvular heart disease [4]. Obesity, a growing global pandemic, is also shown to have a strong association with AF and subsequent clinical outcomes [5]. More than one-third of the population suffers from obesity and targeting this important risk factor has a great potential to reduce the global burden of AF [6]. Hence, current data suggest that the management of obesity should be an

important aspect of care for patients with and at risk for AF.

Obesity and the Risk of AF

Several large-scale studies have established a strong association of obesity with incident AF. In a subanalysis of the Framingham Heart Study, increase in obesity status as measured by 1-unit increase in body mass index (BMI) associated with a 4% increase in the risk of AF (Table 17.1) [7–12]. The adjusted hazard ratios (HR) for AF associated with obesity status were 1.52 for men (95% confidence interval [CI] 1.09–2.13; $p = 0.02$) and 1.46 for women (95% CI 1.03–2.07, $p = 0.03$). Similarly, an analysis of the Women's Health Study found a significant association between BMI and incident AF, which persisted after accounting for hypertension, diabetes, and the interim development of cardiovascular disease [8]. In this study, BMI was found to be associated linearly with the risk of incident AF with a 4.7% (95% CI 3.4–6.1, p 30 kg/m^2), and 12.2% increased risk of incident AF was attributable to obesity independent of other cardiovascular risk factors [8]. In addition to obesity as measured by BMI, the Guangzhou Biobank Cohort Study demonstrated an association between obesity as measured by waist circumference and incident AF [13]. Obesity is also shown to have an association with postoperative AF following cardiac

M. Nishimura · J. C. Hsu (✉)
Cardiac Electrophysiology Section, Division of Cardiology, Department of Medicine, University of California, San Diego, La Jolla, CA, USA
e-mail: manishimura@health.ucsd.edu;
Jonathan.hsu@health.ucsd.edu

© Springer Nature Switzerland AG 2021
M. J. Wilkinson et al. (eds.), *Prevention and Treatment of Cardiovascular Disease*, Contemporary Cardiology, https://doi.org/10.1007/978-3-030-78177-4_17

Table 17.1 Selected studies on obesity and AF

Author	Title	Study size and design	Findings
Wang et al. [7]	Obesity and the risk of new-onset atrial fibrillation	Community based, observational cohort, $n = 5282$	Subanalysis of the Framingham Heart Study. Increase in 1-unit increase in BMI was associated with a 4% increase in the risk of AF. Adjusted HRs for AF associated with obesity status were 1.52 for men and 1.46 for women
Tedrow et al. [8]	The long and short term impact of elevated body mass index on risk of new atrial fibrillation in the women's health study	Observational cohort, $n = 34,309$	Subanalysis of the Women's Health Study. Found significant association between BMI and incident AF. Linear association between BMI and risk of incident AF with 4.7% increase in risk with each 1-unit increase in BMI; 1.65–1.77-fold increase in the risk of incident AF with obesity (compared to normal weight), and 12.2% of the increase in risk was attributable to obesity
Chatterjee et al. [9]	Genetic obesity and the risk of atrial fibrillation – Causal estimates from Mendelian randomization	Mendelian randomization, $n = 51,646$	Causal relationship between obesity and incident AF (HR 1.15 and 1.11 for two genetic instruments analyzed)
Abed et al. [10]	Effect of weight reduction and cardiometabolic risk factor management on symptom burden and severity in patients with atrial fibrillation – a randomized clinical trial	Randomized controlled study, $n = 150$	Obese patients with symptomatic AF randomized to prescription of either a weight-management program or general lifestyle advice. Weight loss with a prescribed weight-management program resulted in significant reduction in AF burden and improvement in symptoms
Pathak et al. [11]	Long-term effect of goal-directed weight management in an atrial fibrillation cohort, a long-term follow-up study (LEGACY)	Observational cohort, $n = 355$	10% weight loss resulted in a six-fold increase in arrhythmia-free survival at 5 years. Weight fluctuation >5% led to two-fold increase in risk of arrhythmia recurrence
Middeldorp et al. [12]	PREVEntion and regressive effect of weight loss and risk factor modification on atrial fibrillation: REVERSE-AF study	Observational cohort, $n = 355$	Subanalysis of the LEGACY study. Weight loss associated with reduction in AF disease progression. Three percent progressed from paroxysmal to persistent AF and 88% reversed from persistent to paroxysmal or no AF at follow-up with 10% weight reduction, compared to 41% progression from paroxysmal to persistent AF and 26% reversal from persistent to paroxysmal in those without significant weight loss

BMI Body mass index, *AF* atrial fibrillation, *HR* hazard ratio, *LEGACY* Long-Term Effect of Goal-Directed Weight Management on Atrial Fibrillation Cohort: a 5-Year follow-up

surgery (adjusted OR [aOR] for obese I compared to normal weight 1.36, 95% CI 1.14–1.63; aOR for obese II 1.69, 95% CI 1.35–2.11; aOR for obese III 2.39, 95% CI 1.81–3.17) [14]. Finally, a meta-analysis, including 626,603 subjects from 51 studies, found a 19–29% increased risk of incident AF for every 5 unit increase in BMI [15]. A 10% increase (OR 1.10, 95% 1.04–1.17) in the incidence of postoperative AF was also seen for every 5 kg/m² increase in BMI [15]. In line with the findings from the observational studies, a study employing mendelian randomization analysis suggested a causal relationship between obesity and incident AF (HR 1.15 [95% CI 1.04–1.26] and 1.11 [95% CI 1.05–1.17] for two genetic instruments analyzed) [9]. Hence, available data strongly suggest an association between obesity and incident AF and underscore the plausibility of obesity management for those at risk for AF.

Mechanisms Linking Obesity and AF

Obesity may result in a wide range of structural, hemodynamic, and electrophysiological changes that promote the development and persistence of AF. In a sheep obesity model, sustained obesity resulted in bi-atrial enlargement with diastolic dysfunction, increased profibrotic transforming growth factor (TGF)-beta-1 expression, and increased interstitial fibrosis and fatty infiltration of the atrial myocardium, which may contribute to dysrhythmia [16]. The myocytes of obese animals demonstrated slowed and heterogeneous conduction and increased complex fractionated electrograms, resulting in a higher AF burden [16]. Another animal study showed an association of obesity with adverse remodeling of the left atrium, as demonstrated by an increase in left atrial volume with left atrial fibrosis, lipidosis, inflammatory infiltrates, and expression of profibrotic mediators all noted [17]. Electrical changes such as a decrease in conduction velocity and an increase in conduction heterogeneity were also observed, as well as an increase in inducible and spontaneous AF in obese animals [17]. In a pig model, high-fat diet led to a reduction in pulmonary vein effective refractory period and an increase in AF vulnerability [18].

Epicardial fat associated with obesity may also be implicated in the pathogenesis of AF. In a study of patients undergoing cardiac computed tomography (CT), peri-atrial epicardial fat thickness was found to be a significant predictor of AF burden (aOR 5.30, 95% CI 1.39–20.24, $p = 0.015$) [19]. Another study using cardiac CT similarly found an association between thickness of epicardial fat and presence of AF, as well as AF severity [20]. Epicardial fat is a source of several proinflammatory mediators which may play a role in AF pathogenesis. In sheep atrial myocytes, the arrhythmogenic effect of epicardial fat may be mediated by free fatty acids through disruption of T-tubule architecture and

alteration of ionic currents to reduce action potential duration [21].

Finally, in addition to the independent role obesity may play in the pathogenesis of AF, some of the adverse effect may also be mediated by its association with other established AF risk factors such as diabetes, hypertension, and obstructive sleep apnea [4, 22].

Obesity and Outcomes in AF

In addition to AF incidence, obesity is also associated with AF progression. An observational study involving 1385 patients demonstrated an association between more severe obesity with progression of paroxysmal AF into permanent AF (aHR for BMI >40 kg/m² 1.79, 95% CI 1.13–2.84) [23]. Furthermore, obesity may also be associated with failure of rhythm control. In a meta-analysis including 51 studies, a 5-kg/m² increase in BMI was associated with a 13% (OR 1.13, 95% CI 1.06–1.22) greater excess risk of AF recurrence following AF ablation [11]. Similarly, in a secondary analysis of the AFFIRM trial (Atrial Fibrillation Follow-Up Investigation of Rhythm Management), higher BMI associated with a greater number of cardioversions (OR 1.183 for 10 kg/m² increase of BMI, 95% CI 1.049–1.334, $p = 0.006$) and a higher likelihood of rhythm control failure at follow-up (OR 1.218 for 10 kg/m² increase of BMI, 95% CI 1.021–1.452, $p = 0.0283$) [24].

Obesity may also lead to worse outcomes among patients with AF aside from its association with AF burden. In an analysis of the Danish Diet, Cancer, and Health Study, the composite endpoint of ischemic stroke, thromboembolism, or death was found to be significantly higher in overweight (HR 1.31, 95% CI 1.09–1.56) and obese patients (HR 1.55, 95% CI 1.27–1.90) compared to those with normal weight [25]. Importantly, the study also found that the association remained significant after adjustment for CHA$_2$DS$_2$-VASc score (OR for overweight 1.31, 95% CI 1.10–1.56; OR for obese 1.36, 95% CI 1.11–1.65) [25]. For this reason, following AF diagnosis, comorbid obesity may have important implications affecting subsequent clinical outcomes.

Weight Loss and AF

If obesity is associated with incident AF and subsequent clinical outcomes, can weight loss lead to an improvement in AF-related outcomes? In the LEGACY study (Long-Term Effect of Goal-directed weight management on Atrial Fibrillation Cohort: a 5-Year follow-up), 355 patients with AF and BMI >27 kg/m^2 were offered a weight-management program with subsequent weight loss and AF recurrence assessed [11]. The authors found that a 10% weight loss resulted in a sixfold (95% CI 3.4–10.3, $p < 0.001$) increase in arrhythmia-free survival at 5 years. Furthermore, another analysis of the LEGACY study demonstrated that degree of weight loss correlated with a reduction in AF progression [12]. Among subjects who achieved 10% weight reduction, only 3% progressed from paroxysmal to persistent AF while 88% reversed from persistent to paroxysmal or no AF at follow-up, compared to 41% progression from paroxysmal to persistent AF and 26% reversal from persistent to paroxysmal in those without significant weight loss [12]. Furthermore, weight loss may also improve the success of a rhythm control strategy in AF patients. In a study of 239 morbidly obese patients that underwent AF ablation, those that underwent bariatric surgery prior to ablation were found to have a lower risk of AF recurrence compared to those without (20% vs. 61%, $p < 0.0001$) [26]. There was also a significant reduction in the need for repeat ablation among those that underwent bariatric surgery prior to AF ablation (12% vs. 41%, $p < 0.0001$) [26]. In line with the findings of observational studies, Abed et al. randomized obese patients with symptomatic AF to either a weight-management program or general lifestyle advice [10]. Weight loss with a prescribed weight-management program resulted in a significant reduction in AF burden and symptom improvement [10]. Hence, current evidence suggests a suc-

cessful improvement in AF-related outcomes with weight loss.

Caffeine and Supraventricular Tachycardia

Caffeine is ubiquitously consumed around the world and is mostly widely consumed behaviorally active substance worldwide [27]. Caffeine is a stimulant that affects excitatory transmitter release via actions on adenosine receptors and commonly consumed in the forms of coffee, tea, chocolate, and energy drinks [27].

Mechanism of action of caffeine is via sympathetic nervous system activation. Historically, practioners believed that high caffeine intake leads to palpitations and tachycardia. Hence, health-care providers commonly prescribed reductions in caffeine intake for patients suffering from arrhythmias such as SVT [28]. In fact, prior American College of Cardiology/ American Heart Association/European Society of Cardiology guidelines on the management of supraventricular arrhythmias suggested that behavioral risk factors including excessive caffeine intake be reduced in patients with a history consistent with premature ectopic beats [29]. Yet, most studies analyzing the effect of caffeine on arrhythmia burden are largely negative.

In a population study involving 130,054 patients, the association between coffee drinking and the risk of cardiac arrhythmia was analyzed [30]. The study found an inverse association between the amount of coffee intake and risk of hospitalization for SVT (aHR 0.63 for those >4 cups/day, 95% CI 0.41–0.98, $p < 0.05$). Of note, the inverse relation of coffee drinking to arrhythmia-related hospitalization was found to be consistent across genders, races, and age groups [30]. Furthermore, in an analysis of the Cardiovascular Health Study, there was no statistically significant difference in the number of SVT runs across different levels of caffeine product intake (coffee, tea, or chocolate) [31]. Finally, in a study of patients with SVT undergoing electrophysiologic study, patients were randomized to either receiving oral caffeine or placebo prior to the procedure [32]. Caffeine intake was not found to significantly affect atrial/ventricular refractory period or AV node conduction. Caffeine intake also did not affect SVT inducibility or the cycle length of induced tachycardia [32]. Hence, despite common perceptions, studies do not suggest the presence of an association between caffeine intake and SVT.

Dietary Electrolytes in the Management of Arrhythmia

Serum and intracellular electrolytes play central roles in the electrophysiologic environment of the myocardium, and electrolyte derangements can contribute to development of arrhythmia. Potassium and magnesium are most commonly implicated electrolytes, and they affect multiple physiologic parameters including the resting membrane potential, action potential, and refractory period duration [33, 34].

The effect of hypokalemia and hypomagnesemia on ventricular electrophysiology and arrhythmogenesis is well characterized. Hypokalemia predisposes patients to ventricular tachycardia (VT), ventricular fibrillation (VF), and torsades de pointes, especially in the context of concurrent myocardial infarction or heart failure [34, 35]. Hypomagnesemia also predisposes patients to premature ventricular contraction, VT, and VF and plays a central role in the pathogenesis and in the acute management of patients with torsades de pointes [36–38].

On the other hand, the effect of hypokalemia and hypomagnesemia on atrial arrhythmias, including atrial fibrillation, is not well characterized. Studies have suggested an association of hypomagnesemia with risk of incident AF, with the majority of evidence in the context of cardiac surgery with mixed findings outside the postoperative setting [39–43]. Prophylactic magnesium, most often administered intravenously in studies, may be beneficial in reducing the incidence of postoperative AF following cardiac surgery [41–43]. The effect of hypokalemia and potassium supplementation on the risk of AF is less clear with mixed findings [35, 44–46].

Nevertheless, despite the evidence of an association between serum electrolytes and arrhythmia, much less is known about the role of dietary electrolytes. In an analysis of the ARIC (Atherosclerosis Risk in Communities) study, 14,232 patients were followed for 12 years, and the serum levels of magnesium, amount of dietary magnesium, and incidence of sudden cardiac death (SCD) were analyzed [47]. The study found that subjects with the highest quartile of serum magnesium were at significantly lower risk of SCD (HR 0.62, 95% CI 0.42–0.93), most of which likely resulted from ventricular arrhythmias. The association between serum magnesium and the risk of SCD persisted after adjustment for potential confounders. However, despite the association between serum magnesium and SCD, the study did not observe an association between dietary magnesium and SCD. Similarly, analysis of the data from the Women's Health Initiative also did not find a statistically significant association between dietary magnesium and the risk of SCD [48].

Studies exploring the role of dietary electrolyte intake and the incidence of AF is also scarce. In another analysis of the ARIC study, although serum hypomagnesemia was found to be associated with risk of AF, a similar association was again not found between dietary magnesium intake and AF [49]. A study of oral magnesium supplementation in patients with persistent AF with or without sotalol therapy did not demonstrate a reduction in AF [50]. Hence, although evidence suggests the role of serum electrolyte intake and the development of arrhythmia, further studies are needed to elucidate the effect of dietary electrolyte supplementation in the management of patients with arrhythmia.

Conclusion

Diet is an important modifiable risk factor with multiple implications in the management of patients with arrhythmia. Studies have suggested association between obesity and incidence of AF, as well as its association with disease progression and worse outcomes. Given its high prevalence, obesity may be a highly relevant clinical target that can be addressed to reduce the global disease burden of AF. While reduction of caffeine intake is a common recommendation made for patients suffering from palpitations, available evidence do not seem to suggest a clear association between caffeine intake and SVT. Although studies suggest an association between serum electrolyte levels and the development of certain arrhythmias, further studies are needed to elucidate the role of dietary electrolyte supplementation in the management of patients with arrhythmia.

References

1. Lloyd-Jones DM, Wang TJ, Leip EP, Larson MG, Levy D, Vasan RS, et al. Lifetime risk for development of atrial fibrillation: the Framingham heart study. Circulation. 2004;110:1042–6.

2. Si S, Hart CL, Hole DJ, McMurray JJV. A population-based study of the long-term risks associated with atrial fibrillation: 20-year follow-up of the Renfrew/Paisley study. Am J Med. 2002;113:359–64.

3. Go AS, Hylek EM, Phillips KA, Chang Y, Henault LE, Selby JV, et al. Prevalence of diagnosed atrial fibrillation in adults. JAMA. 2001;285(18):2370.

4. Benjamin EJ, Levy D, Vaziri SM, D'agostino RB, Belanger AJ, Wolf PA. Independent risk factors for atrial fibrillation in a population-based cohort: the Framingham heart study. JAMA. 1994;271(11):840–4.

5. Kelly T, Yang W, Chen CS, Reynolds K, He J. Global burden of obesity in 2005 and projections to 2030. Int J Obes. 2008;32(9):1431–7.

6. Hales CM, Fryar CD, Carroll MD, Freedman DS, Ogden CL. Trends in obesity and severe obesity prevalence in US youth and adults by sex and age, 2007-2008 to 2015-2016. JAMA. 2018;319(16):1723–5.

7. Wang TJ, Parise H, Levy D, D'Agostino RB, Wolf PA, Vasan RS, et al. Obesity and the risk of new-onset atrial fibrillation. JAMA. 2004;292(20):2471–7.

8. Tedrow UB, Co D, Ridker PM, Cook NR, Koplan BA, Manson JE, et al. The long and short term impact of elevated body mass index on risk of new atrial fibrillation in the women's health study. J Am Coll Cardiol. 2010;55(21):2319–27.

9. Chatterjee NA, Giulianini F, Geelhoed B, Lunetta KL, Misialek JR, Niemeijer MN, et al. Genetic obesity and the risk of atrial fibrillation. Circulation. 2017;135(8):741–54.

10. Abed HS, Wittert GA, Leong DP, Shirazi MG, Bahrami B, Middeldorp ME, et al. Effect of weight reduction and cardiometabolic risk factor management on symptom burden and severity in patients with atrial fibrillation: a randomized clinical trial. JAMA. 2013;310(19):2050–60.

11. Pathak RK, Middeldorp ME, Meredith M, Mehta AB, Mahajan R, Wong CX, et al. Long-term effect of goal-directed weight management in an atrial fibrillation cohort: a long-term follow-up study (LEGACY). J Am Coll Cardiol. 2015;65(20):2159–69.

12. Middeldorp ME, Pathak RK, Meredith M, Mehta AB, Elliott AD, Mahajan R, et al. PREVEntion and regRessive effect of weight-loss and risk factor modification on atrial fibrillation: the REVERSE-AF study. Europace. 2018;20(12):1929–35.

13. Long MJ, Jiang CQ, Lam TH, Xu L, Sen ZW, Lin JM, et al. Atrial fibrillation and obesity among older Chinese: the Guangzhou Biobank Cohort Study. Int J Cardiol [Internet]. 2011;148(1):48–52. https://doi.org/10.1016/j.ijcard.2009.10.022.

14. Zacharias A, Schwann TA, Riordan CJ, Durham SJ, Shah AS, Habib RH. Obesity and risk of new-onset atrial fibrillation after cardiac surgery. Circulation. 2005;112(21):3247–55.

15. Wong CX, Sullivan T, Sun MT, Mahajan R, Pathak RJ, Middledorp M, et al. Obesity and the risk of post-operative, and post-ablation atrial fibrillation: A meta analysis of 626,603 individuals in 51 studies. JACC Clin Electrophisiol. 2015;1(3):139–54.

16. Mahajan R, Lau DH, Brooks AG, Shipp NJ, Manavis J, Wood JPM, et al. Electrophysiological, electroanatomical, and structural remodeling of the atria as consequences of sustained obesity. J Am Coll Cardiol. 2015;66(1):1–11.

17. Abed HS, Samuel CS, Lau DH, Kelly DJ, Royce SG, Alasady M, et al. Obesity results in progressive atrial structural and electrical remodeling: implications for atrial fibrillation. Heart Rhythm. 2013;10(1):90–100.

18. Okumura Y, Watanabe I, Nagashima K, Sonoda K, Sasaki N, Kogawa R, et al. Effects of a high-fat diet on the electrical properties of porcine atria. J Arrhythm. 2015;31(6):352–8.

19. Batal O, Schoenhagen P, Shao M, Ayyad AE, Van Wagoner DR, Halliburton SS, et al. Left atrial epicardial adiposity and atrial fibrillation omar. Circ Arrhythm Electrophysiol. 2010;3(3):230–6.

20. Yorgun H, Canpolat U, Aytemir K, Hazırolan T, Şahiner L, Kaya EB, et al. Association of epicardial and peri-atrial adiposity with the presence and severity of non-valvular atrial fibrillation. Int J Cardiovasc Imaging. 2015;31(3):649–57.

21. O'Connell RP, Musa H, Gomez MSM, Avula UM, Herron TJ, Kalifa J, et al. Free fatty acid effects on the atrial myocardium: membrane ionic currents are remodeled by the disruption of T-tubular architecture. PLoS One. 2015;10(8):1–18.

22. Huxley RR, Filion KB, Konety S, Alonso A. Meta-analysis of cohort and case-control studies of type 2 diabetes mellitus and risk of atrial fibrillation. Am J Cardiol. 2011;108(1):56–62.

23. Thacker EL, McKnight B, Psaty BM, Longstreth WT, Dublin S, Jensen PN, et al. Association of body mass index, diabetes, hypertension, and blood pressure

levels with risk of permanent atrial fibrillation. J Gen Intern Med. 2013;28(2):247–53.

24. Guglin M, Maradia K, Chen R, Curtis AB. Relation of obesity to recurrence rate and burden of atrial fibrillation. Am J Cardiol. 2011;107(4):579–82.

25. Overvad TF, Rasmussen LH, Skjøth F, Overvad K, Lip GYH, Larsen TB. Body mass index and adverse events in patients with incident atrial fibrillation. Am J Med. 2013;126(7):640.e9–640.e17.

26. Donnellan E, Wazni OM, Kanj M, Baranowski B, Cremer P, Harb S, et al. Association between pre-ablation bariatric surgery and atrial fibrillation recurrence in morbidly obese patients undergoing atrial fibrillation ablation. Europace. 2019;21(10):1476–83.

27. Fredholm BB, Bättig K, Holmén J, Nehlig A, Zvartau EE. Actions of caffeine in the brain with special reference to factors that contribute to its widespread use. Pharmacol Rev. 1999;51(1):83–133.

28. Hughes JR, Amori G, Hatsukami DK. A survey of physician advice about caffeine. J Subst Abus. 1988;1(1):67–70.

29. Blomström-Lundqvist C, Scheinman MM, Aliot EM, Alpert JS, Calkins H, Camm AJ, et al. ACC/AHA/ESC guidelines for the management of patients with supraventricular arrhythmias – executive summary: a report of the American College of Cardiology/American Heart Association Task Force on Practice Guidelines and the European Society of Cardiology. J Am Coll Cardiol Elsevier Masson SAS. 2003;42:1493–531.

30. Klatsky A. Coffee, caffeine, and risk of hospitalization for arrhythmias. Perm J. 2011;15(3):19–25.

31. Dixit S, Stein PK, Dewland TA, Dukes JW, Vittinghoff E, Heckbert SR, et al. Consumption of caffeinated products and cardiac ectopy. J Am Heart Assoc. 2016;5(1):1–10.

32. Lemery R, Pecarskie A, Bernick J, Williams K, Wells GA. A prospective placebo controlled randomized study of caffeine in patients with supraventricular tachycardia undergoing electrophysiologic testing. J Cardiovasc Electrophysiol. 2015;26(1):1–6.

33. Agus M, Agus Z. Cardiovascular actions of magnesium. Crit Care Clin. 2001;17(1):175–86.

34. Schulman M, Narins RG. Hypokalemia and cardiovascular disease. Am J Cardiol. 1990;65(10):E4.

35. Nordrehaug JE, Von Der Lippe G. Serum potassium concentrations are inversely related to ventricular, but not to atrial, arrhythmias in acute myocardial infarction. Eur Heart J. 1986;7(3):204–9.

36. Ceremuzyński L, Gębalska J, Wołk R, Makowska E. Hypomagnesemia in heart failure with ventricular arrhythmias. Beneficial effects of magnesium supplementation. J Intern Med. 2000;247(1):78–86.

37. Gottlieb S, Baruch L, Kukin M, Bernstein J, Fisher M, Packer M. Prognostic importance of the serum magnesium concentration in patients with congestive heart failure. JACC. 1990;16(4):827–31.

38. Al-Khatib SM, Stevenson WG, Ackerman MJ, Bryant WJ, Callans DJ, Curtis AB, et al. 2017 AHA/ACC/HRS guideline for management of patients with ventricular arrhythmias and the prevention of sud-

den cardiac death: executive summary. Circulation. 2018;138(13):e210–71.

39. Khan AM, Lubitz SA, Sullivan LM, Sun JX, Levy D, Vasan RS, et al. Fibrillation in the community : the Framingham heart study. Circulation. 2014;127(1):33–8.

40. Markovits N, Kurnik D, Halkin H, Margalit R, Bialik M, Lomnicky Y, et al. Database evaluation of the association between serum magnesium levels and the risk of atrial fibrillation in the community. Int J Cardiol. 2016;205:142–6.

41. Alghamdi AA, Al-Radi OO, Latter DA. Intravenous magnesium for prevention of atrial fibrillation after coronary artery bypass surgery: a systematic review and meta-analysis. J Card Surg. 2005;20(3):293–9.

42. Chaudhary R, Garg J, Turagam M, Chaudhary R, Gupta R, Nazir T, et al. Role of prophylactic magnesium supplementation in prevention of postoperative atrial fibrillation in patients undergoing coronary artery bypass grafting: a systematic review and meta-analysis of 20 randomized controlled trials. J Atr Fibrillation. 2019;12(1):1–7.

43. Miller S, Crystal E, Garfinkle M, Lau C, Lashevsky I, Connolly SJ. Effects of magnesium on atrial fibrillation after cardiac surgery: a meta-analysis. Heart. 2005;91(5):618–23.

44. Auer J, Weber T, Berent R, Lamm G, Eber B, MacDonald JE, et al. Serum potassium level and risk of postoperative atrial fibrillation in patients undergoing cardiac surgery [3] (multiple letters). JACC. 2004;44(4):938–9.

45. Madias JE, Shah B, Chintalapally G, Chalavarya G, Madias NE. Admission serum potassium in patients with acute myocardial infarction: its correlates and value as a determinant of in-hospital outcome. Chest. 2000;118(4):904–13.

46. Krijthe BP, Heeringa J, Kors JA, Hofman A, Franco OH, Witteman JCM, et al. Serum potassium levels and the risk of atrial fibrillation: the Rotterdam study. Int J Cardiol. 2013;168(6):5411–5.

47. Peacock JM, Ohira T, Post W, Sotoodehnia N, Folsom AR. Serum magnesium and risk of sudden cardiac death in the atherosclerosis risk in communities (ARIC) study. Am Heart J. 2011;160(3):464–70.

48. Li J, Hovey KM, Andrews CA, Quddus A, Allison MA, Van Horn L, et al. Association of Dietary Magnesium Intake with fatal coronary heart disease and sudden cardiac death. J Women's Health. 2020;29(1):7–12.

49. Misialek JR, Lopez FL, Lutsey PL, Huxley RR, Peacock JM, Chen LY, et al. Serum and dietary magnesium and incidence of atrial fibrillation in whites and in african americans – atherosclerosis risk in communities (ARIC) study. Circ J. 2013;77(2):323–9.

50. Frick M, Darpö B, Östergren J, Rosenqvist M. The effect of oral magnesium, alone or as an adjuvant to sotalol, after cardioversion in patients with persistent atrial fibrillation. Eur Heart J. 2000;21(14):1177–85.

Index

A

Acquired immunodeficiency syndrome (AIDS), 186
Adenosine triphosphate (ATP), 2
Albumin, 36
Allostatic load (AL), 66
α-linolenic acid (ALA), 198
Alpha-tocopherol beta-carotene (ATBC) cancer
    prevention study, 5
Alternate day fasting (ADF), 144, 148–151, 165
Arachidonic acid (AA), 198
Arrhythmia
    atrial fibrillation and obesity
        clinical outcomes, 267, 268
        mechanisms, 267
        risk factors, 265–267
        weight loss, 268
    caffeine, 268, 269
    dietary electrolytes, 269
    supraventricular tachycardia, 268, 269
Arteriosclerosis, 171
Atherosclerosis, 180, 181
    gut microbiota, 226, 227
    LDL, 193
Atherosclerotic cardiovascular disease (ASCVD), 47,
    49–51, 194, 196, 211
Atherosclerotic heart disease, 257
Atkins diet, 80, 81
Atrial fibrillation (AF)
    clinical outcomes, 267, 268
    mechanisms, 267
    risk factors, 265–267
    weight loss, 268

B

Berberine, 218
Beta-hydroxybutyrate (BOHB), 73
Bile acids, 230, 231
Blood pressure, 31
BOHB dehydrogenase (BDH1), 74
B12 deficiency, 103
Buchinger fasting method, 154–156
Bupropion, 135

C

Caffeine, 268, 269
Calcium, 8, 9
Caloric restriction (CR), 130
Calorie-containing substances, 88
Carbohydrate-insulin model (CIM), 74
Cardiovascular biomarkers
    albumin and prealbumin, 36
    blood pressure, 31
    BMI/body composition, 29–30
    HbA_{1c} and fasting glucose, 37–38
    HDL, 32
    hs-CRP, 34
    LDL, 32
    lipoprotein (a), 33–34
    magnesium, 37
    major food group, 30
    non-HDL cholesterol, 33
    TMAO, 34–36
    total cholesterol, 31
    triglyceride, 33
    vitamin B12 and folate, 39–40
    vitamin D, 38, 39
Cardiovascular disease (CVD), 62, 129
Carnitine palmitoyltransferase, 73
Cerebrovascular accident (CVA), 65, 96
Chromium, 12
Chronic kidney disease (CKD), 62
Chronic low-grade inflammation, 55
Cinnamon, 217, 218
Circadian rhythms, 235, 236
Classic southern diet, 68, 69
Clostridium difficile infection (CDI), 227
CoA Q10 (CoQ10), 13
Coconut oil, 122, 123
Coenzyme Q10 (CoQ10), 13, 260
Cognitive behavioral intervention (CBI) program, 67
Congestive heart failure (CHF), 65
Continuous glucose monitoring (CGM), 172
Copper, 11, 12
Corn oil, 117
Coronary artery disease (CAD), 96, 97, 257
Coronary heart disease (CHD), 65, 194

C-reactive protein (CRP), 34
Crohn's disease, 185
Curcumin, 16, 218
Cyanocobalamin (B12), 2

D
Diabetes mellitus (DM), heart failure, 256, 257
Diabetic ketoacidosis (DKA), 75
Dietary approaches to stop hypertension (DASH) trial,
       164, 165, 215
   beneficial cardiometabolic effects, 65–66
   benefits of, 62
   blacks/african americans, 64–65
   classic southern diet, 68, 69
   control diet, 61
   current evidence-based guideline recommendations,
      62–63
   effectiveness of, 63–64
   LDL-C, 201, 202
   oldways african heritage diet, 69
   persons with diabetes and CKD, 64–65
   prevent and control BP, 61
   SDOH, 67, 68
   translating into real-world setting, 69–70
   WHEELS app, 67
   youth, 64–65
Dietary cholesterol, 197
Dietary composition, 171, 172
Dietary electrolytes, 269
Dietary fat
   dietary cholesterol, 197
   MUFA, 199
   PUFA, 198, 199
   saturated fatty acids, 197, 198
   TFA, 199, 200
Dietary fibers, 201, 236, 237
Dietary habits, 235, 236
Dietary intervention
   dietary fiber, 236, 237
   Mediterranean diet, 237
   TMAO, 237–239
Dietary management
   alcohol, 214
   DASH, 215
   fructose, 214
   low-carbohydrate diets, 215
   marine omega-3 fatty acids, 216, 217
   MCT, 214
   Mediterranean diet, 214, 215
   plant-based diets, 215, 216
   strategies, 212
   TFAs, 214
Dietary sugars, 200, 201
Dietary supplements
   berberine, 218
   cinnamon, 217, 218
   cocoa products, 217
   fiber, 217
   nuts, 217

   RYR, 218
   spirulina, 218
   turmeric, 218
Diet-heart hypothesis, 74
Docosahexaenoic acid (DHA), 14, 116, 198
Dr. Barnard's vegan diet, 108
Dr. Esselstyn's plant-based diet, 107–108
Dual energy absorptiometry (DEXA) scans, 29
Dyslipidemia, 172–174, 186

E
Eicosapentaenoic acid (EPA), 14, 116, 198, 216
Elemental minerals
   calcium, 8, 9
   chromium, 12
   copper, 11, 12
   magnesium, 7
   manganese, 8
   phosphorus, 9
   potassium, 10
   selenium, 10, 11
   zinc, 6, 7
Endothelial dysfunction, 13
Estimated glomerular filtration rate, 64
Euglycemic ketoacidosis, 85

F
Farnesoid X receptor (FXR), 230, 231
Fasting
   ADF, 148, 150, 151
   FMD, 156
   history, 143
   intermittent fasting, 146, 148
   periodic fasting, 154–156
   physiology of, 143–144
   TRE, 151, 153, 154
Fasting-Mimicking Diet (FMD), 144, 156
Fatty acids, structure of, 115
Fecal microbiota transplantation (FMT), 231, 235
Flavin monooxygenases (FMO), 231
Fluid restriction, 257, 258
Folate (B9), 2
Fortified foods, 40
Fridewald equation, 33
Fructose, 214

G
Gamma-aminobutyric acid (GABA), 134
Garlic (*allium sativum*), 14
Gastric banding, 137
Gastrointestinal (GI) tract, 185
Ginkgo biloba, 15
GLUT1 deficiency syndrome, 80
Glycemia, 171, 172
Gut microbiota
   composition, 240
      atherosclerosis, 226, 227

heart failure, 227, 228
hypertension, 227
insulin resistance, 228
obesity, 228
metabolites, 228, 229, 240
bile acids, 230, 231
PAGln, 234
SCFAs, 228–230
TMAO, 231–234
morbidity and mortality, 225
physiology, 225, 226
therapeutic target
dietary habits and circadian rhythms, 235, 236
dietary intervention, 236, 237, 239
FMT, 235
prebiotics, 235
probiotics, 234, 235
TCM, 239
TMA lyase Inhibitors, 239, 240

H

Heart failure (HF), 85
atherosclerotic heart disease, 257
diabetes mellitus, 256, 257
diet, 253, 254
gut microbiota, 227, 228
hypertension, 255, 256
medical management, 251
metabolism, 252, 253
obesity, 254, 255
prevalence, 251
treatment and prevention, 258
CoQ10, 260
fluid restriction, 257, 258
iron deficiency, 259, 260
nutrition, 258
sodium restriction, 257
thiamine, 260
vitamin D, 259
Hemoglobin A1C levels, 174
High-density lipoprotein cholesterol
(HDL-C), 52, 144
High-density lipoproteins (HDL), 32
High-sensitivity C-reactive protein (hs-CRP), 34
High sodium-control diet, 66
Homocysteine metabolism (pyroxidine (B6), 2
Human immunodeficiency virus (HIV)
ART, 186
dietary consideration, 187
lifestyle management, 187
morbidity and mortality, 186
Hyperinsulinemia, 85
Hyperketonemia, 75
Hypertension
gut microbiota, 227
heart failure, 255, 256
Hypertriglyceridemia (HTG), *see* Triglyceride (TG)
Hypokalemia, 269
Hypomagnesemia, 269

I

Inflammatory bowel disease (IBD)
dietary consideration, 186
incidence, 185
lifestyle management, 185, 186
upregulated cytokines, 185
VTE, 185
Insulin deficiency, 171
Insulin resistance, 228
Intermittent fasting (IF), 144, 146–148, 165, 166, 204
Iron, 102
Iron deficiency, 259, 260

K

Keshan disease, 11
Ketogenic diets (KD), 82–84, 174, 175, 204
benefits of, 75–80
calorie intake, 88
controlling macronutrient, 88
heart failure, 85
hyperinsulinemia, 85
lack of placebo, 88
LCHADD, 86
MCADD, 86
NAFLD, 85
nutrition and dietary clinical trials, 87
obesity, 84
RCT or cross-over, 87–88
saturated Versus unsaturated fats, 86–87
SGLT2i, 85
type 2 diabetes, 84
Ketone bodies (KB)
acetoacetate, 73
physiological uses of, 74
Ketonemia-inducing diets, 80

L

LDL-cholesterol, 117
Left anterior descending (LAD) occlusion, 144
Linoleic acid (LA), 198
Lipoprotein (a), 33–34
Liraglutide, 135
Long-chain 3-hydroxyacyl-CoA dehydrogenase
deficiency (LCHADD), 86
Lorcaserin (Belviq), 133
Low-carbohydrate (LC) diets, 73, 80, 215
atkins, 80, 81
ketogenic diet, 82–84
paleo diet, 81, 82
Low carbohydrate-based nutrition, 74, 75
Low-carbohydrate, high-fat (LCHF) diets, 73
Low-density lipoprotein-cholesterol
(LDL-C), 62, 115, 144
atherosclerosis, 193
dietary fat, 200
dietary cholesterol, 197
MUFA, 199
PUFA, 198, 199

Low-density lipoprotein-cholesterol (*cont.*)
    saturated fatty acids, 197, 198
    TFA, 199, 200
  dietary fibers, 201
  dietary patterns, 205
    DASH, 201, 202
    intermittent fasting, 204
    ketogenic diet, 204
    Mediterranean diet, 202, 203
    plant-based vegetarian diet, 203, 204
  dietary sugars, 200, 201
  phytosterols, 201
  primary prevention, 193–195
  secondary prevention, 194, 196
Low-density lipoproteins (LDL), 32
Low sodium-DASH diet, 66

M

Macronutrient supplement compounds
  CoQ10, 13
  curcumin, 16
  fish oil, 14–15
  garlic (*allium sativum*), 14
  ginkgo biloba, 15
  macronutrient supplement compounds
    RYR, 15
    RES, 15
Magnesium, 7, 37
Manganese, 8
Marine omega-3 fatty acids, 216, 217
Martin-Hopkins equation, 33
Medi-RIVAGE study, 163
Mediterranean diet, 131, 132, 214, 215
  dietary intervention, 237
  LDL-C, 202, 203
Mediterranean diet (MedDiet), 30
  communal gatherings, 47
  components of, 47–48
  effect on blood pressure, 53
  effect on glucose/insulin resistance, 52
  effect on lipids, 52
  effect on weight loss/obesity, 53
  evidence for ASCVD reduction, 49, 50
  impact on biomarkers, 54–57
  MDS, 48
  MetS, 53
  physical activity, 47
  prevention of MetS, 53–54
  risk of T2D, 52
  sharing of meals, 47
  treatment of MetS, 54
Mediterranean diet pyramid, 48
Mediterranean diet score (MDS), 48
Mediterranean dietary pattern (MDP), 162, 163
Mediterranean-style diet, 49
Medium chain triglyceride (MCT), 214
Medium-chain acyl-CoA dehydrogenase deficiency
    (MCADD), 86
Metabolic syndrome (MetS), 51, 53

classifications, 161
DASH, 164, 165
heart-healthy dietary patterns, 162, 167
intermittent fasting, 165, 166
Mediterranean dietary pattern, 162, 163
PBD, 163, 164
risk factors, 162
stages of, 161
Mild-moderate hypertriglyceridemia, 211
Mitochondrial 3-hydroxymethylglutaryl-CoA synthase
    (HMGCS2), 73
Monounsaturated fatty acid (MUFA), 115, 199
Multivitamin and B vitamins
  vitamin A, 3
  vitamin C, 2
  vitamin D, 3, 4
  vitamin E, 4, 5
  vitamin K, 5

N

Naltrexone, 135
National heart, lung, and blood institute (NHLBI), 61
Nicotinamide adenine dinucleotide (NAD), 2
Non-alcoholic fatty liver disease (NAFLD), 84
Non-alcoholic steatohepatitis (NASH), 150
Non-HDL cholesterol, 33
Nutrition counseling, 175
Nutritional ketosis, 75
Nutritional therapy, 29

O

Obesity, 228
  bariatric surgery
    gastric banding, 137
    RYGB, 137
    sleeve gastrectomy, 137
  clinical outcomes, 267, 268
  dietary approaches
    caloric restriction, 130
    food processing, 131
    intermittent fasting, 130–131
    meal replacements, 131
    Mediterranean diet, 131, 132
    plant-based diets, 132–133
  heart failure, 254, 255
  mechanisms, 267
  pharmacologic approaches, 134
    liraglutide, 135
    naltrexone SR-bupropion SR, 135
    orlistat, 133, 134
    phentermine, 134, 135
  risk factors, 265–267
  weight loss, 268
Obesity paradox, 254
Obesity-related comorbidities, 129
Olive oil, 120
Omega-3 (ω-3) fatty acids, 198
Omega-6 (ω-6) fatty acid, 198

Optimal diet, diabetes
  diabetes and weight management, 175
  dietary composition and glycemia, 171, 172
  dyslipidemia, 172–174
  fat diabetes, 171
  hypertension, 174
  ketogenic diets, 174, 175
  monitoring and evaluation, 175
  nutrition counseling, 175
  nutrition intervention, 174
  registered dietitian/nutritionists, 174
  risk factors, 171, 172
  strategies, 174
Orlistat, 133, 134
Ornish diet, 105–107

P
Paleo diet, 81, 82
Palm kernel oil, 122
Palm oil, 121
Peanut oil, 121
Periodic fasting, 154–156
Phentermine, 134, 135
Phenylacetylglutamine (PAGln), 234
Phosphatidylcholine, 35
Phosphorus, 9
Phytosterols, 201
Plant-based diet (PBD), 38, 163, 164, 215, 216
  animal-based products, 95
  animal products, 96
  beneficial effect on
    atherogenic lipids, 99–100
    cardiovascular and all-cause
      mortality, 98–99
    coronary artery disease, 97
    HDL-C and triglycerides, 100
    heart failure, 98
    hypertension, 97
    stroke, 98
    type 2 diabetes mellitus, 99
  cardiovascular risk outcomes, 107
  components of total caloric intake, 104
  Dr. Barnard's vegan diet, 108
  Dr. Esselstyn's plant-based diet, 107–108
  folic acid, 95
  iron, 95
  magnesium, 95
  Ornish diet, 105–107
  phytochemicals, 95
  polyphenols and fiber, 101
  pritikin diet, 103, 104
  pro-atherogenic compounds, 101
  shortfalls of
    iron, 102
    protein deficiency, 101
    vitamin B12, 102, 103
    vitamin D, 102
    zinc, 102
  vitamin C and E, 95

Plant-based oils
  cis and trans configuration, 116
  fatty acids, 115, 116
  hydrogenated vegetable oils, 123–124
  monounsaturated fatty acids
    canola and rapeseed oil, 118–119
    olive oil, 120
    peanut oil, 121
    sunflower and safflower oil, 119–120
  polyunsaturated fatty acids
    corn oil, 117
    soybean oil, 116–117
    walnut oil, 117–118
  saturated fatty acids
    coconut oil, 122, 123
    palm and palm kernel oil, 121–122
    trans fatty acids, 123
Plant-based vegetarian diet, 203, 204
Polyphenols, 101
Polyunsatuated fatty acids
    (PUFA), 14, 115, 198, 199
Post-operative dumping syndrome, 137
Potassium, 10
Prealbumin, 36
Prebiotics, gut microbiota, 235
Pritikin diet, 103, 104
Probiotics, gut microbiota, 234, 235
Pro-inflammatory diseases
  atherosclerosis, 180, 181
  clinical cardiovascular disease, 180, 181
  HIV
    ART, 186
    dietary consideration, 187
    lifestyle management, 187
    morbidity and mortality, 186
  IBD
    dietary consideration, 186
    incidence, 185
    lifestyle management, 185, 186
    upregulated cytokines, 185
    VTE, 185
  innate and adaptive immunity, 179
  psoriasis
    biomarkers, 183
    dietary consideration, 183
    incidence, 182
    lifestyle management, 183
  rheumatoid arthritis
    dietary considerations, 182
    incidence, 180
    lifestyle management, 182
    mortality and ischemic heart
      disease, 180
    synovium, 180
  SLE
    dietary consideration, 185
    lifestyle management, 184, 185
    morbidity and mortality, 184
    pathogenesis, 184
    prevalence, 184

Proopiomelancortin (POMC) stimulation, 135
Prophylactic magnesium, 269
Proprotein convertase subtilisin/kexin type 9
    (PCSK9), 194
Prostate-specific antigens (PSA), 38
Protein deficiency, 101
Psoriasis
    biomarkers, 183
    dietary consideration, 183
    incidence, 182
    lifestyle management, 183

Q

Quantitative coronary angiography
    (QCA), 97, 106

R

Red yeast rice (RYR), 15, 218
Resveratrol (RES), 15
Retinoic acid (RA), 3
Rheumatoid arthritis (RA)
    dietary considerations, 182
    incidence, 180
    lifestyle management, 182
    mortality and ischemic heart disease, 180
    synovium, 180
Roux-en-Y gastric bypass (RYGB), 137

S

S-allyl-L-cysteine (SAC), 14
Saturated fatty acids, 115, 197, 198
Selenium, 10, 11
Severe hypertriglyceridemia, 212
Short-chain fatty acids (SCFAs), 228–230
Single-pill MVI supplements, 1
Sleeve gastrectomy (SG), 137
Social determinants of health (SDOH), 67
Sodium restriction, 257
Sodium-glucose co-transporter 2 inhibitors (SGLT2i),
    85–86
Soybean oil, 116–117
Spirulina, 218
SR+bupropion SR, 135
Stroke, 98
Sudden cardiac death (SCD), 269
Supplement dietary sources, 16–18
Supraventricular tachycardia (SVT), 268, 269
Systemic lupus erythematosus (SLE)
    dietary consideration, 185
    lifestyle management, 184, 185
    morbidity and mortality, 184
    pathogenesis, 184
    prevalence, 184
Systolic BP (SBP), 62

T

Thiamine deficiency, 260
Time-restricted eating (TRE), 144, 151–154,
    165, 166
Time-restricted feeding (TRF), 151
Total cholesterol, 31
Traditional Chinese medicine (TCM), 239
Trans fatty acids, 116, 199, 200, 214
Triglycerides (TGs), 33, 52, 172, 173
    dietary management
        alcohol, 214
        DASH, 215
        fructose, 214
        low-carbohydrate diets, 215
        marine omega-3 fatty acids, 216, 217
        MCT, 214
        Mediterranean diet, 214, 215
        National Lipid Association, 212, 213
        plant-based diets, 215, 216
        strategies, 212
        TFAs, 214
    dietary supplements
        berberine, 218
        cinnamon, 217, 218
        cocoa products, 217
        fiber, 217
        nuts, 217
        RYR, 218
        spirulina, 218
        turmeric, 218
    epidemiological studies, 211
    HTG, 211
    lifestyle modifications, 218
        exercise, 212
        treatment, 212
        weight loss, 212
    mild-moderate hypertriglyceridemia, 211
    severe hypertriglyceridemia, 212
Trimethylamine N-oxide (TMAO),
    34–36, 101, 231–234, 237–239
Type 2 diabetes, 75, 129
Type 2 diabetes mellitus (DM), 99, 133

U

Ulcerative colitis (UC), 185
Ursodeoxycholic acid (UDCA), 231

V

Venous thromboembolism (VTE), 185
Ventricular fibrillation (VF), 269
Ventricular tachycardia (VT), 269
Vitamin A, 3
Vitamin B1 (*thiamine*), 2
Vitamin B3, 2
Vitamin B5 (*pantothenic acid*), 2

Vitamin B12, 102, 103
Vitamin C, 2
Vitamin D, 3, 4, 38, 39, 102, 259
Vitamin E, 4, 5
Vitamin K, 5
VLDL-cholesterol, 117

W
Walnut oil, 117–118
Weight loss, 173, 212

Western diet, 47
WHEELS DASH app, 67

Z
Zinc, 6, 7, 102

Printed in the United States
by Baker & Taylor Publisher Services